CONTEMPORARY MANAGEMENT IN CRITICAL CARE

MARTIN J. TOBIN, MD, Editor-in-Chief

Professor of Medicine
Division of Pulmonary and Critical Care Medicine
Stritch School of Medicine
Loyola University of Chicago
Chicago, Illinois

AKE GRENVIK, MD, PhD, Editor-in-Chief

Professor of Anesthesiology, Medicine & Surgery
Director, Multidisciplinary CCM Training Program
University of Pittsburgh Medical Center
Pittsburgh, Pennsylvania

CHURCHILL LIVINGSTONE
New York, Edinburgh, London, Melbourne, Tokyo 1991

RECENT AND FORTHCOMING ISSUES

RESPIRATORY MONITORING

MARTIN J. TOBIN, MD, Editor

Professor of Medicine
Division of Pulmonary and Critical Care Medicine
Stritch School of Medicine
Loyola University of Chicago
Chicago, Illinois

CHURCHILL LIVINGSTONE
New York, Edinburgh, London, Melbourne, Tokyo 1991

Copyright © 1991 by Churchill Livingstone Inc.
Contemporary Management in Critical Care is published quarterly. Annual subscription rates (1992): U.S., $65 individual, $85 institution; foreign, add $35 for airmail or $20 for surface mail; single copy, $32.50.

ISSN 1050-9623
ISBN 0-443-08831-4

Direct subscription orders, changes of address, and claims for missing issues (within five months of publication) to Churchill Livingstone Inc. (650 Avenue of the Americas, New York, NY 10011). In Japan, contact Nankodo Co., Ltd., 42-6, Hongo 3-chome, Bunkyo-ku, Tokyo 113, Japan.

The authors, editors, and publisher have exerted every effort to ensure that drug selection and dosage and descriptions of instruments and recommendations for their use set forth in all articles appearing in *Contemporary Management in Critical Care* are in accord with current recommendations and practice at the time of publication. However, many considerations necessitate caution in applying in practice any information appearing in *Contemporary Management in Critical Care*. The reader is advised to check package inserts for each drug for indications and dosages and the descriptions provided by instrument manufacturers for warnings and precautions.

Printed in the United States of America

Volume 1 Number 4
First published in 1991

CONTRIBUTING AUTHORS

KENNETH R. CHAPMAN, MD, FRCPC
Acting Director
Asthma Centre of the Toronto Hospital
Assistant Professor of Medicine
University of Toronto
Toronto, Ontario, Canada

PATRICK J. FAHEY, MD
Chief, Pulmonary and Critical Care Medicine
Loyola University Medical Center
Maywood, Illinois

REED M. GARDNER, PhD
Professor of Medical Informatics
University of Utah
Co-Director of Medical Computing
LDS Hospital
Salt Lake City, Utah

BARRY J. GRAY, MD, MRCP
Department of Thoracic Medicine
King's College School of Medicine and Dentistry
London, United Kingdom

DUNCAN C. S. HUTCHISON, BM, FRCP
Department of Thoracic Medicine
King's College School of Medicine and Dentistry
London, United Kingdom

AMAL JUBRAN, MD
Staff Physician
Division of Pulmonary and Critical Care Medicine
Edward Hines Jr. Veterans Administration Hospital
Assistant Professor
Loyola University of Chicago Stritch School of
   Medicine
Hines, Illinois

STEVEN KESTEN, MD, FRCPC
Assistant Professor of Medicine
University of Toronto
Division of Respiratory Medicine
The Toronto Hospital
Toronto, Ontario, Canada

BRUCE P. KRIEGER, MD
Associate Professor of Medicine
University of Miami School of Medicine
Chief, Pulmonary Intensive Care
Mount Sinai Medical Center
Miami Beach, Florida

C. KEES MAHUTTE, MD, PhD
Associate Professor of Medicine
University of California, Irvine
Chief, Pulmonary and Critical Care Section
VA Medical Center
Long Beach, California

JOHN J. MARINI, MD
Professor of Medicine
University of Minnesota
Director, Pulmonary and Critical Care Medicine
St. Paul-Ramsey Medical Center
Minneapolis/St. Paul, Minnesota

ALAN H. MORRIS, MD
Director of Research
Pulmonary Division
LDS Hospital
Professor of Medicine
University of Utah
Salt Lake City, Utah

WILLIAM T. PERUZZI, MD
Associate in Clinical Anesthesia
Department of Anesthesia
Northwestern University Medical School
Chicago, Illinois

BARRY A. SHAPIRO, MD
Professor and Vice Chairman
Chief, Section of Respiratory and Critical Care
Department of Anesthesia
Northwestern University Medical School
Chicago, Illinois

MARTIN J. TOBIN, MD
Professor of Medicine
Division of Pulmonary and Critical Care Medicine
Stritch School of Medicine
Loyola University of Chicago
Chicago, Illinois

JOHN M. WALSH, MD, MS
Assistant Professor of Medicine and Physiology
Division of Pulmonary and Critical Care Medicine
Loyola University Medical Center
Maywood, Illinois

INTRODUCTION

In today's world of medicine, the amount of new research and new concepts is growing at an exponential rate. This makes it extremely difficult for the busy physician to keep pace with new advances. Due to its multidisciplinary nature and high technology base, the field of Critical Care Medicine may be affected more than any other subspecialty. Accordingly, the availability of timely and pertinent reviews in a convenient form becomes an essential tool for the achievement of excellence in the practice of Critical Care Medicine.

The aim of *Contemporary Management in Critical Care* is to provide the practitioner with concise surveys of major topics in Critical Care Medicine. The Guest Editors and authors are leaders in their respective fields, and the orientation is clinical and practical. The *contemporary* nature of the series is emphasized, as we strive to cover the most current topics and keep the reader abreast of the latest issues and advances in Critical Care Medicine.

As Editors of the series, we look forward to suggestions and comments from our readers.

Martin J. Tobin, MD
Ake Grenvik, MD, PhD

To Kieran

RESPIRATORY MONITORING

CONTENTS

RESPIRATORY MONITORING

PREFACE

An issue of *Contemporary Management in Critical Care* devoted to respiratory monitoring is particularly pertinent to the management of critically ill patients for two reasons. One, the vast majority of patients in an intensive care unit are admitted because of a primary respiratory problem or because they develop a respiratory complication at some stage during their illness. Two, approximately half of the patients admitted to an intensive care unit are admitted for the purposes of monitoring rather than interventional therapy. Yet, until recently, techniques for monitoring the respiratory system were rudimentary in nature and lagged behind the ability to monitor the function of other organ systems. In the last decade, major advances have been made in respiratory monitoring with the introduction of new techniques and the refinement of previously existing techniques. As this is a relatively young field, most attention has been focused on validating the various techniques. Hopefully, in the next decade, we will also learn how best to apply the various techniques in clinical decision making and how to use them in a cost-effective manner.

The eleven chapters in this issue deal with the many new and exciting developments in respiratory monitoring. Topics discussed include arterial blood gas monitoring, the use of intraarterial electrodes such as optodes, transcutaneous oxygen and carbon dioxide electrodes, pulse oximetry, continuous monitoring of mixed venous oxygen saturation, capnometry, control of breathing and respiratory muscle function, pulmonary mechanics and work of breathing, computerization and quality control of monitoring techniques, use of monitoring information in clinical decision making, and the cost-effectiveness of respiratory monitoring. The authors were selected because of their known expertise in the area, and I believe that their efforts have resulted in a state-of-the-art review of each topic.

I am grateful to each author for his/her contributions, and I can only hope that the reader learns as much as I did from reviewing each chapter. Finally, I wish to thank Ms. Jane Grochowski and Ms. Camille Gogol of Churchill Livingstone Inc., for their constant support throughout the production of this issue.

Martin J. Tobin, MD

ARTERIAL BLOOD GAS MONITORING

BARRY A. SHAPIRO, MD[†]
WILLIAM T. PERUZZI, MD[††]

Critically ill patients often require therapeutic interventions to support respiratory homeostasis, a process dependent to a large extent upon proper interpretation of arterial "blood gas values" (pH, PCO₂, and PO₂).

Numerous technologies have been developed to provide noninvasive and continuous reflections of arterial PO₂ and PCO₂, emphasizing the central importance of arterial blood gas measurements in critical care.

Respiratory homeostasis refers to the vital balance between CO_2 and O_2 exchange at the lung and cellular levels. Critically ill patients often require therapeutic interventions to support respiratory homeostasis, a process dependent to a large extent upon proper interpretation of arterial "blood gas values" (pH, PCO_2, and PO_2). This gold standard for respiratory monitoring involves an analytic method requiring intermittent blood specimens and significant delay in obtaining results. This proffers such an unsuitable milieu for obtaining clinically vital information that numerous technologies have been developed to provide noninvasive and continuous *reflections* of arterial PO_2 and PCO_2. A significant portion of this publication is devoted to in-depth discussions of such technologies—a testament, rather than a refutation, for the central importance of arterial blood gas measurements in critical care. This chapter addresses the essential factors involved in the proper interpretation of serial arterial blood gas measurements for the purpose of supporting ventilation and oxygenation in the critically ill patient.

ASSESSMENT OF VENTILATION

Ventilation is gas movement in and out of the pulmonary system and is most readily measured in critically ill patients as the gas volume exhaled in one minute (V_E). The portion of the V_E that respires (removes CO_2 from the blood and transfers O_2 to the blood) is referred to as alveolar venti-

[†] Professor and Vice Chairman, Chief, Section of Respiratory and Critical Care, Department of Anesthesia, Northwestern University Medical School, Chicago, Illinois
[††] Associate in Clinical Anesthesia, Department of Anesthesia, Northwestern University Medical School, Chicago, Illinois

lation (V_A); the portion of the V_E that does not respire is designated as dead space ventilation (V_D).

ALVEOLAR VENTILATION AND P_aCO_2

The arterial PCO_2 reflects the adequacy with which the V_A balances the CO_2 production. It is imperative that significantly abnormal CO_2 production be identified when interpreting the P_aCO_2 in critically ill patients.

Since metabolism determines the rate of CO_2 diffusion into the blood and alveolar ventilation determines the rate of CO_2 diffusion out of the blood, the arterial PCO_2 reflects the adequacy with which the V_A balances the CO_2 production. It is imperative that significantly abnormal CO_2 production be identified when interpreting the P_aCO_2 in critically ill patients. Common circumstances of abnormal CO_2 production are: (1) temperature deviation that alters CO_2 production approximately 10% per °C change; (2) excessive muscular activity (shivering, rigor, seizure) that can increase CO_2 production three- to five-fold; (3) generalized "stress" responses are known to increase CO_2 production; (4) sepsis, which is known to alter CO_2 production; and (5) total parenteral nutrition with glucose providing more than 50% of the nonprotein calories can increase CO_2 production two- to eight-fold. The following presentation assumes a reasonably normal CO_2 production.

Dead Space Ventilation

Increases in V_D will require an increase in V_E to maintain a consistent V_A.

Ventilation is the sum of alveolar and dead space components: $V_E = V_A + V_D$. Increases in V_D will require an increase in V_E to maintain a consistent V_A. Common circumstances that increase V_D are: (1) acutely diminished cardiac output, which creates a greater portion of lung that is poorly perfused (high V/Q); (2) acute pulmonary emboli, which create ventilated/unperfused alveoli (infinite V/Q); (3) acute pulmonary hypertension, which creates less perfusion of nongravity-dependent lung (high V/Q); (4) severe acute lung injury (ARDS), which creates both zero V/Q and high V/Q pathology causing both significant intrapulmonary shunting and dead space ventilation; and (5) positive pressure ventilation (PPV), which favors distribution of ventilation to nongravity-dependent lung.

V_E–P_aCO_2 Disparity   Clinical observation that minute ventilation (V_E) is increased without an appropriate decrease in arterial PCO_2 raises the possibility of increased V_D. Table 1 shows the expected V_E–P_aCO_2 relationships when CO_2 production remains normal and consistent. In our clinical experience: (1) when the measured V_E is associated with a P_aCO_2 significantly greater than predicted

TABLE 1   Expected Minute Volume to Arterial Carbon Dioxide
Tension Relationships in the Normal Nonexercising
Human

V_E	P_aCO_2	Range (mmHg)
Normal	40	35–45
Twice Normal	30	25–35
Quadruple Normal	20	15–25

in Table 1 and an increased CO_2 production can be reasonably ruled out, increased V_D is the most likely explanation; and (2) when the V_E is associated with a P_aCO_2 significantly less than predicted in Table 1, diminished CO_2 production or depleted CO_2 stores should be suspected.

$P_{(a-et)}CO_2$ Disparity   In the absence of significant pulmonary disease, the "end-tidal" PCO_2 ($P_{et}CO_2$) is several mmHg less than the arterial PCO_2. Acute increases in this $P_{(a-et)}CO_2$ gradient reflect increases in dead space ventilation. This technique can prove useful in the intensive care unit and operating room provided baseline values are available for comparison.

ACUTE VENTILATORY FAILURE

Arterial PCO_2s > 50 mmHg reflect a clinically significant failure of the cardiopulmonary system to adequately satisfy the metabolic requirements for CO_2 excretion. Traditional physiology terms this process *respiratory acidosis;* however, since the life-threatening process that must be treated is inadequate alveolar ventilation, a more clinically relevant term is *ventilatory failure.*[1]

Respiratory failure is a clinical diagnosis inferring that the pulmonary system is failing to provide adequate O_2 and/or CO_2 exchange to meet metabolic requirements. Ventilatory failure (respiratory acidosis) is a blood gas diagnosis that refers only to failure of the pulmonary system to provide adequate CO_2 excretion. As defined in Table 2, when the arterial pH < 7.30 in concert with an arterial PCO_2 > 50 mmHg, an acute ventilatory failure (acute respiratory acidosis) exists that represents a directly life-threatening circumstance.

When acute ventilatory failure is present, the following factors must be immediately considered: (1) the need for ventilatory assistance if the patient is spontaneously breathing; (2) the adequacy of ventilatory assistance if the patient is on a ventilator, especially the presence of significant dead space ventilation; (3) tissue hypoxia should be assumed if concurrent severe hypoxemia is present; and

Respiratory failure is a clinical diagnosis inferring that the pulmonary system is failing to provide adequate O_2 and/or CO_2 exchange to meet metabolic requirements. Ventilatory failure (respiratory acidosis) is a blood gas diagnosis that refers only to failure of the pulmonary system to provide adequate CO_2 excretion.

TABLE 2   Interpretive Guidelines for Critically Ill Patients

	pH	PCO$_2$ (mmHg)	Bicarb (mEq/l)	Base Excess mEq/l
Mean	7.40	40	25	0
Normal range	7.35–7.45	35–45	23–27	±3
Clinically acceptable	7.30–7.50	30–50	20–30	±10
Alkalemia	>7.50			
Acidemia	<7.30			
Ventilatory failure (respiratory acidosis)		>50		
Alveolar hyperventilation (respiratory alkalosis)		<30		
Acute ventilatory failure	<7.30	>50		

(4) concomitant acute metabolic acidosis is most likely secondary to inadequate perfusion or detrimental work of breathing.

Impending Ventilatory Failure

If work of breathing places demands on the cardiopulmonary system that exceed functional reserves, the result is often detrimental to the maintenance of respiratory homeostasis.

Breathing is the process by which the ventilatory pump creates ventilation by cyclic muscle contractions. In essence, we breathe to ventilate and ventilate to respire. Work of breathing (WOB) provided within the limits of cardiopulmonary reserves improves matching of ventilation to perfusion and augments venous return to the heart, factors that can be considered beneficial to the maintenance of respiratory homeostasis. However, if WOB places demands on the cardiopulmonary system that exceed functional reserves, the result is often detrimental to the maintenance of respiratory homeostasis.[2]

Extreme degrees of detrimental WOB are clinically recognized as acute respiratory distress (progressive tachypnea, tachycardia, dyspnea, hypertension, intercostal retraction, use of accessory muscles of ventilation, diaphoresis, and mental status changes); the patient is often described as appearing "fatigued" or "tired out." Lesser degrees of detrimental WOB are manifested by progressive increases in respiratory rate, heart rate, and systolic blood pressure, onset of diaphoresis and mental confusion, delirium, or even obtundation. Patients able to communicate will invariably complain of dyspnea. The progression of clinical signs is an important element in the diagnosis of detrimental WOB.

The clinical suspicion of detrimental WOB in a patient with an acceptable P$_a$CO$_2$ suggests that if no therapeutic interventions to reduce WOB are instituted, acute ventilatory failure (rising P$_a$CO$_2$ and falling pH) will eventually ensue—a circumstance often referred to as *impending ventilatory failure*. Metabolic acidemia and/or hypoxemia are common in patients with impending ventilatory failure and are rapidly reversed when appropriate ventilatory assistance is instituted.

ACUTE RESPIRATORY ALKALOSIS

Clinically significant acute respiratory alkalosis (P_aCO_2 < 30 mmHg; pH > 7.50) represents an acute alveolar hyperventilation and usually indicates an increased WOB. The three common causes of acute alveolar hyperventilation in the critically ill patient are: (1) response to arterial hypoxemia, (2) response to metabolic acidosis, and (3) central nervous system (CNS) malfunction. The latter two are seldom concomitant with hypoxemia. In fact, acute respiratory alkalosis without hypoxemia is most commonly secondary to intracranial pathology, anxiety, or pain. However, severe anemia, carbon monoxide poisoning, and methemoglobinemia should be ruled out.

Acute Respiratory Alkalosis With Hypoxemia

Blood gas findings of acute respiratory alkalosis with hypoxemia are almost always attributable to cardiopulmonary pathology. When the hypoxemia is due to a pulmonary process that is responsive to oxygen therapy (asthma, bronchitis, noncardiogenic edema, retained secretions, early pneumonia), administering oxygen should decrease the work of breathing, increase the P_aCO_2 toward normal, and decrease the heart rate and blood pressure toward normal. The P_aO_2 will approach 70 mmHg but seldom exceed that tension until the cardiopulmonary work has been significantly reduced. When the hypoxemia is due to a pulmonary process that is refractory to oxygen therapy (consolidated pneumonia, lobar atelectasis, ARDS), the blood gases and WOB will not significantly change with oxygen administration.

Acute reductions in cardiac output result in decreased mixed venous oxygenation because the tissues must extract oxygen from less blood per unit time. Therefore, any magnitude of preexisting intrapulmonary shunting will have greater hypoxemic effects on the arterial blood because the "shunted" blood is relatively less oxygenated than the nonshunted blood. In response to the hypoxemia, the pulmonary system may increase minute ventilation in an attempt to decrease alveolar PCO_2s and increase alveolar

When the hypoxemia is due to a pulmonary process that is responsive to oxygen therapy, administering oxygen should decrease the work of breathing, increase the P_aCO_2 toward normal, and decrease the heart rate and blood pressure toward normal.

PO_2s, resulting in an acute alveolar hyperventilation with hypoxemia. The hypoxemia attributable to acute myocardial infarction, acute heart failure, and interstitial pulmonary edema is low V/Q in type. Such hypoxemia should respond to oxygen therapy by increasing P_aO_2s and significantly decreasing cardiopulmonary work. Pulmonary edema involving alveolar fluid may be refractory to oxygen therapy.

ABNORMAL PERIPHERAL CO_2 STORES

Intracellular water must have partial pressures of nitrogen (N_2), oxygen (O_2), and carbon dioxide (CO_2), which are referred to as "gas tissue stores." N_2 stores change when the inspired fraction of N_2 is altered (as with oxygen therapy), and O_2 stores change at such rapid rates that steady-state conditions are almost always present within the confines of biologic viability.[3] However, CO_2 stores change at a relatively slow pace and are influenced by several clinically relevant physiologic mechanisms, making their consideration clinically significant in the interpretation of blood gases.

Peripheral CO_2 stores are estimated to be approximately 110 liters in a 70 kg individual. The vast majority (up to 100 l) is stored in bone and fat, which have relatively poor perfusion, thus, significant changes would be expected to take days. Skeletal muscle represents the next largest component (approximately 5 l), in which significant changes can occur in hours; visceral tissue stores account for the remainder, in which significant changes can occur within minutes.

The CO_2 content of blood constitutes the "central" CO_2 stores. When the alveolar PCO_2 changes, the central CO_2 stores are immediately affected; however, the peripheral CO_2 stores are essentially unaffected over several hours. Thus, the arterial and mixed venous PCO_2s will rapidly return to baseline following relatively transient changes in alveolar ventilation. Assuming a normal CO_2 production, Table 3 demonstrates the relationships between CO_2

TABLE 3 Theoretical Relationship of PCO_2 Changes When Peripheral CO_2 Stores Are Altered*

CO_2 Stores	Tissue PCO_2	P_vCO_2	P_ACO_2	P_aCO_2
Normal	50	46	40	40
Decreased	40	36	30	30
Increased	60	56	50	50

* CO_2 production and minute ventilation are assumed normal.

stores, minute ventilation, and arterial PCO_2. It should be noted that depleted CO_2 stores allow a normal minute ventilation to result in an unexpectedly low P_aCO_2; conversely, increased CO_2 stores allow a normal minute ventilation to result in a greater P_aCO_2 than expected.

Depletion of Peripheral CO_2 Stores

Depletion of peripheral stores occurs when CO_2 excretion exceeds CO_2 production for significant periods of time; skeletal muscle depletion is seen in a few hours and bone depletion within several days.[4] With depletion of peripheral CO_2 stores, a normal minute ventilation and normal dead space ventilation result in a diminished alveolar and arterial PCO_2. This is commonly seen in patients with CNS disease who spontaneously hyperventilate to arterial PCO_2s of 28–30 mmHg for > 48 hours, during which time more CO_2 is being excreted than produced. As the CO_2 stores are depleted, the P_aCO_2 remains constant as the minute ventilation decreases. This situation emphasizes the necessity for measuring minute ventilation in conjunction with arterial blood gas measurements in critically ill patients.

The peripheral CO_2 stores tend to be repleted within several days after reversal of the underlying pathology.[4] The reversal process is important because as the stores are repleted either the P_aCO_2 must increase back toward normal or the minute ventilation must increase to maintain the lower P_aCO_2; if the patient is unable to readily increase ventilatory work, significant cardiopulmonary and CNS deterioration may result. Appropriate interpretation of the blood gas values can alert the clinician to these potential dangers.

Increased Peripheral CO_2 Stores— the "CO_2 Retainer"

Chronic hypercarbia ($P_aCO_2 > 50$ mmHg; $pH_a > 7.35$) is most commonly seen in patients with chronic obstructive pulmonary disease (COPD), but it is also seen with chronic restrictive pulmonary disease, morbid obesity (pickwickian syndrome), and rare CNS disorders. The increased peripheral CO_2 stores allow the patient to maintain CO_2 homeostasis (lung excretion equal to cellular production) while maintaining an increased alveolar PCO_2. Since inspired gas is essentially void of CO_2, in any steady-state circumstance a smaller minute ventilation is required to

Depleted CO_2 stores allow a normal minute ventilation to result in an unexpectedly low P_aCO_2; conversely, increased CO_2 stores allow a normal minute ventilation to result in a greater P_aCO_2 than expected.

Increased peripheral CO_2 stores allow the patient to maintain CO_2 homeostasis (lung excretion equal to cellular production) while maintaining an increased alveolar PCO_2.

maintain an increased alveolar PCO_2 than to maintain a normal alveolar PCO_2.

Chronic hypercarbia (chronic respiratory acidosis, chronic ventilatory failure) involves intracellular adaptation to increased PCO_2. It appears that such adaptation involves maintenance of mitochondrial function despite significantly diminished oxygen delivery. Extracellular acid–base balance is maintained by accumulating an increased bicarbonate ion concentration and a chloride ion deficiency. Available data suggests that water and chloride ion shifts between intracellular and extracellular spaces result in a slightly greater extracellular pH than the normal population.[5] Chronic hypercarbia is most commonly seen in conjunction with arterial pHs above 7.40.

Chronic hypercarbic patients have a limited capability to increase cardiopulmonary work in response to stress. Although a significant proportion of these patients will not acutely hypoventilate when given oxygen, the drug must be carefully administered since many will significantly hypoventilate in response to excessive oxygen administration.[6]

Although a significant proportion of chronic hypercarbic patients will not acutely hypoventilate when given oxygen, the drug must be carefully administered since many will significantly hypoventilate in response to excessive oxygen administration.

Chronic Hypercarbia and Acute Ventilatory Failure

Typical room air blood gas levels in the case of chronic hypercarbia and acute ventilatory failure are as follows: pH < 7.35; $PCO_2 > 60$ mmHg; $PO_2 < 40$ mmHg. The severity of this condition must be judged by the degree of acute acidemia. Regardless of the PCO_2 level, a pH above 7.30 usually denotes a tolerable change from baseline. If the pH falls below 7.20, evaluation for ventilatory assistance is mandatory. Although lactic acidosis is common in these patients, sodium bicarbonate administration is contraindicated prior to supporting ventilation because of the added CO_2 load.

Chronic Hypercarbia and Acute Hyperventilation

Typical room air blood gas levels in the case of chronic hypercarbia and acute hyperventilation are as follows: pH > 7.50, $PCO_2 > 40$ mmHg, $PO_2 < 50$ mmHg. These blood gas values should be initially interpreted as a "partly compensated metabolic alkalosis with significant hypoxemia." However, diseases causing metabolic alkalemia rarely cause significant hypoxemia! When presented with these blood gas values, consideration should be given to the probability that a patient with chronic hypercarbia may transiently respond to an acute stress by hyperventilating, thus unmasking the preexisting base excess.

Diseases causing metabolic alkalemia rarely cause significant hypoxemia.

ASSESSMENT OF OXYGENATION

The tissue oxygenation status is a global concept that cannot be directly measured. No single or combination of measurements can reliably reflect the oxygenation status of vital tissues in critically ill patients. Therefore, all clinical assessments of the oxygenation status must begin with an evaluation of the arterial blood.

No single or combination of measurements can reliably reflect the oxygenation status of vital tissues in critically ill patients. All clinical assessments of the oxygenation status must begin with an evaluation of the arterial blood.

ARTERIAL OXYGENATION

The milliliters of oxygen contained in 100 ml of blood is defined as oxygen content (ml/dl). The traditional calculation ($1.34 \times \%HbO_2 + PO_2 \times 0.003$) requires measurement of the PO_2 (mmHg), $\%HbO_2$, and the total Hb (g/dl). The vast majority of oxygen in the blood exists in chemical combination with hemoglobin, while less than 5% is dissolved in the plasma. The quantity of oxygen that moves into (or out of) the blood depends on three factors: (1) the amount of dissolved oxygen (PO_2), (2) the amount of oxygen combined to the hemoglobin ($\%HbO_2$), and (3) the degree to which the hemoglobin attracts the oxygen (Hb-O_2 affinity).

The $\%HbO_2$ is the portion of the total hemoglobin that is oxygenated. The $\%HbO_2$ must be measured by multiwavelength oximetry that measures oxyhemoglobin, reduced hemoglobin, carboxyhemoglobin, and methemglobin. When the oxyhemoglobin is measured by dual wavelength oximetry or calculated from the arterial pH and PO_2, the assumption is made that only oxy- and reduced hemoglobin exist.

Hemoglobin has a strong affinity for oxygen that can be altered by numerous factors. A decreased Hb-O_2 affinity (shift to the right, increased P_{50}) results in a diminished oxygen content that may further limit oxygen delivery; an increased Hb-O_2 affinity will increase the oxygen content but potentially inhibit oxygen unloading to the tissues. Since numerous factors in critically ill patients modify the Hb-O_2 affinity, the presence of hypoxemia demands that both PO_2 and $\%HbO_2$ be assessed. A shift to the left or right should never diminish clinical concern when significant hypoxemia is present.

DEFINING ARTERIAL HYPOXEMIA

Oxygen delivery (DO_2) is defined as the volume of oxygen presented to the tissues in one minute ($C_aO_2 \times$ cardiac output $\times$ 10). Oxygen consumption (VO_2) is defined as the volume of oxygen consumed in 1 minute. Data support the assumption that when DO_2 is 3–4 times greater than VO_2, tissue oxygen needs are reasonably satisfied in non-septic patients.[7]

Deficiencies in arterial oxygen content that demand increased cardiac work to assure tissue oxygenation are significant arterial oxygenation deficits. Significant hypoxemia is defined as P_aO_2s < 60 mmHg or $\%HbO_2$s < 90%. When the P_aO_2 is greater than 60 mmHg (> 90 $\%HbO_2$), the blood oxygen content is close to the maximum for that hemoglobin content and cellular oxygenation will depend upon cardiac output and capillary perfusion, that is, little will be gained by further increase of the PO_2.

Arterial PO_2s less than 40 mmHg (most often associated with $\%HbO_2$s below 75%) reflect not only a significantly decreased oxygen content, but also imply hemoglobin molecules less willing to release oxygen to tissues. Such severe hypoxemia is a direct threat to tissue oxygenation despite increases in cardiac output. PO_2s from 40–60 mmHg may threaten tissue oxygenation if other functions such as cardiac output or total hemoglobin cannot sufficiently compensate for the diminished oxygen content.

Correction of arterial hypoxemia greatly depends on delineation of the degree to which each of three essential functions are contributing to the hypoxemia: (1) oxygen transfer in the lungs, (2) cardiac output, and (3) oxygen consumption.

OXYGENATION DEFICITS

Correction of arterial hypoxemia greatly depends on delineation of the degree to which each of three essential functions are contributing to the hypoxemia: (1) oxygen transfer in the lungs, (2) cardiac output, and (3) oxygen consumption. Specific identification and quantification of these factors requires blood gas analysis of both arterial and pulmonary arterial blood plus cardiac output measurement. Obtaining these values allows calculation of DO_2, oxygen extraction $[C_{(a-v)}O_2]$ and the intrapulmonary shunt fraction (Q_{sp}/Q_t).

Oxygen Extraction

Oxygen extraction represents the oxygen transferred to the tissues from 100 ml (dl) of blood. This relationship can be quantified on a global scale as the oxygen content difference between arterial and mixed venous blood $[C_{(a-v)}O_2]$. When the VO_2 is constant, the $C_{(a-v)}O_2$ will vary inversely to the cardiac output. As shown in Table 4, critically ill patients with adequate cardiac reserves have $C_{(a-v)}O_2$s in the 3–4 ml/dl range.[8] In the absence of anemia and sepsis in a patient with clinically adequate peripheral perfusion, a $C_{(a-v)}O_2$ of 3–4 ml/dl suggests adequate cardiac reserves

TABLE 4 Pulmonary Arterial Oxygenation Values

Cardiovascular Status	P_vO_2	S_vO_2	$C_{(a-v)}O_2$
Healthy resting human volunteer	40 (37–43)	75 (70–76)	5.0 (4.5–6.0)
Critically ill, adequate cardiovascular	27 (35–40)	70 (68–75)	3.5 (2.5–4.5)
Critically ill, borderline cardiovascular	32 (30–35)	60 (56–68)	5.0 (4.5–6.0)
Critically ill, inadequate cardiovascular	<30	<56	>6.0

to meet further stress if required, whereas a $C_{(a-v)}O_2$ of 5 ml/dl suggests inadequate cardiac response to the stress.

The relationship between the oxygen supply and oxygen demand can also be reflected in the mixed venous oxygen saturation (S_vO_2) when the hemoglobin content is greater than 10 g/dl.[9] The availability of technology to continuously measure S_vO_2 and its clinical application are discussed elsewhere in this publication.

The Lung as an Oxygenator

Blood that goes from the right to left heart without contacting alveolar gas (zero V/Q, true shunt) will create hypoxemia by mixing in the left heart with blood that has been oxygenated in the lung. The resultant degree of hypoxemia will be determined by both the amount of blood that shunts and the oxyhemoglobin saturation of the shunted blood. Alveoli that are poorly ventilated in relation to perfusion (low V/Q, shunt effect) will have less than ideal alveolar PO_2s, and blood that respires with these alveoli will be oxygenated to a lesser degree than if exposed to a perfect alveoli, causing arterial hypoxemia.

Blood that goes from the right to left heart without contacting alveolar gas (zero V/Q, true shunt) will create hypoxemia by mixing in the left heart with blood that has been oxygenated in the lung.

Shunt Calculation The topic of shunt calculation and its nomenclature is controversial, confused, and arbitrary. However, we believe the following is a reasonable overview: Q_s/Q_t represents measurement of the intrapulmonary shunt at an F_IO_2 of 1.0 and is traditionally considered to reflect the "true shunt" (zero V/Q); Q_{sp}/Q_t (the physiologic shunt) represents measurement of the intrapulmonary shunt at less than 100% inspired oxygen concentrations, therefore including both the "true shunt" and "low V/Q" (shunt effect); Q_{va}/Q_t (venous admixture) is exactly the same as the physiologic shunt but is preferred by some to avoid using the term "physiologic" when addressing abnormal states.

The shunt equation is:

$$\frac{Q_{sp}}{Q_t} = \frac{C_cO_2 - C_aO_2}{C_cO_2 - C_vO_2}$$

C_cO_2 is the ideal end pulmonary capillary oxygen content that is calculated using the ideal alveolar gas equation to determine the ideal PO_2. The equation calculates that portion of the cardiac output that transverses from the right heart to the left heart without increasing oxygen content. The mathematics assume that the nonshunting blood perfectly oxygenates by exchanging with perfect alveolar gas. Although the intrapulmonary shunt measurement does not reflect regional relationships as does the V/Q concept, it does reflect the degree to which the lung deviates from ideal as an oxygenator of pulmonary blood. It is this quantitative ability to evaluate the lung as an oxygenator that makes this measurement unique and valuable in the clinical setting.

Interpretive Guidelines

1. A calculated shunt less than 10% is clinically compatible with normal lungs.

2. A calculated shunt of 10–19% denotes a degree of pathology that seldom requires significant support.

3. A calculated shunt of 20–29% may be life-threatening in a patient with limited cardiovascular or nervous system function.

4. A calculated shunt greater than 30% is potentially life-threatening and usually requires significant cardiopulmonary supportive therapy.

5. When significant shunt effect (low V/Q) mechanisms are present, the shunt calculation will significantly increase as the F_1O_2 is decreased from 0.5.

Alternatives to the Shunt Calculation Shunt calculations require analysis of pulmonary artery blood. Oxygen tension-based indices ($P_{[A-a]}O_2$, P_AO_2/P_aO_2, P_aO_2/F_1O_2, etc) do not require mixed venous oxygen analysis but have significant limitations in reliably reflecting shunt fractions in critically ill patients.[10] In our opinion, the popularity of these indices is not based on their accuracy or reliability, but rather the fact that mixed venous oxygen measurements are not required.

Oxygen tension-based indices do not require mixed venous oxygen analysis but have significant limitations in reliably reflecting shunt fractions in critically ill patients.

The estimated shunt:

$$EST\ Q_{sp}/Q_t = \frac{C_cO_2 - C_aO_2}{(C_cO_2 - C_aO_2) + C_{(a-v)}O_2}$$

is an oxygen content-based index derived by mathematical manipulation of the shunt equation that places the $C_{(a-v)}O_2$ in the denominator. As shown in Table 5, the estimated shunt has been demonstrated to be far superior to oxygen tension-based indices in reflecting changes in the Q_{sp}/Q_t.[11] We are not suggesting that the estimated shunt is an adequate substitute for Q_{sp}/Q_t measurement, but rather that it is a far more reliable alternative than the oxygen tension-based indices when pulmonary artery blood is not available.

HYPOXEMIA AND O_2 THERAPY

Alveolar PO_2s result from the dynamic equilibrium between the oxygen molecules delivered to the alveolus (ventilation and F_IO_2) and the oxygen molecules diffusing into the pulmonary capillary blood. All other factors remaining constant, increasing the F_IO_2 will increase the delivery of oxygen molecules to the alveolus and thereby increase the alveolar PO_2.

Increasing the F_IO_2 will increase the delivery of oxygen molecules to the alveolus and thereby increase the alveolar PO_2.

The hypoxemia caused by true intrapulmonary shunting (zero V/Q) will be relatively refractory to increased F_IO_2 because the non-shunting blood is well oxygenated, so that increasing the alveolar PO_2s will add insignificant quantities of oxygen to the pulmonary capillary blood.[12] Hypoxemia secondary to shunt effect mechanisms (low V/Q) is due to diminished alveolar PO_2s, therefore, the arterial hypoxemia is responsive to increasing F_IO_2s.[12] The therapeutic range of oxygen administration is essentially limited to less than 50% because the alveolar PO_2s of low V/Q alveoli are usually greater than 80 mmHg with F_IO_2s of 0.5 and denitrogenation atelectasis becomes significant at F_IO_2s $\geq$ 0.5.

The therapeutic range of oxygen administration is essentially limited to less than 50%.

TABLE 5   Comparison of Gas Exchange Indices

Parameter	Mean ($\pm$SD)	Range (min–max)	r Value
Q_{sp}/Q_T	22.3 (11.2)	3.0–53.0	
Estimated shunt	27.6 (11.3)	2.7–62.3	+0.94
R.I.	3.1 (2.6)	0.3–14.0	+0.74
P_aO_2/P_AO_2	0.3 (0.2)	0.06–0.77	−0.72
P_aO_2/F_IO_2	1.8 (0.9)	0.1–4.3	−0.71
$P_{(A-a)}O_2$	222.8 (141.7)	32–611	+0.62

R.I. = respiratory index ($P_{[A-a]}O_2/P_aO_2$).

ABERRANT INTRACELLULAR METABOLISM

Arterial blood gas interpretation requires additional considerations when aberrant metabolism is present, particularly with sepsis, lactic acidosis, and parenteral hyperalimentation.

Alterations in metabolic rate predictively accompany temperature variation, thyroid dysfunction, and physical activity. Such changes in metabolic rate do not alter the relationship of CO_2 production to O_2 consumption, therefore the general rules applied to interpretation of arterial pH, PCO_2, and PO_2 remain valid. However, arterial blood gas interpretation requires additional considerations when aberrant metabolism is present, particularly with sepsis, lactic acidosis, and parenteral hyperalimentation.

Sepsis

Typical room air blood gas levels in the case of sepsis are pH > 7.35, PCO_2 < 35 mmHg, and PO_2 > 80 mmHg. Hyperdynamic sepsis ("warm shock") involves a decreased oxygen extraction $[C_{(a-v)}O_2]$, which is most likely secondary to decreased oxidative metabolism,[13] resulting in an increased S_vO_2 and thereby an improved arterial oxygenation status. A P_aCO_2 below normal is most commonly seen with the hyperdynamic phase of septic shock, probably due to a decreased CO_2 production.[13] Blood lactate levels are seldom significantly increased so that a significant component of metabolic acidosis is uncommon. Most of the guidelines for assessing oxygenation are not applicable with sepsis because the oxygen extraction is decreased independent of the adequacy of cellular oxygenation, making the relationship between arterial PO_2 and tissue oxygenation unpredictable and unreliable. "Cold septic shock" involves cellular hypoperfusion and manifests blood gases similar to all hypoperfusion states.

Lactic Acidosis

The cellular production of lactic acid is unreliably reflected in arterial or central venous blood because specific-organ system perfusion and hepatic function are variable.

Anaerobic metabolism produces lactic acid, a nonvolatile metabolite. The most common cause of anaerobic metabolism is cellular hypoperfusion. Severe hypoxemia or anemia may produce anaerobic metabolism, but most commonly a concurrent element of cellular hypoperfusion is present. The cellular production of lactic acid is unreliably reflected in arterial or central venous blood because specific-organ system perfusion and hepatic function are variable. An adequately oxygenated and perfused liver is dramatically capable of rapidly metabolizing lactic acid to carbonic acid. Thus, while certain organ systems (eg, skeletal muscle, gastrointestinal tract, skin) may produce lactic acid, normal hepatic function can prevent significant accumulation of lactic acid in the core circulation.

The presence of increased blood lactate levels documents the presence of anerobic metabolism, however, the absence of blood lactate does not infer the absence of anaerobic metabolism. Metabolic acidosis in a patient with severe hypoxemia and/or poor perfusion status must be assumed to be lactic acidosis until proven otherwise. The presence of metabolic acidemia secondary to lactic acid in a patient with shock, seizures or shivering is a dire circumstance. The absence of metabolic acidemia infers that vital organs may still be reasonably oxygenated, but by no means is that a certainty.

Metabolic acidosis in a patient with severe hypoxemia and/or poor perfusion status must be assumed to be lactic acidosis until proven otherwise.

Parenteral Hyperalimentation

Patients with increased CO_2 production are required to increase minute ventilation to maintain a normal alveolar PCO_2, producing a V_E–P_aCO_2 disparity similar to that seen with increased dead space ventilation. The respiratory quotient (RQ) is measured as the relationship of the CO_2 production to the O_2 consumption in 1 minute and averages 0.8. Total parenteral nutrition (TPN) usually provides nonprotein calories via hypertonic glucose solutions, calling for the excess glucose to be stored as lipid. Lipogenesis involves a high respiratory quotient (approaching 8.0), causing the overall respiratory quotient to significantly increase independent of the relatively stable intracellular process, producing metabolic energy. Patients receiving TPN in which the nonprotein source is primarily glucose will have an increased CO_2 production that can be reduced by providing sufficient nonprotein calories as lipid.

ARTERIAL BLOOD GASES DURING CPR

Lung function normally determines CO_2 excretion and maintains a venous-to-arterial PCO_2 gradient [$P_{(v-a)}CO_2$] of 8 mmHg or less. However, with significant diminishment of cardiac output as seen with cardiogenic shock and cardiopulmonary resuscitation (CPR), blood flow becomes the limiting factor of CO_2 excretion despite lung function. The acid–base abnormalities coincident with CPR are unique and demand separate consideration when interpreting arterial blood gases.

With significant diminishment of cardiac output as seen with cardiogenic shock and cardiopulmonary resuscitation (CPR), blood flow becomes the limiting factor of CO_2 excretion despite lung function.

ACID–BASE BALANCE
DURING CPR

During CPR with normal lungs and increased minute ventilation, venous respiratory acidosis occurs in conjunction with an arterial respiratory alkalosis.[14] In spontaneously breathing patients with poor cardiac output, the $P_{(v-a)}CO_2$ has been observed to increase 50–100%; a three- to tenfold increase has been observed in patients receiving CPR. An acute increase in venous PCO_2 results in a decreased venous pH with little change in plasma bicarbonate concentration. Since systemic capillary blood is similar to the venous blood, it is inferred that tissue PCO_2 and pH will be similar to the venous values.

Inadequate tissue perfusion inevitably leads to anaerobic metabolism and the production of lactic acid. This lactate production has traditionally been considered the primary cause of acidosis during CPR, however, it is now clear that a significant plasma bicarbonate depletion due to lactic acid accumulation is seldom present in the first 10–15 minutes of CPR.[15] The best explanation for this observation is that hepatic function metabolizes lactate to CO_2 as long as liver oxygenation is adequate; as liver oxygenation gradually diminishes the lactic acid gradually accumulates. Early lactate production probably increases CO_2 production by the liver and thereby contributes to the venous respiratory acidosis.

The plasma bicarbonate deficit attributable to metabolic acidosis is essentially equal in both the venous and arterial blood, which means that the paradoxic venous and arterial pHs seen in early CPR are due to the differences in PCO_2s. The degree of metabolic acidosis in arterial blood is reflective of total body metabolic acidosis.

A significant plasma bicarbonate depletion due to lactic acid accumulation is seldom present in the first 10–15 minutes of CPR. The paradoxic venous and arterial pHs seen in early CPR are due to the differences in PCO₂s.

Arterial pH and PCO$_2$

Mixed venous pH (pH_v) is always less than the arterial pH (pH_a). During CPR, a pH_a of less than 7.20 reflects severe tissue acidosis and is a poor prognostic sign.[16] An alkalemic pH_a during CPR is almost always due to low P_aCO_2s and does not reflect the tissue acid–base state.[17] The poor cardiac output coincident with CPR greatly increases physiologic dead space. Therefore, a significant increase in total ventilation (minute ventilation) will be required to maintain a "normal" $PaCO_2$ of 40 mmHg. In CPR dog models with normal lungs, it is possible to avoid arterial acidemia for up to 18 minutes by providing the required increase in minute ventilation.

Since the $P_{(v-a)}CO_2$ greatly increases during CPR, blood going from the right heart to the left heart without exchanging with alveolar gas (true shunt mechanisms, zero V/Q) will enter the left heart with a PCO_2 significantly greater than the blood that has exchanged with alveolar gas. If the lungs have shunting in excess of 20%, the P_aCO_2 may be greatly increased despite adequate minute ventilation. No particular comfort can be validly derived from a P_aCO_2 less than 40 mmHg, while P_aCO_2s greater than 40 mmHg reflect either inadequate minute ventilation or intrapulmonary shunting.

ARTERIAL PO$_2$ DURING CPR

Arterial oxygen content should be as high as possible to deliver maximal oxygen to the heart and brain during CPR. Arterial PO$_2$s less than 100 mmHg with F_IO_2s greater than 0.60 suggest either inadequate lung ventilation or significant intrapulmonary shunting. True shunting in excess of 25% will be associated with hypoxemia despite high F_IO_2s.

TEMPERATURE CORRECTION

Transport of CO_2 and O_2 involves gases in solution that are affected by temperature variation. Simply stated, a blood sample of given O_2 and CO_2 contents will manifest different gas tensions when analyzed at various temperatures. An open system allows for gas exchange with the adjacent environment, for example, capillary blood or a blood sample exposed to the air. A closed system does not allow mass exchange of gas content, for example, arterial blood or a gas-tight syringe. Blood samples are in a closed system where changes in temperature induce alteration of gas tensions. *In vivo* gas tension alterations due to temperature variation occur in an open system where gas contents can, and do, change.

To obtain "true" *in vivo* blood gas values, the measuring electrode's temperature would have to be adjusted to that of the patient, a process that would add at least 30 minutes to each analysis as well as complicate quality assurance. To avoid these undesirable factors, the pH, PCO_2, and PO_2 electrodes are encased in a constant 37°C environment to which the blood sample chamber is also exposed. Thus, independent of the patient's temperature, the pH, PCO_2, and PO_2 are analyzed in a closed system at 37°C.

The term "temperature correction" refers to applying mathematical adjustments to the measured 37°C values for the purpose of obtaining a more accurate reflection of the *in vivo* gas tensions. Although the derivation of temperature correction formulae is quite empiric in reference in *in*

Arterial PO$_2$s less than 100 mmHg with F_IO_2s greater than 0.60 suggest either inadequate lung ventilation or significant intrapulmonary shunting. True shunting in excess of 25% will be associated with hypoxemia despite high F_IO_2s.

vitro changes in a closed system, it is generally agreed that they are reasonably accurate within the clinically relevant ranges.[18]

CLINICAL RELEVANCE OF TEMPERATURE CORRECTION

The popularity of temperature-correcting pH, PCO_2, and PO_2 values is based on the observation that large differences in the blood gas values are present when the patient's temperature is profoundly hypo- or hyperthermic. This observation leads many to conclude that the 37°C values are "wrong." The danger in this logic is the unfounded conclusion that temperature-corrected values are "right." The scientific truth is that with significant changes in patient temperature we do not fully understand the complexity of effects on metabolism, vascular function, and respiration. Therefore, both corrected and uncorrected blood gas values are of uncertain usefulness in patients with significant deviations in body temperature. There is no logical or scientific basis for assuming that temperature-corrected values are better than the 37°C values. In fact, the available technical and biologic data leads to the conclusion that no clinical advantage to using values other than those at 37°C exists.[19]

Although temperature correction of blood gases cannot be considered wrong, several realities lead to the conclusion that blood gas values should only be temperature corrected when specifically requested by the clinician. First, acid–base balance is always best judged by the 37°C values since available data suggests that the "normal" pH is not constant with temperature variation but varies in a predictable fashion that allows the 37°C values to reliably reflect *in vivo* imbalances. Second, oxygenation is best evaluated with the 37°C values; for example, a temperature-corrected P_aO_2 of 42 mmHg in a 30°C patient does not mean severe hypoxemia exists because the 37°C value is 65 mmHg, which is acceptable for a normal VO_2 and is probably acceptable for a VO_2 diminished by 50%. Third, the assumption that the laboratory has received the patient's true temperature at the time of sampling is not borne out in our experience. Finally, temperature-corrected values can be confused with uncorrected values and vice versa.

With significant changes in patient temperature we do not fully understand the complexity of effects on metabolism, vascular function, and respiration. Therefore, both corrected and uncorrected blood gas values are of uncertain usefulness in patients with significant deviations in body temperature.

Acid–base balance and oxygenation are best evaluated with the 37°C values.

Interpretation of End-tidal PCO_2

Exhaled gas measurements will reflect the *in vivo* (temperature-corrected) P_aCO_2. With normal alveolar ventilation and a body temperature of 30°C, the end-tidal PCO_2

would be 28 mmHg while the uncorrected arterial PCO_2 would be 40 mmHg. The clinician must be aware of this circumstance so that the end-tidal PCO_2 will not be inappropriately interpreted. The P_aCO_2 must be temperature corrected to assure that the two values are being considered at the same temperature.

Oxygen Tension Indices

When oxygen tension indices are utilized, the P_aO_2 must be temperature corrected to reflect the true difference with the calculated alveolar tension.

FUTURE DIRECTIONS

Despite recent sophistications of blood gas machine technology, it remains associated with four clinically undesirable factors: (1) arterial invasion, (2) intermittent measurements, (3) removal of a blood sample with each measurement, and (4) a 5–10-minute delay in obtaining the values. It is not surprising that continuous, noninvasive techniques that can potentially reflect the arterial blood gas values, such as transcutaneous electrodes, capnography, and pulse oximetry, have gained much popularity. Detailed discussion of these technologies appears elsewhere in this issue.

FLUORESCENT OPTODES

The technology of fluorescent optode microsensing promises to introduce a new and exciting generation of bedside monitors that may revolutionize our ability to assess respiratory homeostasis at the bedside with minimally invasive techniques.

Fluorescent dyes experience molecular excitation when exposed to a light source and emit their own light (fluorescence) when the external light source is removed. Fluorescence chemistry has two characteristics that enhance adaptability for bedside monitoring: (1) fluorescence consumes so little substrate that small amounts of dye can function for long periods of time without replenishment, and (2) these dyes linearly augment or quench fluorescence activity in response to altered concentrations of specific moieties within the dye.

When fluorescence chemistry is combined with fiberoptics, optical microsensors (optodes) can be produced that are capable of detecting changes in oxygen, carbon dioxide,

The technology of fluorescent optode microsensing promises to introduce a new and exciting generation of bedside monitors that may revolutionize our ability to assess respiratory homeostasis at the bedside with minimally invasive techniques.

and hydrogen ion concentrations. Our group at Northwestern reported evaluation of a microprocessor-controlled fluorescence optode system intended to continuously and reliably measure arterial pH, PCO_2, and PO_2.[20] Although such devices are several years from being commercially available, our data confirms that this technology is capable of either continuously, or at frequent intervals, measuring the arterial blood gases without taking blood from the patient.

The continuous, or very frequent, availability of blood gas and pH values should detect significant respiratory changes prior to perturbation of clinical signs, thereby ensuring more timely therapeutic interventions. Further, when combined with transcutaneous oxygen measurement and capnography, it may be possible to trend cardiac output, categorize the perfusion status, and quantify intrapulmonary shunting without requiring pulmonary artery catheterization.[21]

The continuous, or very frequent, availability of blood gas and pH values should detect significant respiratory changes prior to perturbation of clinical signs, thereby ensuring more timely therapeutic interventions.

Transcutaneous PO_2 Index

Since the transcutaneous PO_2 ($tcPO_2$) is affected by both the arterial PO_2 and skin perfusion, it should provide a sensitive reflection of changes in skin perfusion. In fact, the $tcPO_2$ index ($tcPO_2/P_aO_2$) has been shown to correlate with cardiac output and clinical signs of peripheral perfusion in post-resuscitation patients.[22] While skin perfusion per se is of limited importance, a diminution in skin blood flow is an early sign of decreasing cardiac output and overall peripheral perfusion in most patients. Frequent monitoring of the transcutaneous PO_2 Index may provide a reliable early detection of global decreases in the perfusion status.

P_aCO_2–$P_{et}CO_2$ Gradient

A normal capnograph shows an end-tidal PCO_2 ($P_{et}CO_2$) approximately 2–3 mmHg below the arterial PCO_2. The slope and appearance of the PCO_2 rise is primarily influenced by changes in the sequence of alveolar emptying, making lung disease the most common cause of changes in the appearance of the capnograph. In the presence of an abnormal capnograph, no reliability can be placed on the extent to which the $P_{et}CO_2$ reflects the P_aCO_2, severely limiting the circumstances in which the $P_{et}CO_2$ can be considered a reliable reflection of the P_aCO_2. However, the arterial to end-tidal CO_2 gradient ($P_{[a-et]}CO_2$) is known to be a reliable indicator of changes in dead space ventilation.[23]

The most common causes of alterations in dead space ventilation are: (1) lung disease, (2) changes in cardiac output, and (3) pulmonary embolic phenomena. When the $P_{(a-et)}CO_2$ changes in conjunction with changes in the capnographic configuration, it is reasonable to assume that the dead space change is secondary to lung pathology. When the capnographic configuration is unchanged, alteration of the $P_{(a-et)}CO_2$ is most likely attributable to changes in cardiac output.[24] With frequent measurement of P_aCO_2, this concept offers the possibility of trending cardiac output changes in response to therapeutic interventions such as intravenous fluid challenge, inotropic therapy, or diuretics.

Applying the Estimated Shunt Calculation

Monitoring of the $tcPO_2$ index and the $P_{(a-et)}CO_2$ should allow for verification of the adequacy of cardiac output and peripheral perfusion, thereby confirming the reliability of the estimated shunt to quantify changes in Q_{sp}/Q_T.[21]

SUMMARY

Frequent bedside analysis of arterial blood gases without removing blood samples from the patient, combined with continuous $tcPO_2$ and $P_{et}CO_2$ measurements, promises to provide moment-to-moment trending of changes in cardiac output, the peripheral perfusion status, and oxygen transfer capability of the lungs. This might enable rapid and accurate titration of most therapies used to support cardiopulmonary function in critically ill patients. Additionally, this minimally invasive combination of monitors may provide an objective means of identifying those patients in whom more invasive monitoring, such as pulmonary artery catheterization, is warranted. Further study and development promises to make all this a clinical reality in the not too distant future.

However, despite technologic advances, the value of arterial blood gas monitoring remains with the bedside practitioner's ability to interpret and apply the values for the benefit of the patient.

References

1. Shapiro BA, Harrison RA, Cane RD, Templin R: Respiratory acid–base balance. p. 38. In: Clinical application of blood gases. 4th ed. Year Book Medical Publishers, Chicago, 1989

2. Shapiro BA, Kacmarek RM, Cane RD et al: Acute respiratory failure. p. 252. In Shapiro BA (ed): Clinical applications of respiratory care. 4th ed. Mosby-Year Book, St. Louis, 1991

3. Farhi LE, Rahn H: Gas stores of body and unsteady states. J Appl Physiol 7:472, 1955

4. Farhi LE, Rahn H: Dynamics of changes in carbon dioxide stores. Anesthesiology 21:604, 1960

5. Robin ED: Abnormalities of acid–base regulation in chronic pulmonary disease, with special reference to hypercapnia and extracellular alkalosis. N Engl J Med 268:917, 1963

6. Milic-Emili J, Aubier M: Some recent advances in the study of the control of breathing in patients with chronic obstructive lung disease. Anesth Analg 59:865, 1980

7. Shoemaker WC, Appel PL, Waxman K et al: Clinical trial of survivors' cardiorespiratory patterns as therapeutic goals in critically ill postoperative patients. Crit Care Med 10:398, 1982

8. Harrison RA, Davison R, Shapiro BA, Meyer NS: Reassessment of the assumed A-V oxygen content difference in the shunt calculation. Anesth Analg 54:198, 1975

9. Stock MC, Shapiro BA, Cane RD: Reliability of S_vO_2 in predicting the A-VDO$_2$ and the effect of anemia. Crit Care Med 14:402, 1986

10. Shapiro BA: Assessment of oxygenation: today and tomorrow. Scand J Clin Lab Invest 50(Suppl)203:197, 1990

11. Cane RD, Shapiro BA, Templin R et al: The unreliability of oxygen tension based indices in reflecting intrapulmonary shunting in critically ill patients. Crit Care Med 16:1243, 1988

12. Shapiro BA, Kacmarek RM, Cane RD et al: Limitations of oxygen therapy. p. 135. In Shapiro BA (ed): Clinical applications of respiratory care. 4th ed. Mosby-Year Book, St. Louis, 1991

13. Nishijima H, Weill MH, Shubin H et al: Hemodynamic and metabolic studies on shock associated with Gram negative bacteremia. Medicine 52:287, 1973

14. Weill MH, Rackow EC, Trevino R et al: Difference in acid–base state between venous and arterial blood during cardiopulmonary resuscitation. N Engl J Med 315:153, 1986

15. Sanders AB, Ewy GA, Taft TV: Resuscitation and arterial blood gas abnormalities during prolonged cardiopulmonary resuscitation. Ann Emerg Med 13:676, 1984

16. Suljaga-Pechtel K, Goldberg E, Strickon P et al: Cardiopulmonary resuscitation in a hospitalized population: prospective study of factors associated with outcome. Resuscitation 12:77, 1984

17. Ornato JP, Gonzalez ER, Coyne MR et al: Arterial pH in and out of hospital cardiac arrest: response time as a determinant of acidosis. Am J Emerg Med 3:498, 1985

18. Ashwood ER, Kost G, Kenny M: Temperature correction of blood gas and pH measurement. Clin Chem 29:1977, 1983

19. Shapiro BA, Harrison RA, Cane RD, Templin R: Temperature correction of blood gases. p. 176. In: Clinical application of blood gases. 4th ed. Year Book Medical Publishers, Chicago, 1989

20. Shapiro BA, Cane RD, Chomka CM et al: Preliminary evaluation of an intra-arterial blood gas system in dogs and humans. Crit Care Med 17:455, 1989

21. Shapiro BA, Cane RD: Blood gas monitoring: yesterday, today, and tomorrow. Crit Care Med 17:573, 1989

22. Tremper KK, Shoemaker WC: Transcutaneous oxygen monitoring of critically ill adults, with and without low flow shock. Crit Care Med 9:706, 1981

23. Shapiro BA, Harrison RA, Cane RD, Templin R: Capnography. p. 220. In: Clinical application of blood gases. 4th ed. Year Book Medical Publishers, Chicago, 1989

24. Smallhout B, Kalenda Z: An atlas of capnography. Vol I. Kerckebosch, Zeist, The Netherlands, 1975

ON-LINE BLOOD GAS MONITORING

C. KEES MAHUTTE, MD, PhD[†]

Intermittent arterial blood sampling for blood gas analysis is one of the most frequently performed and important laboratory tests used in the evaluation and management of patients with pulmonary or acid–base disorders. Despite the importance of this test, the indications for performing arterial blood gas analysis are rather broad and nonspecific.[1] Even though a wide variety of cardiorespiratory and metabolic disorders are associated with blood gas abnormalities, a perusal of these disorders gives little insight into the question of when a blood gas determination should be made. In the intensive care unit (ICU), clinicians usually order a blood gas analysis when clinical signs suggesting acute respiratory failure are present, when a change in management is made, or *after* an acute change in the patient's status has occurred. At present, a paucity of information on the optimal frequency of blood gas sampling that would be associated with minimal patient morbidity exists. In the near future it will become feasible to monitor blood gases on a continuous or nearly continuous basis, which has been a long sought objective[2]; hence, sudden precipitous changes in the patient's blood gas status could be managed more rapidly. Hopefully, this more rapid interaction would result in reduced morbidity and mortality.

In this chapter, the potential benefits of continuous blood gas monitoring will be reviewed, as well as the desirable features such a system should have. The methods for continuous intraarterial blood gas monitoring, that is, diffusion, ion-selective field-effect transistors, polarographic electrodes, and fluorescence, will also be examined. With regard to the fluorescent method, the intravascular blood gas probe, on-demand extravascular blood gas sensors, and continuous on-line extracorporeal blood gas analysis will be discussed.

In the near future it will become feasible to monitor blood gases on a continuous or nearly continuous basis.

[†] Associate Professor of Medicine, University of California, Irvine, Chief, Pulmonary and Critical Care Section, VA Medical Center, Long Beach, California

POTENTIAL BENEFITS OF CONTINUOUS BLOOD GAS ANALYSIS

A major reason for continuous monitoring of blood gases is to rapidly detect significant changes in patient ventilatory, oxygenation, or acid–base status.

A major reason for continuous monitoring of blood gases is to rapidly detect significant changes in patient ventilatory, oxygenation, or acid–base status (Table 1). A significant change would then prompt a rapid therapeutic response. Potentially catastrophic events, such as a cardiac arrest caused by hypoxemia, could presumably be prevented by continuous monitoring, which would reduce the associated morbidity and mortality.

Continuous monitoring would also allow more rapid identification of trends in blood gases. Thorson et al. have shown considerable spontaneous variability in blood gases in ICU patients, who otherwise appear to be clinically stable.[3] In this study, the authors analyzed gases at 10-minute intervals over 1 hour. The average variation ($\pm$SD) was 16.2 ± 10.9 mmHg in PO_2, 3.0 ± 1.9 mmHg in PCO_2, and 0.03 ± 0.02 in pH. As a result of this considerable spontaneous variation, the authors[3] suggested that therapeutic decisions should not be made on the basis of an isolated blood gas, but rather be based on trends in blood gases. Monitoring of trends might also suggest the possible etiology of the observed changes at an earlier time and thus help diagnostically.

The availability of continuous blood gas data would presumably also decrease the therapeutic decision time. Therapeutic decision time has been defined as: the total time from the ordering of a test until a therapeutic action is taken, based on the testing result.[4] Reducing the therapeutic decision time would allow more rapid optimization of ventilator, oxygen, and drug therapy and could potentially reduce hospital stay. Although many problems will need to be solved before this can become reality, eventually the ventilator adjustments can be tailored automatically to changes in blood gases. Thus, a patient's desired blood gases would be "dialed" into the ventilator and further ventilator adjustments would be made under feedback control of the continuously monitored blood gases.

TABLE 1   Benefits of Continuous Blood Gas Monitoring

Provides alarms and thereby reduces patient morbidity
Enables trends in blood gases to be followed
Decreases therapeutic decision time and allows more rapid
  optimization of ventilator, oxygen, or drug therapy
Reduces the risks of infection to both patient and operator
Reduces blood loss
Reduces cost

Another advantage to an indwelling blood gas sensor is that the necessity of withdrawing frequent blood samples, with the attendant blood loss, would be avoided. One might also expect a decreased risk in nosocomial line sepsis with an indwelling blood gas sensor since this would be part of a closed system. Because the operator would have less contact with blood than with intermittent sampling, the risk to the operator of acquiring infection from the patient would also be reduced. A reduction in billing due to intermittent blood gas analysis could make continuous blood gas monitoring cost-effective. Finally, continuous monitoring would allow one to better follow the patient's progress and might aid in determining the prognosis.

DESIGN REQUIREMENTS OF BLOOD GAS BIOSENSORS

A monitoring system that provides continuous blood gases has to have a number of important features (see Table 2). The system would have to be reliable and rugged enough to perform well in the demanding and unforgiving critical care environment. Preferably, it should not interfere with conventional practice, that is, the blood gas probe needs to be sufficiently small to fit through a cannula—preferably a 20-gauge radial artery cannula. At the same time, the capability of pressure monitoring and blood withdrawal needs to be preserved. The presence of the probe should neither increase the rate of occlusion of the probe-cannula system nor increase the rate of intravascular thrombosis. The probe has to be biocompatible, in order to avoid an accumulation over time of deposits of blood products that would interfere with diffusion and measurement of gases. The failure rate of the probe, for example, due to breakage, should be low enough to be clinically acceptable. The sensors should be stable over time and drift should be clinically acceptable. The response time of the system has to be suf-

A monitoring system that provides continuous blood gases has to be small, rugged, and reliable, and its accuracy needs to be preserved under a wide variety of clinical conditions.

TABLE 2   Design Requirements of Intravascular Blood Gas Sensor

---

Should measure all parameters (pH, PCO_2, PO_2, and temperature)
Should be small enough to fit in a 20-gauge radial artery cannula
Has to be biocompatible and nonthrombogenic
Needs to be stable and have rapid response time
Needs to be consistently accurate, rugged, and reliable
Should not be affected by reduced blood flow
Needs to work under all clinical extremes, eg, hypotension
Needs to be inexpensive and simple to operate

ficiently rapid to warn of life-threatening sudden hypoxemia or hypoventilation (for example, 90% response time $\leq$ 2 min). Accuracy of the system should be comparable to that of conventional blood gas analysis and this accuracy should be preserved over the clinically observed ranges of PO_2, PCO_2, and pH. Most importantly, the accuracy of the system should be preserved under a wide variety of clinical conditions. Particularly important conditions include hypotension, intermittent arterial spasm that can decrease perfusion, atherosclerosis, and radial artery temperature variations. Considerable progress has been made in developing systems that satisfy most of these stringent requirements. However, as will be discussed, satisfactory performance on the test bench, in animals, normal volunteers, or carefully selected stable patients does not necessarily imply satisfactory performance in unstable critically ill patients.

A biosensor may be defined as a small probe-like device that, without the addition of a reagent, gives a rapid and specific response to an analyte of biological interest.[5] The technologies that can be sufficiently miniaturized[2,5–8] to allow intravascular placement and continuous monitoring of one or more blood gases include: indwelling gas-permeable sampling catheters connected to gas chromatographs or mass spectrometers (diffusion method), field-effect transistors gated by ions, electrochemical sensors, and fluorescent sensors. Of these methods, fluorescent sensor technology appears to be the most promising,[5,9–13] however, a brief discussion of the other methods will also be included.

Methods based on diffusion, transistors, electrochemistry, and fluorescence can all be used for intravascular continuous monitoring of one or more blood gases.

PO$_2$ AND PCO$_2$ MEASUREMENT VIA DIFFUSION INTO INDWELLING PROBE

Intermittent aspiration of O$_2$ and CO$_2$, diffused into an indwelling probe, and in vitro analysis on a mass spectrometer enable semicontinuous on-line measurement of arterial PO$_2$ and PCO$_2$.

In 1960, Woldring et al.[14] stretched latex over a catheter tip and were able to show that PO_2 and PCO_2 equilibrated across the semipermeable membrane in quantities proportional to the partial pressures in the arterial blood. Intermittent aspiration of the diffused O_2 and CO_2, by entraining it in a carrier gas, and *in vitro* analysis on a gas chromatograph or mass spectrometer enabled semicontinuous on-line measurement of arterial PO_2 and PCO_2.[14–22] Thrombosis at the catheter tip was an early problem.[14] More sophisticated catheter probes that allowed faster equilibration and aspiration of gases were developed.[15–17,21] Yet a number of unresolved problems remain with this approach. The early probes required insertion of 18-gauge or larger radial artery cannulae.[16–20] Eighteen-gauge radial artery cannulae have been associated with an increased incidence of radial artery thrombosis compared to 20-gauge cannulae.[23] The probes were also expensive, and fragile, and therefore had a high failure rate.[19] Performance tended to deteriorate over time. The gases were aspirated and calculated at 4-minute intervals, and the 90% response time to changes in inspired oxygen concentration was 8–12 minutes. Thus, the system response was very slow.

Vasospasm and thrombosis were common and deleteriously affected performance.[20] These effects were evidenced by diminished waves of arterial pressure, results of angiograms, and the aspiration of thrombi.[20] Other studies using external (finger probe) blood pressure devices also have shown variations in blood pressure, presumably due to intermittent radial artery spasms caused by indwelling arterial cannulae.[24–26] Interestingly, PO_2 values obtained by the device at the radial artery site tended to be less than the simultaneously obtained blood PO_2.[19,20] This difference probably occurred because the accuracy of the probe depends on the blood velocity at the probe tip.[15,17,18] At low flows (as may occur in the radial artery, particularly when vasospasm or hypotension is present), gas depletion in the blood surrounding the probe tip might occur. Thus, better accuracy might be expected if the probe tip were located in a high flow area such as the axillary artery.[20]

The accuracy of the system was not as good as one might desire. Standard errors of the estimate of the linear regression of device versus blood gas variables were 15 mmHg for PO_2 and 5.1 mmHg for PCO_2.[19]

More recently,[21,22] probes that can pass through 22-gauge arterial cannulae have been described. The accuracy of these smaller probes should be less dependent on flow since a smaller amount of gas is aspirated. The gas diffusion through this probe membrane is analyzed on a mass spectrometer, and data display is updated every 2 minutes.[21,22] However, no human data are available as of yet with these smaller probes.

The cost associated with the instrumentation is substantial since it includes a mass spectrometer. In addition, the relatively slow response time, the dependence of the PO_2 accuracy on blood flow, thrombosis, and the fact that only two parameters (PO_2 and PCO_2) are obtained all limit the clinical applicability of this approach.

Slow response times, lack of accuracy, two parameter measurement (PO_2 and PCO_2), and cost of a mass spectrometer all limit the clinical applicability of the diffusion approach.

pH AND PCO$_2$ MEASUREMENT VIA TRANSISTORS

Ion-selective field-effect transistors can be used to measure intravascular pH and PCO$_2$, but they are still in the developmental stage.

An ion-selective field-effect transistor (ISFET) is a type of electrochemical sensor.[5,6,27] In this solid-state device, current is carried across a silicon substrate. The magnitude of the current can be influenced by the voltage, or electric field, applied to a "gate." Usually the gate is merely a metal applied to, but insulated from, the silicon substrate. If the gate is replaced by an ion-selective membrane, voltage changes caused by the accumulation of ions then influence the current. Therefore, the current can be used as a measure of the ion concentration. In this fashion, it is feasible to design a pH sensor.[28,29] Incorporation of such a pH sensor into a Severinghaus electrode[30] allows construction of a small PCO$_2$ electrode.[28,31] These devices have not yet been combined into a single pH-PCO$_2$ probe, nor can a PO$_2$ ISFET be easily developed.

ISFET devices may become clinically useful in the future because they have a high signal-to-noise ratio and can be sufficiently miniaturized to pass through 20-gauge cannulae.[31] Problems with the sensors' design, thrombus formation and protein adsorption on the surface, and stability of the sensors still remain. Thus, the devices are yet in the developmental stage, clinical data are relatively sparse,[28,29,31] and introduction in clinical practice is distant.

INTRAARTERIAL ELECTROCHEMICAL O$_2$ ELECTRODE

The development of the polarographic oxygen sensor by Clark in 1956 was followed by numerous attempts to adapt this electrode so that it could be placed on a catheter to allow continuous in vivo PO$_2$ monitoring.

The development of the polarographic oxygen sensor by Clark in 1956[32] was followed by numerous attempts to adapt this electrode so that it could be placed on a catheter to allow continuous *in vivo* PO$_2$ monitoring.[33] In the Clark type of oxygen sensor, an electrode, such as platinum, is maintained at a negative potential relative to a reference electrode, such as silver, and both of these electrodes are immersed in a potassium chloride electrolyte solution. This system is enclosed by a membrane selectively permeable to oxygen. Oxygen diffuses through the membrane and is reduced at the platinum cathode. A current proportional to the amount of oxygen is then generated and measured. Such a sensor, suitable for intravascular use,[34] was originally developed by Hoffman La-Roche laboratories and subsequently marketed by Kontron and more recently by Shiley Laboratories (Continucath, Shiley, Irvine, CA). With this device, the electrolyte solution, anode, and cathode (both consisting of silver wires) are enclosed by an oxygen-permeable polyethylene membrane. The electrode is approximately 8 cm long and has a diameter of 0.66 mm. Thus, it can pass easily through an 18-gauge cannula and barely through a 20-gauge cannula. More recently, a monopolar platinum PO_2 electrode that can pass through a 22-gauge arterial cannula has been developed.[35] Clinical data with this latter electrode are limited, and this review will therefore be confined to the more extensively studied Continucath.[36–41]

Initial studies with this electrode demonstrated that it was necessary to heparinize the electrode surface in order to prevent thrombus formation.[42] With surface heparinization, subsequent good long-term performance was shown.[37,39] To optimize pressure monitoring, it is preferable that the probe be passed through an 18-gauge arterial cannula, larger than that conventionally inserted at the radial artery site. Once the electrode is inserted, it needs time to stabilize (about 10 min) and must be calibrated against a simultaneously obtained arterial blood gas. Temperature is not measured by the probe itself and has to be entered manually based on a separate temperature measurement obtained elsewhere on the body. The sensor has a 90% response time of less than 2 minutes. The values of intravascular PO_2 have been reported to correlate well with simultaneously sampled arterial PO_2, with correlation coefficients greater than 0.96.[36–38,40,41] However, the standard errors of the estimate of the regression of intravascular PO_2 versus arterial PO_2 are substantial and of the order of 18 mmHg.[41] Similarly, although changes in intravascular probe PO_2 follow changes in arterial PO_2 with a correlation coefficient of 0.94, the standard error of the estimate associated with the regression is 28 mmHg.[41] Because these standard errors are substantial, it was concluded that this instrument was valuable as a trend monitor of PO_2 but that any acute and significant change in probe PO_2 should be confirmed by a conventional blood gas analysis.[41,43] During hypotension, the intravascular PO_2 was shown to be less than the arterial PO_2.[38] This and other data suggest that decreased blood flow at the radial artery site[36,38,43] may also deleteriously affect the accuracy of this probe. Malfunction,[36,41] drift,[39,40] and pressure damping and thrombosis[40] have also been reported.

The intravascular PO_2 probe has not found widespread acceptance. Factors that contribute to this are the above-mentioned problems: lack of accuracy and temperature correction, drift, pressure damping and thrombosis, flow dependence, and single parameter (PO_2) measurement. Per-

The intravascular PO_2 probe has not found widespread acceptance due to lack of accuracy, lack of a temperature correction, thrombosis, and single parameter measurement (PO_2).

haps most important for this lack of acceptance is the widespread availability of easy noninvasive measures of arterial oxygen saturation via pulse oximetry.

FLUORESCENT INTRAARTERIAL BLOOD GAS MONITORING

The most promising technique for continuous intraarterial blood gas measurement utilizes thin optical fibers to conduct light to and from certain chemical dyes located within or at the fiber tip.[7,9,10-13,44-46] The intensity of the fluorescent light from the dyes can yield blood gas values (*vide infra*). These optochemical sensors have also been termed optodes.[47] Major advantages of optodes are that: (1) they can be easily and inexpensively miniaturized without sacrificing accuracy; (2) patient safety is improved because an electrical connection between the patient and instrument does not exist; (3) no interference from use of electrocautery equipment occurs; (4) no utilization of substrate is present because the fluorescence involves reversible chemical reactions; and (5) enhanced accuracy occurs at low PO_2.[7,9,44,46] Disadvantages include the fragility of the glass fibers and the potential toxicity of the fluorescent indicators—both of which require secure encapsulation.[9,46]

In principle, the concepts involved in fluorescent fiberoptic sensors are simple. Light composed of suitable wavelengths travels down the fiberoptic fiber to the chemical dye, specific wavelengths are absorbed, and thereby electrons in the dye are briefly excited into higher electronic states. Subsequent decay back into the ground state is accompanied by the emission of so-called fluorescent light. The emitted light has a lower frequency than the incident light, and, by manipulating the dye and its matrix, the intensity of the emitted light can be reduced by the presence of oxygen. This quenching of fluorescence by oxygen is the basic principle of the oxygen optode.[47-52] The inverse relationship between intensity and PO_2, according to the Stern-Volmer equation,[48] implies that the oxygen optode is, in principle, more accurate at low PO_2 values. Fluorescent-based pH sensors are founded on the principle that the absorbed wavelengths of certain dyes change as a function of acidity.[53-55] Fluorescent PCO_2 sensors can then be constructed, as usual, by embedding a pH sensor in a bicarbonate solution whose pH varies as a function of the PCO_2.[30]

Based on the above principles, a fluorescent intravascular blood gas system capable of continuous monitoring of pH, PCO_2 and PO_2 has been developed (CDI system

For certain molecules, the decay of electrons, excited into higher states by incident light, back into the ground state is accompanied by emission of fluorescent light. For certain dyes, the intensity of the fluorescent light is inversely proportional to PO_2, and for other dyes can be related to pH and PCO_2.

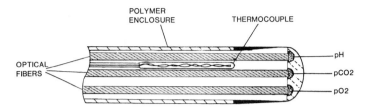

FIGURE 1   The fiberoptic probe tip. The optical fibers conduct light to the fluorescent dyes. The intensity of the light returning from the dyes can be related to the pH, PCO_2, and PO_2. A thermocouple measures temperature. From Mahutte CK, Sassoon CSH, Muro JR et al: Progress in the development of a fluorescent intravascular blood gas system in man. J Clin Monit 6:147, 1990. With permission.

1000, CDI, 3M Healthcare, Irvine, CA).[9,10,12,44,56–60] Other, more limited fluorescent probes capable only of PO_2 measurement[61] or PO_2 and PCO_2 measurement[62] have also been described. A schematic illustration of the pH/PO_2/PCO_2 probe developed by CDI, 3M Healthcare is shown in Figure 1. It consists of three 140 μm diameter optical fibers that conduct light to and from each of the sensors. Together with a thermocouple to measure temperature, these fibers are enclosed by a heparin-coated Teflon sheath. The total diameter is approximately 0.6 mm so that the probe can be passed through a standard 20-gauge radial artery cannula while preserving capability to withdraw blood, monitor pressure, and infuse standard drip solution. The pH, PCO_2, and PO_2 chemistries at the probe tip are proprietary but have been described in some detail elsewhere.[44,57] The optical bundle is sealed in a Y connector to allow fluid infusion, and the proximal end of the fiberoptic cable connects to the so-called "patient interface module." The patient interface module separates the emitted fluorescent light from the excitation light, and via photodiodes converts these emitted optical intensities into electronic signals.[44,56] The microprocessor-based system monitor contains the excitation light source (a pulsed xenon lamp). A display module displays the data, updated every 6 seconds, and the control functions. The system is illustrated in Figure 2. Prior to insertion in a patient, the probe needs to be calibrated against two gases of known O_2, CO_2, and N_2 concentrations.[10]

The above system has progressed from bench testing and animal studies to studies in normal volunteers and patients.[9,10,12] As this chapter will emphasize, success in the first three categories does not necessarily imply uniform success in a wide variety of patients. Results of *in vitro* testing of the system against standard blood gas analyzers or tonometered blood have been reported.[9,44,56,57] Linear

The pH, PCO₂, and PO₂ optode has progressed from bench testing and animal studies to studies in normal volunteers— success in the first three categories does not necessarily imply uniform success in a wide variety of patients.

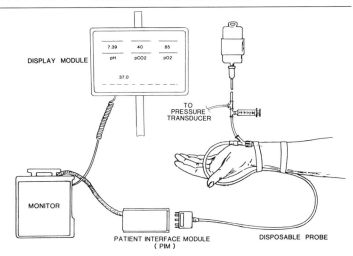

FIGURE 2   Schematic of intravascular monitoring system (CDI system 1000). The probe tip, retracted to just within the arterial cannula tip, is connected with a fiberoptic cable to the patient interface module. The monitor contains the light source and the display module shows the data and contains the control functions. From Mahutte CK, Sassoon CSH, Muro JR et al: Progress in the development of a fluorescent intravascular blood gas system in man. J Clin Monit 6:147, 1990. With permission.

In vitro and animal studies showed excellent accuracy, little drift, and clinically adequate response times for all three sensors.

regression relations of probe versus conventional blood gas values in these studies demonstrated correlation coefficients greater than 0.98 for all sensors.[57] The standard errors of the estimate were: 0.026 for pH in the range of 7.05 to 7.65, 1.9 mmHg for PCO_2 in the range of 10–60 mmHg, and 3.6 mmHg for PO_2 in the range of 20–100 mmHg.[57] Stability of the sensors was excellent with drifts/24 h of 0.005 for pH, 0.9 mmHg for PCO_2, and 2.1 mmHg for PO_2.[57] Typical response times, defined as the time to reach 63% (1/e) of a new equilibrium value, were 0.6 minutes, 1.6 minutes and 1.0 minutes for the pH, PCO_2, and PO_2 sensors, respectively.[57] Thus, *in vitro* results were excellent. *In vivo* studies in dogs also showed excellent performance of the pH and PCO_2 sensors but less accurate PO_2 performance.[9,10] Early clinical studies in patients performed at several sites (Northwestern University, Loma Linda University, Long Beach VAMC) showed poor results with frequent aberrant values.[9,12] These aberrancies tended to fall into two categories: (1) a "down, up, down" pattern in pH, PCO_2, and PO_2 compared to simultaneously obtained blood gases and (2) intermittent down drops in PO_2 only. Post study calibration of these probes showed that these patterns could not be attributed to probe malfunction. Experiments in animals in which clots were generated at the probe tip showed the appearance of the "down, up, down" pattern (Fig. 3).[12] This is consistent

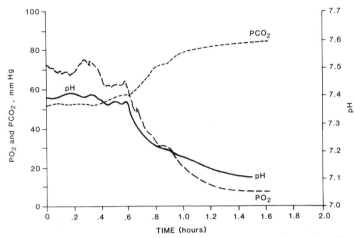

FIGURE 3 A "down, up, down" pattern, consisting of a decrease in pH, increase in PCO_2, and decrease in PO_2, that was associated with thrombus formation at the probe tip. From Mahutte CK, Sassoon CSH, Muro JR et al: Progress in the development of a fluorescent intravascular blood gas system in man. J Clin Monit 6:147, 1990. With permission.

with what might be expected with a localized metabolic process that consumes oxygen (low PO_2), releases carbon dioxide (high PCO_2), and causes increased acidity (low pH). To elucidate the drops in PO_2, experiments were performed in normal volunteers.[12] In these experiments, flow, sensor position, and sensor configuration were all varied. The experiments demonstrated that the drops in PO_2 were most likely explained by the sensor touching the arterial wall and, in effect, measuring tissue gas values (Fig. 4). The simplest way to avoid this "wall effect" consisted of retracting the sensor tip to just within the arterial cannula tip. This probe cannula configuration was studied in normal volunteers, whose blood gases were altered (Figs. 5 and 6) to cover the ranges in pH of 7.2–7.6, in PCO_2 of 20–70 mmHg, and in PO_2 of 50–200 mmHg. Standard errors of the estimate of 0.017, 2.4 mmHg, and 12.6 mmHg were obtained for pH, PCO_2, and PO_2, respectively.[12] The larger standard errors in probe PO_2 were due to an underestimation of arterial PO_2 and were speculated to be due to reduced flow at the sensor. Reduced flow could be caused by intermittent arterial spasm or a clot at the cannula tip. Reduced flow could potentially result in a longitudinal PO_2 along the radial artery with the lowest PO_2 occurring most distally. Evidence for intermittent radial artery spasm has already been cited.[24–26] The retraction of the probe tip within the cannula tip (to keep it away from the arterial wall) created other problems, such as interference of flush solution and decreased response times. These

In humans, increases in sensor PCO_2 accompanied by decreases in sensor pH and PO_2 were due to clots at the probe tip.

In humans, isolated decreases in sensor PO_2 (not accompanied by a decrease in blood gas PO_2) could be caused by the sensor touching the arterial wall or decreased flow past the sensor. To avoid the arterial wall, the probe tip was retracted just within the cannula tip.

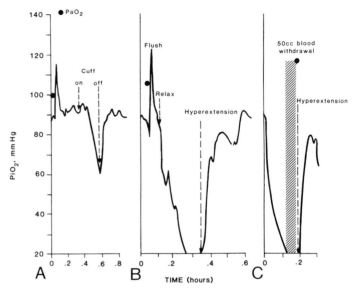

FIGURE 4   Decreases in intravascular PO_2 induced in normal volunteers. (A) The effect of blood pressure cuff elevation above arterial pressure. (B) A decrease and subsequent increase in PO_2 induced by positional changes at the wrist. (C) A positionally induced decrease in PO_2 could not be corrected by blood withdrawal past the probe tip, but only by a subsequent positional change, presumably moving the probe tip away from the arterial wall. From Mahutte CK, Sassoon CSH, Muro JR et al: Progress in the development of a fluorescent intravascular blood gas system in man. J Clin Monit 6:147, 1990. With permission.

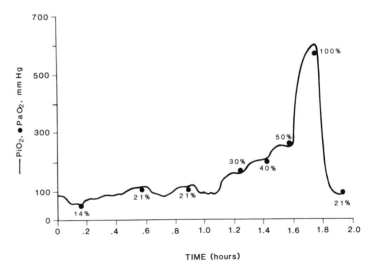

FIGURE 5   Tracing of intravascular PO_2 and arterial PO_2 as inspired oxygen is changed in a normal volunteer. From Mahutte CK, Sassoon CSH, Muro JR et al: Progress in the development of a fluorescent intravascular blood gas system in man. J Clin Monit 6:147, 1990. With permission.

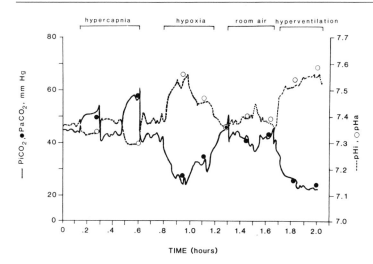

FIGURE 6   Tracings of intravascular PCO_2 and pH as well as the arterial values, as hypercapnia, hypoxia, and hypocapnia are induced in a normal volunteer. From Mahutte CK, Sassoon CSH, Muro JR et al: Progress in the development of a fluorescent intravascular blood gas system in man. J Clin Monit 6:147, 1990. With permission.

factors were dealt with by enhancing the arterial blood's tidal action at the probe tip. Enhancing the blood's oscillatory action ensured continuous exposure of the retracted sensors to arterial blood. Enhanced tidal action was achieved by inserting a variable compliance within the arterial line.[12] With the above described configuration of probe tip retracted to just within the cannula tip, and vari-

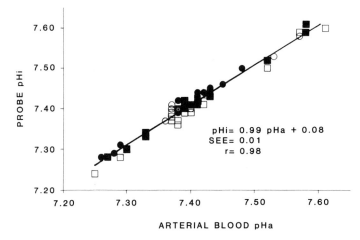

FIGURE 7   Intravascular pH versus arterial pH in four normal volunteers. Data were obtained under optimal conditions with a retracted probe cannula system and enhancement of radial artery blood by PGE_1 infusion.

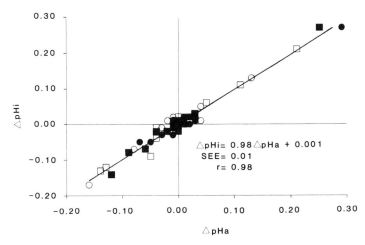

FIGURE 8   Sequential changes in intravascular pH versus the corresponding changes in arterial pH in four normal volunteers. Data were obtained under optimal conditions with a retracted probe cannula system and enhancement of radial artery blood by PGE_1 infusion.

Enhancement of radial artery blood flow with PGE_1 infusion and avoidance of the arterial wall by retracting the probe to just within the cannula tip has resulted in outstanding probe accuracy in normal volunteers.

able compliance within the arterial line circuit, satisfactory preliminary data have been published in a group of carefully selected patients.[10] In these patients, heat packs were applied to the wrist and forearm to assure that probe temperature remained within 2°C of core temperature, which presumably assured adequate radial artery blood flow. We (CK Mahutte and M Yafuso, unpublished data) have used continuous radial artery infusions of the arterial vasodilator PGE_1 to enhance radial artery blood flow[63] in normal volunteers and patients. Normal volunteers had gases and acid–base status altered as described previously.[12] With

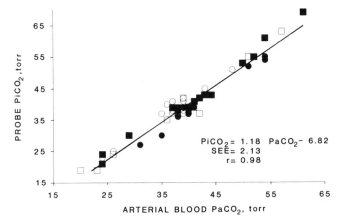

FIGURE 9   Intravascular PCO_2 versus arterial PCO_2 in four normal volunteers. Data were obtained under optimal conditions with a retracted probe cannula system and enhancement of radial artery blood by PGE_1 infusion.

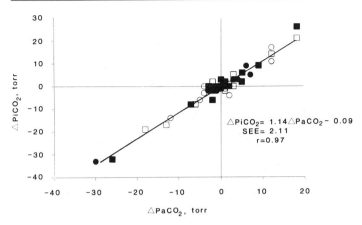

FIGURE 10   Sequential changes in intravascular PCO_2 versus the corresponding changes in arterial PCO_2 in four normal volunteers. Data were obtained under optimal conditions with a retracted probe cannula system and enhancement of radial artery blood by PGE_1 infusion.

PGE_1 in normal subjects, probe performance was outstanding as illustrated in Figures 7–12. However, even with PGE_1, results in patients have so far remained inconsistent.

It is clear that sensor technology has advanced to the point that pH, PCO_2, and PO_2 can be accurately measured with small fluorescent sensors. However, a number of problems remain to be solved before continuous intravascular blood gas monitoring can be performed routinely in critically ill patients. Inaccuracies caused by thrombus formation at the probe tip, by the sensor's contact with the arterial wall, or by low blood flow will need to be solved by innovations in probe cannula design. Intermittent low blood flow, due, for example, to intermittent arterial

Sensor technology has advanced to the point that pH, PCO_2, and PO_2 can be accurately measured with small fluorescent sensors, but innovations in probe cannula design are required to reliably measure these parameters in patients.

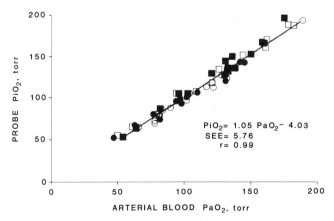

FIGURE 11   Intravascular PO_2 versus arterial PO_2 in four normal volunteers. Data were obtained under optimal conditions with a retracted probe cannula system and enhancement of radial artery blood by PGE_1 infusion.

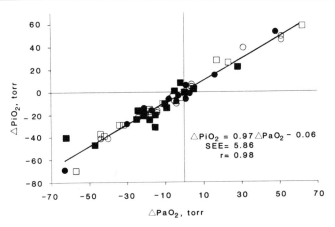

FIGURE 12   Sequential changes in intravascular PO_2 versus the corresponding changes in arterial PO_2 in four normal volunteers. Data were obtained under optimal conditions with a retracted probe cannula system and enhancement of radial artery blood by PGE_1 infusion.

Thrombi, the sensor touching the arterial wall, and intermittent decreases in radial artery blood flow can all interfere with optode accuracy.

spasm, atherosclerotic changes, positional changes at the wrist, or hypotension, may fundamentally interfere with the capability to reliably measure blood gases at the radial artery site. This may necessitate longer probes or the use of arteries with larger flows such as the brachial or femoral. The increased risks associated with the use of these larger arteries might make continuous monitoring less attractive. Long-term drift of the sensors will also need to be studied and minimized. Furthermore, manufacturing capability has to exist for consistent and reliable mass production of these delicate optodes. Finally, reliable and consistent performance will also need to be demonstrated under a wide variety of clinical conditions before these probes can be relied upon in the management of critically ill patients. It is likely to be only a matter of time before these issues are solved.[13]

ON-DEMAND EXTRAVASCULAR FLUORESCENT BLOOD GAS MONITORING

Blood gases can be measured intermittently by drawing blood into a fluorescent sensor chamber placed in the arterial monitoring line.

Fluorescent technology has also been applied to on-demand blood gas measurement.[64] In this system (CDI system 2000, CDI, 3M Healthcare, Irvine, CA), the fluorescent pH, PCO_2, and PO_2 sensors are placed in the arterial monitoring line on the patient's wrist (see Fig. 13). The system thus allows normal pressure monitoring and blood sampling. When a blood gas is desired, blood is drawn into the sensor chamber in a manner similar to current sampling

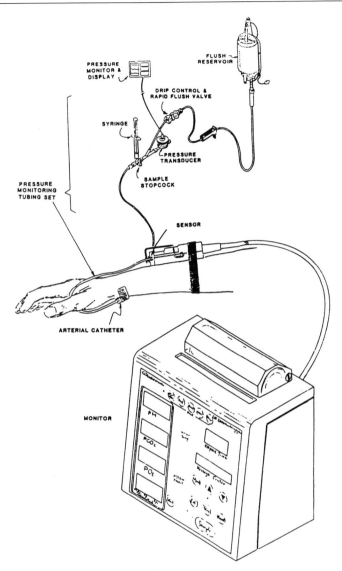

FIGURE 13   Schematic of the extravascular system (CDI system 2000). The sensor of this system is inserted in the pressure tubing line, near the arterial cannula. When a blood gas is desired, blood is drawn into the sensor cuvette. Values are displayed within 2 minutes and blood can then be flushed back into the patient. Sterility and blood pressure monitoring are maintained during the procedure.

techniques except that no break in the sterile fluid path is required. Blood gas values are then obtained within 2 minutes, after which the blood can be flushed back into the patient. Therapeutic decision time is thus reduced. Sampling can be done by nurses, therapists, or physicians and can be performed as frequently as required. Eventually, this system could be automated to give arterial blood gas values at intervals specified by the operator. Although values will not be obtained continuously, this approach avoids the difficulties and problems encountered with intravascular blood gas monitoring.

Performance has been tested in normal volunteers[64] and clinical trials in patients are ongoing. The normal volunteers inspired various steady-state concentrations of O_2 and CO_2 to induce hyperoxia, hypoxia, and hypercapnia with accompanying acidemia. Hypocapnia and alkalaemia were induced by hyperventilation of the subjects using a mechanical ventilator. Blood gases of the sensor were compared to simultaneously obtained arterial gases analyzed with a conventional gas analyzer (IL 1306, Instrumentation Laboratories, Lexington, MA). Bias (mean difference between sensor and arterial value) and precision (SD of differences) were: 0.0001 and 0.016 for pH in the range 7.23–7.60, -0.4 and 2.0 mmHg for PCO_2 in the range 20–71 mmHg, and -3.6 and 7.7 mmHg for PO_2 in the range 45–265 mmHg.[64] Thus, the system yields values close to those obtained by conventional blood gas analysis. Drift of the sensors was not studied in these short-term studies.

The accuracy of the on-demand extravascular fluorescent blood gas system, its rapid response time, the strict maintenance of sterility, and the lack of blood loss may all make this system clinically useful.

The accuracy of this system, its rapid response time, the strict maintenance of sterility, and the lack of blood loss may all make this system clinically useful, particularly in patients requiring frequent blood gases.

CONTINUOUS EXTRACORPOREAL FLUORESCENT BLOOD GAS MONITORING

Fluorescent technology was first applied to continuously monitor arterial and venous blood in the extracorporeal loop during open-heart surgery.

Fluorescent technology was first applied to continuously monitor arterial and venous blood in the extracorporeal loop during open-heart surgery.[58,65–68] During bypass surgery, sudden and large changes can occur in blood gases or acid–base status. Thus, great need for a trend monitor exists. The instrumentation (Gas-STAT, CDI, 3M Healthcare, Irvine, CA), which was introduced in 1982, has gone through several generations of development. Unfortunately, most of the published literature[65–68] has evaluated the earlier models. In all studies it was concluded that the instrument provided adequate trend monitoring of blood gases. Conclusions about accuracy were more variable. Accuracy was found to be comparable to measurements obtained with electrochemical sensors,[66] and by others not accurate enough to supplant conventional laboratory measurements.[68] No significant interference of sensor performance by the drugs typically used during cardiac surgery was found.[67] Accuracy data on the most recent generation instrument (Gas-STAT 400) have not been published, but it is claimed to be considerably improved from the earlier models, particularly with respect to PO_2 accuracy. Acceptance of the instrument by perfusionists has been excellent.

Acceptance of the most recent trend monitor model by perfusionists has been excellent.

SUMMARY

This chapter has reviewed the various methods, available or under development, for on-line blood gas monitoring (Table 3). Diffusion methods yield PO_2 and PCO_2, but only on an intermittent basis. Thrombus formation, flow dependence, and cost associated with a mass spectrometer are additional major drawbacks. Ion-selective field-effect transistors, capable of measuring pH or PCO_2, are still in the developmental stage. Problems with miniaturization, combining pH and PCO_2 ISFETs into one sensor, and adding a PO_2 sensor remain formidable. Polarographic intravascular PO_2 probes yield only PO_2 and preferably are to be inserted through an 18-gauge radial artery cannula. Associated problems are lack of accuracy, sensor drift, flow dependence, and thrombus formation.

Fluorescence appears to be the most promising of the reviewed technologies. In-line devices used for extracoporeal blood gas monitoring have been available for years.

Fluorescence appears to be the most promising of the reviewed technologies.

TABLE 3   Intravascular Blood Gas Sensors

Method	Parameter	Problems
Diffusion	PO_2 and PCO_2	Not continuous (each 2–4 min), requires 18-gauge cannula, slow response, flow-dependent, expensive (mass spectrometer)
ISFET	pH or PCO_2	No PO_2 or combined pH-PCO_2 sensor, developmental
Polaro-graphic	PO_2	Requires 18-gauge cannula, drifts, inaccurate, flow-dependent, temperature is not measured
Intravascular fluorescent	all*	Accuracy affected by thrombi, sensor proximity to wall, and reduced flow
Extravascular fluorescent	all*	On-demand and in-line but not continuous, manual sampling

* all = pH, PCO_2, PO_2, and temperature

Accurate optodes can be built, but intravascular performance remains problematic. Once this is solved, continuous intravascular monitoring will become a reality. Its role and place among the various invasive and noninvasive monitoring modalities will then have to be determined.

A fluorescent device, incorporated in the patient's arterial line circuit, that yields pH, PCO_2, and PO_2 on demand, as frequently as desired, and without blood loss to the patient, is about to be introduced for general clinical use. Fluorescent technology has now also advanced to the point that accurate and very small pH, PCO_2, and PO_2 sensors, suitable for continuous intravascular monitoring, can be built reliably. Interaction of the probe with the intravascular environment appears to be the major stumbling block. In particular, thrombus formation, contact of the sensor with the arterial wall, and decreased blood flow past the probe can all lead to erroneous blood gas values. Once these problems are solved, continuous intravascular monitoring will become a reality. Its role and place among the various invasive and noninvasive monitoring modalities will then have to be determined.

ACKNOWLEDGMENT

Supported in part by the Department of Veterans Affairs Medical Research Service.

References

1. Raffin TA: Indications for arterial blood gas analysis. Ann Intern Med 105:390, 1986

2. Eberhart RC, Weigelt JA: Continuous blood gas analysis: an elusive ideal. Crit Care Med 8:418, 1980

3. Thorson SH, Marini JJ, Pierson DJ et al: Variability of arterial blood gas values in stable patients in the ICU. Chest 84:14, 1983

4. Zaloga GP: Evaluation of bedside testing options for the critical care unit. Chest 97(Suppl):185S, 1990

5. Pickup JC: Biosensors: a clinical perspective. Lancet II:817, 1985

6. Czaban JD: Electrochemical sensors in clinical chemistry: yesterday, today, tomorrow. Anal Chem 57:365A, 1985

7. Peterson JI, Vurek GG: Fiber-optic sensors for biomedical applications. Science 224:123, 1984

8. Misiano DR, Meyerhoff ME, Collison ME: Current and future direction in the technology relating to bedside testing of critically ill patients. Chest 97(Suppl):204S, 1990

9. Hansmann DR, Gehrich JL: Practical perspectives on the in vitro and in vivo evaluation of a fiber optic blood gas sensor. In: Optical fibers in medicine. III. SPIE 906:4, 1988

10. Shapiro BA, Cane RD, Chomka CM et al: Preliminary evaluation of an intra-arterial blood gas system in dogs and humans. Crit Care Med 17:455, 1989

11. Shapiro BA, Cane RD: Blood gas monitoring: yesterday, today, and tomorrow. Crit Care Med 17:573, 1989

12. Mahutte CK, Sassoon CSH, Muro JR et al: Progress in the development of a fluorescent intravascular blood gas system in man. J Clin Monit 6:147, 1990

13. Halbert SA: Intravascular monitoring: problems and promise. Clin Chem 36:1581, 1990

14. Woldring S, Owen G, Woolford D: Blood gases: continuous in vivo recording of partial pressure by mass spectrography. Science 153:885, 1966

15. Brantigan JW, Gott VL, Vestal MS et al: A non thrombogenic diffusion membrane for continuous in vivo measurement of blood gases by mass spectrometry. J Appl Physiol 28:375, 1970

16. Brantigan JW: Catheters for continuous in vivo blood and tissue gas monitoring. Crit Care Med 4:239, 1976

17. Massaro TA, Behrens-Tepper J, Updike SJ: Non-polarographic blood gas analysis. I. In-vitro evaluation of gas chromatograph system. Biomater Artif Cells Artif Organs 4:385, 1976

18. Behrens-Tepper J, Massaro TA, Updike SJ et al: Non-polarographic blood gas analysis. II. In-vivo evaluation of gas chromatograph system. Biomater Artif Cells Artif Organs 5:293, 1977

19. Carlon GC, Kahn RC, Ray C et al: Evaluation of an "in vivo" PaO_2 and $PaCO_2$ monitor in the management of respiratory failure. Crit Care Med 8:410, 1980

20. Hall JR, Poulton TJ, Downs JB et al: In vivo arterial blood gas analysis: an evaluation. Crit Care Med 8:414, 1980

21. Goodwin B, Jumeau EJ, Clapham TR et al: A micro-intravascular probe for blood gas sampling. Anesthesiology 69:A253, 1988

22. Chilcoat RT, Goodwin B, Jumeau EJ et al: In-vivo evaluation of a micro-intravascular blood-gas probe. Anesthesiology 69:A254, 1988

23. Bedford RF: Radial artery function following percutaneous cannulation with 18- and 20-gauge catheters. Anesthesiology 47:37, 1977

24. Smith NT, Wesseling KH, de Wit B: Evaluation of two prototype devices producing noninvasive, pulsatile, calibrated blood pressure measurement from a finger. J Clin Monit 1:17, 1985

25. Kurki TS, Sanford TJ, Smith NT et al: Changes in distal blood flow during radial artery cannulation. Anesthesiology 65:A121, 1986

26. Kurki TS, Smith NT, Head N et al: Noninvasive continuous blood pressure measurement from the fingers: factors affecting the measurement. Anesthesiology 65:A134, 1986

27. Bergveld P: Development, operation and application of the ion selective field effect transistor as a tool for physiology. IEEE Trans Biomed Eng 19:342, 1972

28. Shimada K, Yano M, Shibatani K et al: Application of catheter-tip i.s.f.e.t. for continuous in vivo measurement. Med Biol Eng Comput 18:741, 1980

29. Van Der Starre PJA, Harinck-De Weerd JE, Schepel SJ et al: Use of an arterial pH catheter immediately after coronary artery bypass grafting. Crit Care Med 14:812, 1986

30. Severinghaus JW, Bradley AF: Electrodes for blood PO_2 and PCO_2 determinations. J Appl Physiol 13:515, 1958

31. Kohama A, Nakamura Y, Nakamura M et al: Continuous monitoring of arterial and tissue PCO_2. Crit Care Med 12:940, 1984

32. Clark LC: Monitoring and control of blood and tissue oxygen. Trans Am Soc Artif Intern Organs 2:41, 1956

33. Kreuzer F, Kimmich HP, Brezina M: Polarographic determination of oxygen in biological materials. p. 173. In Koryta J (ed): Medical and biological applications of electrochemical devices. John Wiley & Sons, New York, 1980

34. Mindt W: Sauerstoffsensoren für in vivo messungen. Proc Jahrestagung D Ges Biomed Tech, Erlangen 29, 1973

35. Katayama M, Murray GC, Uchida T et al: Intra-arterial PO₂ monitoring by an ultrafine microelectrode. Crit Care Med 15:357, 1987

36. Rithalia SVS, Bennett PJ, Tinker J: The performance characteristics of an intra-arterial oxygen electrode. Intensive Care Med 7:305, 1981

37. Nilsson E, Edwall G, Larsson R et al: Continuous intra-arterial PO₂ monitoring with a surface heparinized catheter electrode. Scand J Clin Lab Invest 42:331, 1982

38. Kierascewicz HT, Lam AM: Continuous monitoring of oxygenation during hypotensive anaesthesia: evaluation of an intravascular PO₂ electrode. Can Anaesth Soc J 30:S62, 1983

39. Nilsson E, Arnander C: Long-term monitoring of arterial PO₂ in burned patients. Clin Physiol 4:13, 1984

40. Bratanow N, Polk K, Bland R et al: Continuous polarographic monitoring of intra-arterial oxygen in the perioperative period. Crit Care Med 13:859, 1985

41. Green GE, Hassell KT, Mahutte CK: Comparison of arterial blood gas with continuous intra-arterial and transcutaneous PO₂ sensors in adult critically ill patients. Crit Care Med 15:491, 1987

42. Nilsson E, Edwall G, Larsson R et al: Polarographic PO₂ sensors with heparinized membranes for in vitro and continuous in vivo registration. Scand J Clin Lab Invest 41:557, 1981

43. Tremper KK: Comparison of arterial blood gas with intra-arterial and transcutaneous oxygen tension. Crit Care Med 16:1254, 1988

44. Gehrich JL, Lübbers DW, Opitz N et al: Optical fluorescence and its application to an intravascular blood gas system. IEEE Trans Biomed Eng BME 33:117, 1986

45. Delpy DT: Developments in oxygen monitoring. J Biomed Eng 10:533, 1988

46. Tremper KK, Barker SJ: The optode: next generation in blood gas measurement. Crit Care Med 17:481, 1989

47. Opitz N, Lübbers DW: Theory and development of fluorescence-based optochemical oxygen sensors: oxygen optodes. Int Anesthesiol Clin 25:177, 1987

48. Stern O, Volmer M: Über Abklingzeit der Fluoreszenz. Z Phys 20:183, 1919

49. Kautsky H, De Bruijn H: Die Aufklärung der Photoluminescenztilgung fluorescierender Systeme durch Sauerstoff: die bildung aktiver, diffusionsfähiger Sauerstoffmoleküle durch Sensibilisierung. Naturwissenschaften 19:1043, 1931

50. Vaughan WM, Weber G: Oxygen quenching of pyrenebuteric acid fluorescence in water: a dynamic probe of the microenvironment. Biochemistry 9:464, 1970

51. Lübbers DW, Opitz N: Die PCO₂/PO₂-Optode: eine neue PCO₂-bzw. PO₂-Messonde zur Messung des PCO₂ oder PO₂ von Gasen und Flüssigkeiten. Z Naturforsch 30:532, 1975

52. Peterson JL, Fitzgerald RV, Buckhold DK: Fiberoptic probe for in vivo measurement of oxygen partial pressure. Analyt Chem 56:62, 1984

53. Bülow C, Dieck W: β-Methylumbelliferon als fluoreszierender Indikator. Z Anal Chem 75:81, 1928

54. Peterson JL, Goldstein SR, Fitzgerald RV et al: Fiber optic pH probe for physiologic use. Anal Chem 52:864, 1980

55. Saari LA, Seitz WR: pH sensor based on immobilized fluoresceinamine. Anal Chem 54:821, 1982

56. Tusa J, Hacker T, Hansmann DR et al: Fiber optic microsensor for continuous in-vivo measurement of blood gases. In: Optical fibers in medicine. II. SPIE 713:137, 1986

57. Miller WW, Yafuso M, Yan CF et al: Performance of an in-vivo, continuous blood gas monitor with disposable probe. Clin Chem 33:1538, 1987

58. Miller WW, Gehrich JL, Hansmann DR et al: Continuous in vivo monitoring of blood gases. Laboratory Med 19:629, 1988

59. Yafuso M, Arick SA, Hansmann DR et al: Optical pH measurements in blood. In: Optical fibers in medicine. IV. SPIE 1067:37, 1989

60. Greenblott G, Barker SJ, Tremper KK et al: Detection of venous air embolism by continuous intraarterial oxygen monitoring. J Clin Monit 6:53, 1990

61. Barker SJ, Tremper KK, Hyatt J et al: Continuous fiberoptic arterial oxygen tension measurement in dogs. J Clin Monit 3:48, 1987

62. Larson CP, Divers S, Riccitelli S: Evaluation of a continuous blood gas sensor in patients. Anaesthesiology 73:A500, 1990

63. Bevegard S, Oro L: Effect of prostaglandin E_1 on forearm blood flow. Scand J Clin Lab Invest 23:347, 1969

64. Mahutte CK, Sassoon CSH, Zari ZE et al: Performance of fluorescent extravascular blood gas monitor. Am Rev Respir Dis 141(Part 2):A580, 1990

65. Clark CL, O'Brien J, McCulloch J et al: Early clinical experience with Gas-STAT. J Extra-Corpor Technol 18:185, 1986

66. Gøthgen IH, Siggaard-Anderson O, Rasmussen JP et al: Fiber-optic chemical sensors (Gas-STAT) for blood gas monitoring during hypothermic extracorporeal circulation. Scand J Clin Lab Invest 47(Suppl 188):27, 1987

67. Pino JA, Bashein G, Kenny MA: In vitro assessment of a flow-through fluorometric blood gas monitor. J Clin Monit 4:186, 1988

68. Bashein G, Pino JA, Nessly ML et al: Clinical assessment of a flow-through fluorometric blood gas monitor. J Clin Monit 4:195, 1988

TRANSCUTANEOUS AND TRANSCONJUNCTIVAL OXYGEN MONITORING

BARRY J. GRAY, MD, MRCP[†]
DUNCAN C. S. HUTCHISON, BM, FRCP[†]

EARLY TRANSCUTANEOUS GAS MEASUREMENTS

John Abernathy[1] demonstrated in 1793 that carbon dioxide could traverse the intact human skin. Abernathy, Professor of Anatomy and Surgery at the Royal College of Surgeons, London, showed that after immersing his bare forearm and hand in a sealed glass jar of mercury for more than 12 hours a small bubble of carbon dioxide collected over the mercury.

In 1851, Von Gerlach demonstrated an exchange of oxygen and carbon dioxide across the intact skin in man, dogs, and horses. He applied gas-impermeable varnished horse bladders to the skin and, in man, reported a mean decrease in oxygen content of the gas from 21% to 19% and a mean increase in carbon dioxide content from 0% to 2.5% over 24 hours. He concluded that "the cutaneous respiration depended on the quantity of blood streaming through the most superficial skin capillaries and on its flow velocity."[2]

In an experiment conducted over a century later, it was demonstrated[3,4] that skin blood flow and O_2 exchange were dependent on skin temperature, another crucial determinant of skin surface PO_2. The subject immersed one finger in a sealed glass tube filled with a phosphate buffer solution at 45°C. After an equilibrium period of about 20 minutes, the oxygen pressure (PO_2) of the buffer solution attained almost the same value as the arterial oxygen pressure (P_aO_2), provided that the solution was maintained at 45°C.

[†] Department of Thoracic Medicine, King's College School of Medicine and Dentistry, London, United Kingdom

DEVELOPMENT OF TRANSCUTANEOUS MEASUREMENTS USING THE CLARK ELECTRODE

The development by Clark[5] of the covered polarographic electrode was an enormous advance in the measurement of oxygen tension in blood and other fluids and made possible the establishment of the transcutaneous method.

In early experiments, Evans and Naylor[6,7] used a membraned Clark cell to make transcutaneous measurements on human skin. Their electrode did not heat the underlying skin and therefore measured transcutaneous oxygen tension ($tcPO_2$) at normal skin surface temperature. They showed that under these conditions, the $tcPO_2$ is less than 3.5 mmHg and that the amount of oxygen that diffuses from the dermal capillaries to the skin surface is largely governed by skin blood flow and temperature. The oxygen tension gradient across the human epidermis is about 35 mmHg in the adult.[8]

Huch et al.[9] then attempted to measure the $tcPO_2$ on the scalp of newborn infants using a miniaturized Clark electrode. Cutaneous vasodilation was induced with a nicotinic acid derivative, but it soon became clear that the $tcPO_2$ so obtained rarely approached P_aO_2 because the resulting increase in cutaneous blood flow was inadequate and short-lived. Transcutaneous electrodes were then developed, in which a thermostatically controlled heating coil was incorporated within the electrode structure, so that reliable long-term skin heating could produce near-maximum perfusion in the skin beneath the electrode.[10,11] The close relationship between $tcPO_2$ and P_aO_2 in newborns led to the rapid and successful adoption of continuous noninvasive $tcPO_2$ monitoring in neonatal intensive care units.[12–15]

The close relationship between $tcPO_2$ and P_aO_2 in neonates was in a sense due to the fortunate combination of ideal skin structure (thin epidermis and dense capillary network) together with careful electrode design. However, such close agreement could seldom be demonstrated in the differing physiological conditions in the adult.[16,17] As will be discussed later in this chapter, the differences between $tcPO_2$ and P_aO_2 are at their greatest and most unpredictable in adult critically ill patients, particularly those with circulatory failure, hypotension, or hypothermia.[18–21]

The differences between $tcPO_2$ and P_aO_2 are at their greatest and most unpredictable in adult critically ill patients, particularly those with circulatory failure, hypotension, or hypothermia.

PHYSIOLOGY OF THE SKIN

Thermoregulation is a prime function of skin in warm-blooded animals. A complex capillary network at the dermal-epidermal junction has evolved to regulate heat exchange at the skin surface by modulating the exposure of large volumes of blood to heat loss by evaporation and convection. The skin, therefore, possesses the ability to become greatly overperfused relative to local tissue metabolic requirements. It has been established that gas exchange at the skin surface is dependent on skin blood flow and the application of local heat can greatly increase perfusion, allowing flow-dependent skin surface measurements of PO$_2$. Recent studies of gas exchange through the epidermis, using inert gas clearance techniques, have clearly demonstrated that gas exchange obeys simple physical laws and that no active transport of gases through the skin exists.[22]

Recent studies of gas exchange through the epidermis, using inert gas clearance techniques, have clearly demonstrated that gas exchange obeys simple physical laws and that no active transport of gases through the skin exists.

STRUCTURE OF THE EPIDERMIS

The epidermis (Fig. 1) has two distinct layers, an outer keratinized nonliving layer (stratum corneum) and an inner layer of living cells (stratum Malpighi) with a layer of rapidly dividing cells at its base.

STRATUM CORNEUM

The stratum corneum is 10–20 μm in thickness in most parts of the body but is much thicker over the soles, heels, palms, and calluses. Its outer layer consists of flat and disrupted cells, showing a mosaic structure due to the high density of keratin within the cells. Cells and keratin fibers of the stratum corneum are embedded in an amorphous lipid, rich, crystalline matrix.[23] Removal of this layer greatly increases the diffusion rate of gas through the epidermis, suggesting that the dead skin layer is the rate-limiting step in gas transport to the skin surface.[24]

Effects of Heat on the Stratum Corneum

The regular crystalline structure of the lipid component of the stratum corneum melts to a random irregular form at temperatures above 41°C, resulting in an increase in the diffusion constant for gases by a factor between 10^2 and 10^3.[23] A heated transcutaneous electrode therefore causes the formation of a "diffusion window" in the skin immediately below.[25]

The epidermis is thinnest in the fetus and newborn. Little increase in thickness occurs until puberty, but in the 5th and 6th decades, epidermal thinning begins to occur and is associated with a reduction in the size of the dermal

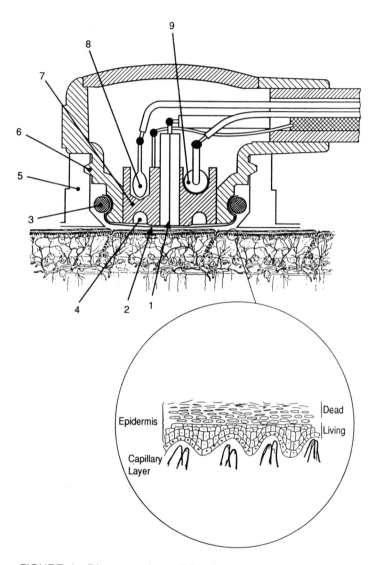

FIGURE 1   Diagram of a tcPO$_2$ electrode (Radiometer type 5243) affixed to the skin and drawn to scale. Only a thin film of fluid is interposed between the electrode and the skin surface, and a large number of dermal capillary loops lie within the electrode heat field. (1) Platinum cathode. (2) Polypropylene membrane held by (3) O-Ring. (4) Electrolyte chamber. (5) Retaining ring attached to skin, into which electrode engages by a (6) screw thread. (7) Silver anode in the form of a ring. (8) Thermistor. (9) Heating element. Inset: The epidermal layers and dermal capillary loops. Modified from Radiometer reprint TC100: Understanding transcutaneous pO$_2$ and pCO$_2$ measurements. Radiometer A/S, Copenhagen. With permission.

papillae.[26] The skin layer deep to the epidermis contains the fat, nerves, blood vessels, sweat glands, and hair follicles, supported by a dense connective tissue matrix. The dermal/epidermal junction is thrown into numerous folds, the dermal papillae. The dermis is highly vascular and the uppermost dermal capillaries rise in convoluted loops within the dermal papillae. The caps of the capillary loops are in contact with the epidermal basement membrane. Blood flow within the capillary loops is closely controlled and capable of undergoing great variation, whereby the blood within the loops acts as a thermoregulatory radiator.

The distance between loops varies between 120 and 220 μm in different regions. Frequent anastomoses between arterial and venous capillary elements are found at all levels. The deeper anastomoses are richly supplied with nerve fibers and play an important role in regulating blood flow. At room temperature and at rest, a dynamic distribution of blood to dermal capillaries exists in the adult, with about 70% of capillaries perfused at any one time, the remainder having very low or absent perfusion due to direct smooth muscle action or to shunting through the anastomoses.[27] The capillary density of all areas of skin declines with age, probably in parallel with degeneration in the supporting connective tissue matrix. In the newborn, the subepidermal capillary network is very dense and lacks mature loop formation.[28,29]

INTRACUTANEOUS PO$_2$

Intracutaneous PO_2 can be measured by a polarographic technique using a bare platinum wire inserted into the skin, although this causes changes in skin blood flow associated with the trauma of skin puncture. Problems of calibration and drift are associated with a bare wire electrode, and such measurements do not accurately reflect P_aO_2.[6]

Problems of calibration and drift are associated with a bare wire electrode, and such measurements do not accurately reflect P_aO_2.

SKIN SURFACE PO$_2$

Using an unheated electrode, $tcPO_2$ is almost zero at room temperature and even breathing 100% O_2 does not significantly increase $tcPO_2$ using this method.[7] Increasing local blood flow, however, raises the skin surface PO_2, and blood flow is itself closely related to the environmental temperature. Digital skin blood flow at a room temperature of 20°–24°C is 0.5–1 ml/100 g/min, which is sufficient to meet metabolic demands.[30] Heat induces vasodilation, and digital skin blood flow increases steadily with rising temperature and reaches about 35 ml/100 g/min between 35°C and

In the heat field under a transcutaneous electrode at 45°C, autoregulation of blood flow and vasoconstrictor responses are completely abolished, and arterial blood pressure is then the principal determinant of local flow.

Oxygen consumption is a significant contributor to the PO_2 gradient that exists between the dome of the dermal capillary loop and the skin surface. Epidermal O_2 consumption is a major determinant of tcPO2 at temperatures above 41°C and accounts for much of the large difference between P_aO_2 and tcPO2 usually seen in adults.

45°C flow.[30,31] Heat application to the skin produces vasodilation by several mechanisms. Local hyperemia may be produced, independently of nerve supply, by a direct inhibitory effect on smooth muscle, but the normal vasomotor control of cutaneous blood vessels is by the sympathetic innervation of smooth muscle in arteriovenous anastomoses.[32,33] In the heat field under a transcutaneous electrode at 45°C, autoregulation of blood flow and vasoconstrictor responses are completely abolished, and arterial blood pressure is then the principal determinant of local flow.[34]

O_2 CONSUMPTION OF THE SKIN

Oxygen consumption is a significant contributor to the PO_2 gradient that exists between the dome of the dermal capillary loop and the skin surface. It is highest in the lower layers of the epidermis, which are thicker and more metabolically active in adults than in neonates. Epidermal O_2 consumption is a major determinant of tcPO2 at temperatures above 41°C and accounts for much of the large difference between P_aO_2 and tcPO2 usually seen in adults; these large differences are less often seen in the newborn.[35]

MODEL OF LOCAL SKIN PERFUSION

A three-layer model (Fig. 2) for determining oxygen profiles in the skin under different conditions of flow has been proposed.[36] The tcPO2 under conditions (a) and (b) are highly dependent on flow. Under conditions (c) and (d), which would be obtained by heating the skin surface to 44°C or 45°C, tcPO2 is virtually independent of blood flow.

The assumptions used in this model relate to the physical and physiological properties of neonatal skin, although they also apply, in principle, to the adult. Larger PO_2 gradients are encountered across the adult epidermis, due to increased thickness and metabolic activity of the living epidermis and a thicker layer of dead epidermal cells. No allowance is made in the model for O_2 consumption at the polarographic electrode cathode, which would further lower tcPO2.

Changes in P_aO_2 can therefore be measured by observing changes in tcPO2. The major determinant of tcPO2 is skin perfusion, and so a "perfusion efficiency factor," which is the ratio tcPO2/P_aO_2 (sometimes called the "transcuta-

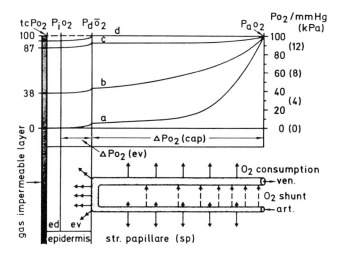

FIGURE 2   A three-layer model for cutaneous oxygen profiles under four different flow conditions. ev: living epidermis; ed: dead epidermis. Values are determined for P$_a$O$_2$, capillary dome PO$_2$ (PdO$_2$), PO$_2$ at ed/ev interface (P$_i$O$_2$), and tcPO$_2$, assuming that the skin surface is covered with a gas impermeable membrane. The flow conditions are: (a) Normal flow with tcPO$_2$ close to zero. (b) Intermediate flow with tcPO$_2$ 38 mmHg. (c) Hyperemia with tcPO$_2$ 87 mmHg (skin surface heated to 44–45°C). (d) Very high skin blood flow where tcPO$_2$ = P$_a$O$_2$ (this state is seldom realized in practice). From Huch R, Huch A, Lübbers DW: Transcutaneous pO$_2$. Georg   Thieme Verlag, Stuttgart, 1981. With permission.

neous index"), has been described.[37] This ratio theoretically approaches unity in high states of flow, when the quantity of O$_2$ delivered to the epidermis greatly exceeds the tissue demand.

EFFECT OF ELECTRODE TEMPERATURE ON HEAT-INDUCED HYPEREMIA AND tcPO$_2$

All modern electrodes are thermostatically heated to a preselected temperature that is uniform throughout the electrode core. Skin surface temperature is usually 1°–2°C below electrode core temperature, which usually needs to be at 44°–45°C to obtain stable tcPO$_2$ measurements in the adult.[38,39]

When heat is applied to the skin surface with an electrode at 45°C, a linear temperature gradient exists from the skin surface (about 43°–44°C) to the subpapillary plexus at a depth of about 1 mm, which is close to the normal body temperature of 37°C. Skin has a high thermal conductivity,

Skin has a high thermal conductivity, and it is therefore essential to design an electrode with a large heating surface.

A plateau of tcPO$_2$ response to increases in electrode temperature must be established; in normoxic conditions in adults, a temperature of 44°–45°C is sufficient to ensure maximal tcPO$_2$ readings.

When skin blood flow is adequate, the tcPO$_2$ signal will rise to an equilibrium during the warm-up period, but where the measurement is compromised by poor skin perfusion, a stable tcPO$_2$ reading may be impossible to achieve, or if it is achieved, the level may be much lower than expected.

and it is therefore essential to design an electrode with a large heating surface. A heating element of diameter 0.6–1.0 cm is the optimum size necessary to achieve a uniform temperature gradient at the center of the element.[40] Heat is conveyed away from the heat field by convection in the blood, by radiation, and by conduction in the surrounding skin and electrode cable. Only about 20% of the heat loss from the electrode is due to blood flow.[17]

With stepwise changes in temperature over the range 38°–45°C, the overall mean increase in tcPO$_2$ is 5.5% per °C,[36] most of which is due to the shift in the oxyhemoglobin dissociation curve to the right. A plateau of tcPO$_2$ response to increases in electrode temperature must be established; in normoxic conditions in adults, a temperature of 44°–45°C is sufficient to ensure maximal tcPO$_2$ readings.[36,38]

A disadvantage of the transcutaneous method is the fact that a period of time (usually 10–20 min) is required for the electrode heater to warm the skin sufficiently to bring about the optimal working conditions. When skin blood flow is adequate, the tcPO$_2$ signal will rise to an equilibrium during the warm-up period, but where the measurement is compromised by poor skin perfusion, a stable tcPO$_2$ reading may be impossible to achieve, or if it is achieved, the level may be much lower than expected.[18] The length of this warm-up period is a definite disadvantage as compared with oximetry, where no such period is required.

PHYSICAL EFFECTS OF SKIN HEATING

An electrode temperature of 45°C usually causes an erythematous burn, followed by separation of the epidermis, blister formation, and an acute inflammatory infiltrate. Length of exposure to heat, skin thickness, and the circulatory state are important factors. The cold, poorly perfused skin of shocked or hypothermic adults and premature infants is especially prone to thermal damage even at electrode temperatures below 45°C.[14,20] Thermal damage leads to low tcPO$_2$ readings because of increased intra-epidermal edema and fluid collection in blister formation (decreasing tissue O_2 conductivity) and increased metabolic consumption of O_2 by the acute inflammatory cells migrating to the area of the burn. The generally accepted maximum safe electrode temperatures are 45°C in adults and 44°C in neonates.[41–43] These temperatures will usually enable safe tcPO$_2$ measurements for up to 6 hours, but skin tolerance to heat varies greatly between subjects.[38]

EFFECT OF CATHODE SIZE AND ELECTRODE MEMBRANE

Oxygen consumption by the cathode is related to its size and surface area. The so-called "macrocathodes" have a high O_2 consumption and influence the O_2 profile within the epidermis, causing large differences between capillary PO_2 and skin surface PO_2. This source of error can be minimized by keeping cathode size and surface area as small as possible. The large oxygen consumption of the macrocathode requires the use of a membrane material of low O_2 conductivity, but this has an adverse effect on the time constant, with 90% response times of 55–60 seconds, compared with 10–15 seconds for microcathode systems.[44] Membranes of low O_2 conductivity also tend to have lower heat conductivity and, consequently, lower skin surface temperatures for a given electrode core temperature, resulting in further lowering of $tcPO_2$ values with slower response times.

Membrane O_2 conductivity and thickness thus have large effects on the absolute skin surface PO_2 signal. Most electrodes currently available have been designed for neonatal work and are not optimally constructed and membraned for a heterogeneous range of subjects with skin factors (such as thickness, heat conductivity, O_2 consumption, and O_2 conductivity) that tend to vary with age.[20,29] For this reason, the ratio of $tcPO_2$ to P_aO_2 varies widely from subject to subject, although the ratio in a single subject tends to remain stable at a constant temperature and skin site.

The so-called "macrocathodes" have a high O_2 consumption and influence the O_2 profile within the epidermis, causing large differences between capillary PO_2 and skin surface PO_2. This source of error can be minimized by keeping cathode size and surface area as small as possible.

EFFECT OF SKIN SITE AND PREPARATION

The absolute level of $tcPO_2$ is affected by skin thickness and capillary density.[37] It is therefore important to place the electrode at a site of high capillary density and minimal thickness for optimal $tcPO_2$ measurements. Site selection presents no particular problem in the newborn where these conditions are usually fulfilled.[29,45] Greater variation is found in adults, and the inside of the upper arm, forearm, infraclavicular regions, and abdomen yield the highest $tcPO_2$ values.

Skin preparation by vigorous rubbing with an alcohol swab, to clean the surface of normal lipid film and induce reactive hyperemia, has been recommended but probably has little effect on the absolute accuracy and response time of subsequent $tcPO_2$ measurements.[46] Another method fre-

It is important to place the electrode at a site of high capillary density and minimal thickness for optimal $tcPO_2$ measurements.

Despite the apparent advantages of epidermis removal, no information on infection rates or other complications exists and suction blister formation is time-consuming and increases the invasiveness of the transcutaneous method.

quently adopted to remove the stratum corneum is the repeated application and removal of adhesive tape to the selected skin site; again, this does not seem to significantly improve the measurement,[46] perhaps because the procedure induces reflex vascular changes and acute inflammation leading to edema and reduction in O_2 conductivity. Epidermal separation in adult subjects was achieved by producing "suction blisters" on the forearm, which was claimed to be a painless procedure.[47] Transcutaneous PO_2 measurements in these experiments increased from a mean of 51 mmHg by the standard technique to a mean of 104 mmHg at the blister base. The method allowed the authors to use the tcPO_2 electrode for longer periods at a lower temperature (42°C), and the response time to changes in tcPO_2 was decreased by 30%. Despite the apparent advantages of epidermis removal, no information on infection rates or other complications exists and suction blister formation is time-consuming and increases the invasiveness of the transcutaneous method.

EFFECTS OF SYSTEMIC AND REGIONAL BLOOD SUPPLY, BLOOD PRESSURE, AND HYPOTHERMIA

The theoretical description of the relationship between tcPO_2 and P_aO_2 has generally assumed a stable circulation with a normal cardiac output and near maximal skin vasodilation below the heated electrode. Under these conditions, the normal adaptive vasoactivity, which regulates blood flow within the outermost parts of the skin vasculature, is largely abolished by the application of heat, and flow in the dermal capillaries is then largely determined by blood pressure and regional blood supply.[34] So long as blood pressure and regional skin perfusion are normal and a state of hyperemia exists in the skin, tcPO_2 will be flow-independent; broadly speaking, tcPO_2 will be related to P_aO_2, but will differ from it by a quantity that is relatively constant and determined by the components of skin and electrode membrane resistance to O_2 flux, skin and electrode O_2 consumption, and temperature-related shifts in the oxyhemoglobin dissociation curve of the blood within the dermal capillaries. In less favorable circumstances of low cardiac output with poor regional perfusion of the skin, the relationship between tcPO_2 and P_aO_2 is less constant. The tcPO_2 then no longer reflects P_aO_2 but is an indicator of regional O_2 tissue delivery to the skin and can be used as a rough guide to the onset of and recovery from low cardiac output shock.[48] In some tcPO_2 measurement systems, the numerical value of the current supplying the electrode heater can be displayed. If skin blood flow falls, one would expect less heat to be removed from the area and thus less current would be required. It has been suggested that the displayed value of the current could also be used as an indicator of skin blood flow, but only 20% of the heat loss is due to blood flow.[17]

The increasing difference between $tcPO_2$ and P_aO_2 in shock states is physiologically explicable by the increasing cutaneous vasoconstriction. Reduction in flow means that skin metabolism consumes an increasing fraction of the total O_2 delivery. It is recognized that $tcPO_2$ is not representative of P_aO_2 in newborns with severe cardiorespiratory distress,[13,14] and the same applies to adults.[49,51] In shocked patients, $tcPO_2$ is more closely related to cardiac output and tissue O_2 delivery and is poorly correlated with P_aO_2.[21] A wide and unpredictable P_aO_2–$tcPO_2$ gradient has also been reported in hypothermic patients following open heart surgery in both newborn infants[52] and adults.[18]

In shocked patients, $tcPO_2$ is more closely related to cardiac output and tissue O_2 delivery and is poorly correlated with P_aO_2.

CALIBRATION METHODS

CALIBRATION USING STANDARD GASES

The polarographic method of measuring $tcPO_2$ requires only a two-point calibration procedure because the signal output from a Clark cell is virtually linear over the physiological range.[5,41] For the lower-point calibration (zero or minimal current), several methods are available, including exposing the electrode to pure nitrogen, placing a drop of reducing solution such as saturated sodium sulphite solution on the electrode membrane, or obtaining electrical zero by disconnecting the electrode cable from the power source. In practice, there is little difference between these methods of lower point calibration in terms of convenience and accuracy.

Calibration of the upper point presents more problems. The conventional calibration method, as recommended by most manufacturers and implemented in the majority of reports, is a two-stage procedure using air or a suitable gas mixture as the upper calibration point. In general, it is essential that the upper point be near the top of the PO_2 range expected during the study and that the electrode is at the working temperature.

The use of dry gases or air for calibration is certainly more convenient than the complicated systems required for calibrating the electrode in thermostatically controlled chambers containing gas mixtures saturated with water vapor

The polarographic method of measuring $tcPO_2$ requires only a two-point calibration procedure because the signal output from a Clark cell is virtually linear over the physiological range.

TABLE 1   Statistical Relationship Between tcPO$_2$ (y axis) and P$_a$O$_2$ (x axis) in Some Reported Studies

Ref. No.	Patient Studies	No. of Patients	No. of Samples	Regression Coefficient	Intercept y Axis (mmHg)	Correlation Coefficient	95% Confidence Limits (mmHg)	Study Range (mmHg)
12	Neonates	22	106	0.81	+12.3	0.94	—	17–180
13	Neonates	30	159	0.96	+ 2.1	0.98	±10	16–145
15	Neonates	12	>100	0.85	+13.0	0.85	±10	35–90
84	Adults and children with lung disease	7	152	0.78	+16.7	0.92	—	43–158
21	ICU adults, no shock	92	934	0.78	+ 4.1	0.9	—	23–495
21	ICU adults, mild shock	74	5	0.5	+ 6.0	0.78	—	
20	ICU adults; hypothermia	18	34	0.29	+50.7	0.52	—	45–200
20	ICU patients	18	24	0.91	+11.2	0.78	—	60–200
17	Adults ICU	—	66	0.52	+19.6	0.63	±37	50–175
18	Adults ICU	14	35	0.69	+14.9	0.9	±24	44–184
18	Adults ambulant	20	20	0.88	+ 5.0	0.93	±10	50–104

The gas calibration method may be sufficient to obtain accurate tcPO$_2$ in neonates, but in older children and adults the electrode properties do not usually compensate for differences in the skin physiology such that tcPO$_2$ usually underestimates P$_a$O$_2$.

In view of the potential errors that can arise from the gas calibration method, it seems more logical to calibrate the upper point using the independently measured PO$_2$ in the subject's own arterial blood.

or electrode membrane/liquid interfaces. It has been shown, moreover, that calibrating tcPO$_2$ electrodes at 45°C in dry gases or ambient air and ignoring vapor pressure introduces only a small and tolerable error of less than 2%.[53]

The gas calibration method may be sufficient to obtain accurate tcPO$_2$ in neonates, but in older children and adults the electrode properties do not usually compensate for differences in the skin physiology such that tcPO$_2$ usually underestimates P$_a$O$_2$.[20,50]

Table 1 shows the result of a selected group of studies in which the P$_a$O$_2$ and tcPO$_2$ are compared in adults and neonates after gas calibration of the upper point. It can be seen that agreement between tcPO$_2$ and P$_a$O$_2$ is not necessarily present in neonatal studies, and in adults, a regression coefficient significantly less than unity is always present as well as a large positive intercept on the tcPO$_2$ axis. The 95% confidence limits further indicate that the statistical reliability that can be placed on an individual tcPO$_2$ result is not high. This has led to the recommendation that tcPO$_2$ should be regarded only as a P$_a$O$_2$ "trend monitor" and not as a reliable measurement of P$_a$O$_2$ itself.[54,55]

CALIBRATION USING AN ARTERIAL BLOOD SAMPLE

In view of the potential errors that can arise from the gas calibration method, it seems more logical to calibrate the upper point using the independently measured PO$_2$ in the subject's own arterial blood. The whole point of the transcutaneous method is, after all, to estimate the arterial PO_2 and not the PO_2 of the ambient air. By this approach, the upper calibration point is obtained after the electrode has been attached to the skin and a stable provisional $tcPO_2$ reading has been obtained. Only the upper point requires recalibration, as the zero point remains unchanged, and this can be achieved either by adjusting the $tcPO_2$ signal gain so that $tcPO_2$ is set to the P_aO_2 obtained from an arterial blood sample or by retrospective derivation of a calibration factor from the ratio of $tcPO_2$ to P_aO_2, also obtained from a single arterial blood sample.[18,50] These two approaches are equivalent since the current is directly proportional to the PO_2 at the platinum cathode.

The use of such a method of recalibration has been criticized on theoretical grounds, with predictions that $tcPO_2$ will not accurately reflect P_aO_2 over a wide range of values.[35,56] In fact, the theoretical background to the arterial calibration method is quite sound. If the skin is sufficiently heated so as to produce near-maximum hyperemia and arterialization of the blood in the dermal capillary loops, $tcPO_2$ will be almost flow-independent.[37] All of the factors contributing to the difference between P_aO_2 and $tcPO_2$ (capillary shunt, diffusion, epidermal O_2 consumption, temperature-related shift in the oxyhemoglobin dissociation curve, and changes in epidermal O_2 conductivity) will remain relatively constant if a constant temperature and heat field can be established in the skin down to the level of the subpapillary plexus.

The two calibration methods were compared in a study of 14 patients in an intensive care unit (ICU).[57] All of the patients had a mean systemic arterial blood pressure greater than 80 mmHg, were not hypothermic (temperature $> 36.5°C$), and appeared to have normal skin circulation (Figs. 3 and 4).

The results demonstrate that by the arterial calibration method, $tcPO_2$ can provide a much more accurate estimate of P_aO_2 than the gas calibration method. The mean $tcPO_2/P_aO_2$ ratio by gas calibration was 0.75; a figure of this order is a common finding in studies involving normal adult subjects and adult ICU patients without evidence of circulatory failure or hypothermia (Table 1), and the wide confidence limits further indicate the lack of precision inherent in this method. In a number of studies, an increasing difference between P_aO_2 and $tcPO_2$ is seen at P_aO_2 values >120 mmHg, which can often be quite simply attributed to the fact that the higher values of P_aO_2 are far outside the original calibration range and are predictably less accurate.

In the ICU, the arterial calibration method offers no ad-

The theoretical background to the arterial calibration method is quite sound. If the skin is sufficiently heated so as to produce near-maximum hyperemia and arterialization of the blood in the dermal capillary loops, $tcPO_2$ will be almost flow-independent.

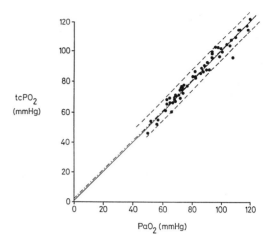

FIGURE 3   Standard gas calibration of $tcPO_2$ in 14 patients in an ICU.[57] A two-point calibration was performed. Lower point: electrical zero; Upper point: air. The relationship between $tcPO_2$ and P_aO_2 is given by: $tcPO_2$ (mmHg) = 0.58 P_aO_2 + 13. 4 (r = 0.82; 95% confidence limits ± 19.6). ⎯⎯ = line of iden- tify; − · − = regression line; − − = 95% confidence limits.

ditional problems if an arterial cannula is already *in situ*. This is seldom the case in ambulant patients or subjects undergoing physiological testing. It might be argued that arterial sampling in these circumstances is unjustified and compromises the noninvasive nature of the transcutaneous measuring technique. A single arterial puncture under ad- equate local anesthesia using a self-filling syringe is a vir-

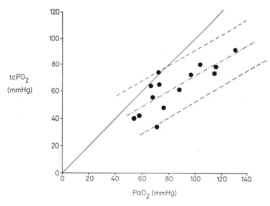

FIGURE 4   Arterial blood calibration in same 14 patients as Fig. 3. Lower calibration point: electrical zero; Upper point: arterial blood. 55 data points are shown and the relationship between $tcPO_2$ and P_aO_2 is given by: $tcPO_2$ (mmHg) = 0.98 P_aO_2 + 1.6 (r = 0.98; 95% confidence limits ± 6.6).

tually painless and trouble-free procedure and is justified by the increased accuracy that it affords. Arterialized capillary blood samples from the earlobe have been shown to yield an accurate estimate of P_aO_2.[58]

It is appropriate to add a note on the methods of statistical analysis undertaken in many of the transcutaneous O_2 studies on adult subjects reported in the literature. Many studies rely heavily on establishing a significant correlation coefficient between the values of P_aO_2 and $tcPO_2$, with much less reliance placed upon regression analysis and estimations of 95% confidence limits. The fact that two methods of measuring the same parameter are significantly correlated should not cause surprise, and indeed it would be astonishing if they were not so related.

ACCURACY AND RESPONSE TIMES

ELECTRODE RESPONSES

The current produced by modern polarographic electrodes when directly exposed to changes in PO_2 in the gas phase is linear from 0 to 100% O_2.[5,41] The response time to a square wave change in PO_2 in the gas phase is rapid, and an equilibrium is usually obtainable within 30 seconds (Fig.

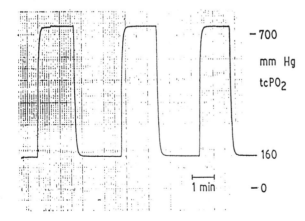

FIGURE 5   Response time of $tcPO_2$ electrode on direct exposure to square wave change in O_2 concentration from and to 100% O_2 and vice versa. The electrode was directly exposed to the gas phase and moved by hand rapidly in and out of a chamber containing continuously flowing 100% O_2. The time taken to establish a plateau is less than 30 seconds in either direction.

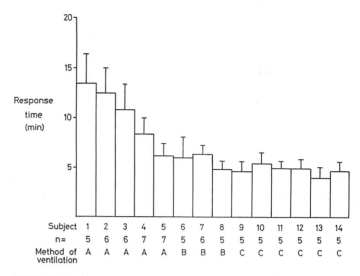

FIGURE 6   Mean response times of tcPO$_2$ (to establishment of a plateau) in 14 patients in an ICU, undergoing a square wave change in F$_I$O$_2$. Bars = 1 SD; n = number of estimations in each patient. Method of ventilation: (A) mechanical ventilation with endotracheal tube; (B) spontaneous ventilation with endotracheal tube; (C) spontaneous ventilation with oxygen mask.

5). The electrode itself is therefore capable of responding faithfully to virtually any physiological change that is likely to occur. In contrast, the *in vivo* response times depend on many physiological variables that are not necessarily constant, including the rate of pulmonary gas mixing and the circulation time, in addition to the delay imposed by the conductivities of the skin and electrode membrane.

RESPONSE TIMES IN INTENSIVE CARE PATIENTS

The tcPO$_2$ responses to sudden changes in F$_I$O$_2$, when they can be measured, are often delayed, especially in the most seriously ill patients, such as those on assisted ventilation.

During studies of any duration in an ICU, it is inevitable that a number of nursing and therapeutic procedures will need to be carried out. Coughing, lifting, catheter drainage, movement, and the general unrest associated with a busy unit make accurate response times difficult to obtain.[61] The tcPO$_2$ responses to sudden changes in F$_I$O$_2$, when they can be measured, are often delayed,[50] especially in the most seriously ill patients, such as those on assisted ventilation. Ventilators and tubing have a large amount of dead space, and patients receiving ventilation are usually those with grossly impaired pulmonary gas exchange, all factors that impose further delay on tcPO$_2$ response to a change in the inspired O$_2$ concentration (Fig. 6).[59]

RESPONSE TIMES IN HYPOXIA

The difficulties of assessing response times in critically ill patients make it necessary to study some of the possible variables in model situations outside the ICU; thus, response times can readily be estimated following a stepwise change in F_IO_2, resulting in hypoxemia or hyperoxemia. The accuracy and response times of end-tidal PO_2, $tcPO_2$, and oxyhemoglobin saturation measurements have been compared in normal subjects at rest and engaged in exercise during changes from normoxic to hypoxic conditions.[59] During exercise, a reduction in circulation time occurs and gas exchange within the lung becomes more efficient due to increased ventilation and better matching of perfusion and ventilation. These factors should all theoretically reduce the response times of end-tidal PO_2, $tcPO_2$, and oxyhemoglobin saturation (S_aO_2) determined by oximetry. Six normal subjects were studied and the $tcPO_2$ electrode was calibrated by setting the initial value to the end-tidal PO_2. The results from a typical subject are shown in Figure 7. The end-tidal PO_2, as expected, changes almost immediately, but a short lag period occurs for $tcPO_2$ and S_aO_2 due to the transmission time from the pulmonary capillaries to the measurement site. The lag period for $tcPO_2$ was slightly longer than for S_aO_2, although the difference is of no clinical importance.

Following the lag period is a quasi-exponential change from which it was shown that the 90% response time for

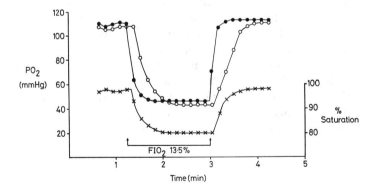

FIGURE 7 Comparison of response times of end-tidal PO_2 (closed circles), $tcPO_2$ (open circles), and S_aO_2 by oximetry (crosses) in a normal subject performing steady-state exercise on a cycle ergometer at 60% of maximal work capacity. The period of hypoxia is introduced and terminated effectively as a square wave. The 90% response times for $tcPO_2$ and S_aO_2 are similar and about 15 seconds longer than for end-tidal PO_2. The lag times for $tcPO_2$ and S_aO_2 are similar (not more than 10 s).

S_aO_2 was on average about 10 seconds faster than $tcPO_2$ during the induction of hypoxia but about 40 seconds faster on recovery. This difference is in part explained by the fact that PO_2 and S_aO_2 are not linearly related. A square wave change in the inspired gas concentration would in theory produce an exponential change in P_aO_2. Consideration of the oxyhemoglobin dissociation curve indicates that P_aO_2 will therefore be in advance of S_aO_2 during induction of hypoxia and will lag behind during the recovery phase. Any comparison of the response times of the two methods must take this into account.

The final equilibrium P_aO_2 was very similar to that of the end-tidal PO_2 indicating that the use of end-tidal PO_2 for calibration is valid in normal subjects, although it would not be an accurate indicator of P_aO_2 in the ICU. The overall results show that hypoxemia could be as readily detected by the transcutaneous method as by oximetry.

RESPONSE TIMES AND ACCURACY DURING EXERCISE

Large changes in cardiac output take place during maximal exercise, and substantial and rapid changes in P_aO_2 occur in emphysematous patients. Six patients with emphysema[60] performed a progressive exercise test to maximal exercise capacity while $tcPO_2$ and P_aO_2 (from an indwelling arterial cannula) were both monitored. The mean $tcPO_2/P_aO_2$ ratio was 0.8 following the conventional preliminary calibration using air as the upper calibration point. The arterial calibration procedure was then performed. $tcPO_2$ was shown to follow P_aO_2 very closely (Fig. 8) both during the slow initial fall and during the very rapid post-exercise increase, which is presumed to be due to the sudden reduction in O_2 consumption leading to a sharp rise in central venous PO_2, while ventilation and cardiac output remain considerably above normal. Sixty-eight paired comparisons were available and the regression equation is given by:

$$tcPO_2 \text{ (mmHg)} = 0.98\, P_aO_2 + 0.7 \text{ (95\% confidence limits 5.7 mmHg)}$$

Both the hypoxia and the exercise studies therefore demonstrate that the physiological response times of the $tcPO_2$ electrodes in common use are sufficiently fast to follow any possible changes in P_aO_2 that are likely to occur, always with the caveat that skin perfusion must be adequate, which of course may not be the case in the ICU.

Both the hypoxia and the exercise studies demonstrate that the physiological response times of the tcPO$_2$ electrodes in common use are sufficiently fast to follow any possible changes in P$_a$O$_2$ that are likely to occur, always with the caveat that skin perfusion must be adequate, which of course may not be the case in the ICU.

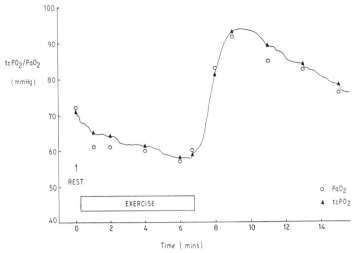

FIGURE 8   Continuous record of tcPO₂ in a patient with emphysema during an exercise test (cycle ergometer), the work load being increased to maximum by 10 watts every minute. The arterial calibration procedure was used; the upper calibration point was obtained from a sample drawn from an indwelling arterial cannula. Circles = arterial PO₂; triangles = tcPO₂ read from digital meter at midpoint of arterial sampling. From Hughes JA, Gray BJ, Hutchison DCS: Changes in transcutaneous oxygen tension in pulmonary emphysema. Thorax 39:424, 1984. With permission.

ELECTRODE DRIFT

Electrodes should be tested for drift by comparison of readings at the beginning and end of any study, against a standard gas or arterial sample if available. In intensive care studies,[59] there was on average a small downward drift of 1.4 mmHg (SD ± 5.3). Larger drifts were observed with combined tcPO₂ and PCO₂ electrodes,[62] although other authors have found this type of electrode to be reliable.[46,63]

THE HALOTHANE EFFECT

Polarographic electrodes are affected by a number of substances other than oxygen, notably the widely used anesthetic gas, halothane.[64] If an electrode is exposed directly (that is, without involving the transcutaneous method) to halothane in the fluid or gas phase, the electrode output is proportional to the halothane concentration[65]; thus the concentrations used in clinical anesthesia (10–20 mg/100 ml) could increase the apparent PO₂ by as much as 150 mmHg. The PO₂ measured by a direct-reading blood gas electrode could therefore be completely misleading in the presence of halothane, even though the effect may be very much smaller when P$_a$O₂ is estimated by the transcuta-

The PO₂ measured by a direct-reading blood gas electrode could be completely misleading in the presence of halothane, even though the effect may be very much smaller when P$_a$O₂ is estimated by the transcutaneous method.

neous method. The drift of a $tcPO_2$ electrode was assessed[66] during anesthesia with a number of agents including halothane and the related substances isoflurane and enflurane. The zero drift was somewhat greater with halothane (mean 1.8 mmHg $\pm$ 3.2) than with the other agents but of little clinical significance. The rate of diffusion of halothane across the skin is therefore probably very low compared with oxygen.

COMPARISON OF $tcPO_2$ MEASUREMENT AND PULSE OXIMETRY

ADVANTAGES OF $tcPO_2$

The $tcPO_2$ provides a direct measurement of P_aO_2 that is more closely related to ventilation than S_aO_2 obtained by oximetry. This advantage is particularly apparent when S_aO_2 is greater than 90%, where a 2% change in S_aO_2 from 97% to 95% would result in a change in P_aO_2 from 95 to 75 mmHg, the limit of accuracy for oximetry being 2% saturation at best. The detection of P_aO_2 values greater than 100 mmHg is of great importance in the monitoring of newborn infants but also has a role in adult monitoring if the patient is breathing an oxygen-enriched mixture. If the lungs are normal, the P_aO_2 should be substantially greater than 100 mmHg—the exact level depending on the F_IO_2. A significant shunt could be detected by the $tcPO_2$ method even though S_aO_2 might remain within the normal range.

ADVANTAGES OF OXIMETRY

No skin heating and therefore no warm-up time are required for oximetry and no danger of skin damage exists. No calibration is required, whereas the calibration of $tcPO_2$ electrode requires a blood sample if the most reliable results are to be obtained.

TRANSCONJUNCTIVAL PO_2

The need to heat the underlying skin and the obligatory warm-up time of transcutaneous electrodes are limitations of this method, consequently, a quest was begun to find a site where measurement of PO_2 at the body surface could be carried out in more advantageous circumstances.

One such site that has been intensively investigated is the conjunctiva. The study of oxygen tension at the conjunctival surface, or transconjunctival O_2 ($cjPO_2$) was begun by the work of Fatt and Kwan.[67,68] The cjPO$_2$ can be measured by a sensor that consists of a miniaturized Clark polarographic cell and a thermistor that are bonded together into an acrylic circular ocular conformer. The conformer fits mainly under the eyelid, allowing the measurement of oxygen tension at the conjunctival surface of the upper eyelid at a point beneath the overlying tarsal plate. The electrode surface is separated from the conjunctiva by a thin film of tear fluid, and the thermistor allows compensation for temperature-dependent variations in output of the electrode. Measurement of PO$_2$ at the conjunctival surface theoretically offers significant advantages compared with the measurement of tcPO$_2$. The conjunctiva is only one or two cells thick and in close approximation to a rich plexus of subconjunctival capillaries. The diffusion path for oxygen is therefore very short, hence heating of the underlying tissue in order to induce hyperemia is not necessary and the oxygen gradients between blood and electrode are therefore small.[69]

The cjPO$_2$ electrode has acceptable response characteristics for the continuous monitoring of P$_a$O$_2$. In vitro the sensor has a 90% response time of less than 40 seconds, sensitivity drift of less than 1% per hour, and absolute temperature-measuring accuracy of $\pm 0.1°C$.[70] The electrode reading is stable within 5 minutes of application to the conjunctiva.

Direct comparisons of cjPO$_2$ and P$_a$O$_2$ have been undertaken.[70–73] The results have usually been expressed as the ratio of cjPO$_2$ to P$_a$O$_2$, or the "transconjunctival index." The transconjunctival index is dependent on cardiac index, tissue oxygen delivery, and oxygen consumption in patients with respiratory failure or low-output shock.[72,74]

It has been suggested that monitoring cjPO$_2$ may provide information about cerebral oxygen delivery because the arterial blood supply to the palpebral conjunctiva is largely derived from the ophthalmic artery, a branch of the internal carotid.[75] However, in a study of 17 patients undergoing carotid endarterectomy under general anesthesia, it was found that low cjPO$_2$/P$_a$O$_2$ ratio existed before anesthesia (mean 0.48), which became lower (mean 0.32) during anesthesia and associated hyperoxia. Large interindividual differences in cjPO$_2$ readings during carotid cross-clamping and carotid endarterectomy were found, and it was concluded from this study that cjPO$_2$ monitoring did not seem to allow early recognition of impending cerebral ischemia.

The role of cjPO$_2$ monitoring in assessing oxygenation in patients with trauma with or without low flow shock has also received some recent attention. The transconjunctival ratio (cjPO$_2$/P$_a$O$_2$) in nonshocked patients varies

The transconjunctival index is dependent on cardiac index, tissue oxygen delivery, and oxygen consumption in patients with respiratory failure or low-output shock.

between 0.5 and 0.7.[73,74,76,77] A study of the value of trans-conjunctival measurements and blood gas measurements in 96 emergency room patients with trauma or cardiores-piratory failure concluded that a low transconjunctival index (less than 0.5) was useful in identifying patients with impending shock. The authors concluded that transcon-junctival monitoring in critically ill surgical and medical patients provided clinically useful information and pro-vided identification of physiological abnormalities in pe-ripheral perfusion and tissue oxygenation as early as con-ventional monitoring methods. The results obtained by measurement of $cjPO_2$ therefore seem very similar to those obtained by the $tcPO_2$ method.

FUTURE TRENDS

COMBINED PO$_2$ AND PCO$_2$ ELECTRODES

Dual O$_2$/CO$_2$ electrodes allow the simultaneous measurement of tcPO$_2$ and tcPCO$_2$, but problems of interpretation arise from the fact that the CO$_2$ electrodes respond much more slowly than the O$_2$ electrodes.

Single transcutaneous PO_2 and PCO_2 electrodes have for some time been available commercially, but the trend has been to combine these two electrodes into a single heated sensor head for ease of application and monitoring.[63,78] The combined dual O_2/CO_2 electrode is more difficult to calibrate, requiring a two-point gas calibration of the PCO_2 electrode. Dual O_2/CO_2 electrodes allow the simultaneous measurement of $tcPO_2$ and $tcPCO_2$, but problems of in-terpretation arise from the fact that the CO_2 electrodes re-spond much more slowly than the O_2 electrodes.

SOLID-STATE ELECTRODES

A solid-state combined transcutaneous PO_2/PCO_2 elec-trode has been designed.[79] The glass section of the PCO_2 electrode has been strengthened by incorporation of ce-ramic material, making it less susceptible to damage. The PO_2 electrode has been designed to reduce O_2 consump-tion; this would reduce O_2 depletion of the tissue at the measuring site, which could improve reliability on skin sites with impaired perfusion.

AVOIDANCE OF HEAT DAMAGE TO THE SKIN

The continuous use of heated electrodes at one skin site has obvious limitations. Tissue damage occurs below the electrode after sustained heating of the skin, so that blister formation and increasingly inaccurate $tcPO_2$ measure-ments are almost inevitable after more than 6 hours of electrode application at temperatures of 44°–45°C. Two possible methods of tackling this problem present themselves for future investigation.

Continued measurement of tcPO$_2$ using a heated electrode is feasible if multiple heated electrode heads are incorporated in one common sensor housing. Such systems have been designed.[80,81] The electrode heads, two or three in number, are positioned close together within the sensor because contiguous areas of skin are likely to have similar characteristics (capillary density and thickness) and are therefore likely to have similar responses to heat. Each electrode head is heated to 44°–45°C in sequence, so that for the most part only one head is heated, with overlap periods of about 15 minutes when two heads are heated. It has thus been possible to obtain accurate tcPO$_2$ recordings for up to 6 hours in normal adult subjects without inducing significant thermal damage to the skin.[81] This approach is promising but requires further evaluation.

It has been proposed[82] that the local application of a tissue respiratory poison would induce maximum hyperemia at normal skin temperatures by paralyzing the vascular smooth muscle sphincters, which normally regulate skin blood flow. In addition, metabolic consumption of oxygen would be greatly reduced, resulting in a smaller P_aO_2–tcPO$_2$ difference. Locally applied dilute solutions of potassium cyanide (KCN) have been reported to produce reversible effects in the skin beneath a tcPO$_2$ electrode, allowing tcPO$_2$ to be measured at a lower temperature (40°C). The local application of KCN is not as dangerous as it might appear, and indeed one of the limitations of the technique is that the KCN is rapidly washed out of the skin tissue. The small quantities of KCN involved are rapidly inactivated in the liver by the enzyme rhodanase and cause no harmful systemic effects.[82] All of the above techniques require further investigation, and perhaps components of each can be combined to produce a tcPO$_2$ method capable of accurately monitoring P_aO_2 for longer periods of time, with a faster response at lower temperatures than that of electrodes currently available.

Continued measurement of tcPO$_2$ using a heated electrode is feasible if multiple heated electrode heads are incorporated in one common sensor housing.

Locally applied dilute solutions of potassium cyanide have been reported to produce reversible effects in the skin beneath a tcPO$_2$ electrode, allowing tcPO$_2$ to be measured at a lower temperature (40°C).

SKIN BLOOD FLOW MEASUREMENTS

Measurements of tcPO$_2$ in intensive care patients become difficult or impossible if any degree of skin underperfusion as seen in shock or hypothermia exists.[18,21] Unless P_aO_2 is directly measured, there are no definite guidelines on the accuracy of the tcPO$_2$ values if skin underperfusion is suspected. Promising experiments have been performed using combined tcPO$_2$ and Laser Doppler techniques.[83] The tcPO$_2$ at an electrode temperature of 37°C is mainly determined by blood flow. The two methods were compared by induction of reactive hyperemia by release of a pressure cuff inflated above arterial pressure. The two methods give similar flow profiles, and future research on these lines could give valuable information on skin perfusion in intensive care patients.

SUMMARY

Transcutaneous oxygen tension measurements are made by means of a polarographic electrode applied to the skin surface. The electrode is provided with a thermostatically controlled heating element designed to enhance the blood flow in the tissues immediately adjacent to the electrode, the purpose being to arterialize the skin circulation, thus allowing the electrode to monitor the arterial oxygen tension. The optimum working electrode temperature is about 45°C. This has a number of additional effects, including a shift of the oxyhemoglobin dissociation curve to the right, with an increase in skin oxygen conductivity and in oxygen consumption. The tcPO$_2$ as measured is significantly influenced by the above factors, the effects of which cannot be estimated with any certainty.

We have therefore recommended a calibration procedure utilizing the subject's own arterial blood (or an equivalent blood or gas sample); this procedure circumvents the majority of the unpredictable "skin factors" and allows a much more accurate estimate of P$_a$O$_2$.

The calibration of a tcPO$_2$ electrode has raised certain problems. A two-point calibration procedure is commonly recommended using a standard gas mixture for the upper point, but the P$_a$O$_2$ so estimated is subject to systematic error and random variability; the results are rather better in newborn infants than in adults. We have therefore recommended a calibration procedure utilizing the subject's own arterial blood (or an equivalent blood or gas sample); this procedure circumvents the majority of the unpredictable "skin factors" and allows a much more accurate estimate of P$_a$O$_2$. The electrode response times to changes in inspired oxygen concentration are sufficiently fast for any likely physiological changes to be accurately followed. The heating requirement is a disadvantage in that a warm-up time of 10–20 minutes is required. In addition, a small burn is likely to arise at the electrode temperature of 45°C, so monitoring is limited to 6 hours at any one site.

Measurement of PO$_2$ at the surface of the conjunctiva requires no local heating, and stable readings can be obtained 5 minutes after application of a specially designed electrode. Apart from this advantage, the conjunctival PO$_2$ behaves in a very similar way to tcPO$_2$ in its ability to monitor P$_a$O$_2$, and like tcPO$_2$, is ineffective in states of low cardiac output or shock. The hope that reduction in cerebral blood flow could be detected by the use of cjPO$_2$ has not been borne out.

Measurement of oxyhemoglobin saturation by oximetry has an advantage over tcPO$_2$ measurement in that no warm-up time or calibration is required; on the other hand, P$_a$O$_2$ values at or above normal cannot be accurately measured. Neither method will give satisfactory results in shock or hypothermic patients.

ACKNOWLEDGMENTS

The authors are grateful for valuable assistance from many members of the clinical, technical, and nursing staff in the Department of Thoracic Medicine and in the Intensive Care Unit at King's College Hospital. Particular thanks are owed to Tracey Fleming who carried out much of the technical work and prepared the typescript.

References

1. Abernathy J: An essay on the nature of the matter perspired and absorbed from the skin. Surgical and Physiological Essays. Part II. London, 1793

2. Von Gerlach: Uber das hautathmen. Arch Anat Physiol (Leipzig) 431, 1851.

3. Baumburger JP, Goodfriend RB: Determination of arterial oxygen tension in man, by equilibration through intact skin. Fed Proc 10:10, 1951

4. Rooth G, Sjorstedt S, Caligara F: Bloodless determination of arterial oxygen by polarography. Science Tools 4:37, 1957

5. Clark LC: Monitor and control of blood and tissue oxygen tensions. Trans Am Soc Artif Intern Organs 2:41, 1956

6. Evans NT, Naylor PF: Steady state oxygen tension in the human dermis. Respir Physiol 2:46, 1967

7. Evans NT, Naylor PF: The dynamics of changes in dermal oxygen tension. Respir Physiol 2:61, 1967

8. Evans NT, Naylor PF: The systemic oxygen supply to the surface of human skin. Respir Physiol 3:21, 1967

9. Huch A, Huch R, Lübbers DW: Quantitative polarographische sauerstoffdruckmessung auf der kopfhaut des neugeborenen. Arch Gynak 207:443, 1969

10. Eberhard P, Hammacher K, Mindt W: Perkutane messung des sauerstoffpartial drukkes: methodik und anwerdungen. Stuttgart Proc Medizin-Technik 26, 1972

11. Huch A, Huch R, Meinzer K: Eine schnelle, beheizte Ptoberflachenelektrode zur kontinuierlichen Uberwachung des pO$_2$ beim Menschen. Stuttgart Proc Medizin-Technik 26, 1972

12. Huch R, Huch A, Albini M et al: Transcutaneous pO$_2$ monitoring in the routine management of infants and children with cardiorespiratory problems. Pediatrics 57:681, 1976

13. Peabody JL, Willis MM, Gregory GA et al: Clinical limitations and advantages of transcutaneous oxygen electrodes. Acta Anaesthesiol Scand Suppl 68:76, 1978

14. Le Souëf PN, Morgan AK, Souttar LP et al: Comparison of transcutaneous oxygen tension with arterial oxygen tension in new born infants with severe respiratory illness. Pediatrics 62:692, 1978

15. Pollitzer MJ, Whitehead MD, Reynolds EO, Delpy D: Effect of electrode temperature and in vivo calibration on accuracy of transcutaneous estimation of arterial oxygen tension in infants. Pediatrics 63:515, 1980

16. Huch A, Huch R: Transcutaneous non-invasive monitoring of pO_2. Hosp Pract 11:43, 1976

17. Eberhard P, Mindt W, Schafer R: Cutaneous blood gas monitoring in the adult. Crit Care Med 9:702, 1981

18. Hutchison DCS, Rocca G, Honeybourne D: Estimation of arterial oxygen tension in adult subjects using a transcutaneous electrode. Thorax 36:473, 1981

19. Strasser K, Goeckenjan G: The monitoring of adult intensive care patients by transcutaneous pO_2 measurements. Birth Defects 15:525, 1979

20. Rithalia SV, Rozkovec A, Tinker J: Characteristics of transcutaneous oxygen tension monitors in normal adults and critically ill patients. Intensive Care Med 5:147, 1979

21. Tremper KK, Shoemaker WC: Transcutaneous oxygen monitoring of critically ill adults, with and without low flow shock. Crit Care Med 9:706, 1981

22. Hansen NT, Sonoda Y, McIlroy MB: Transfer of oxygen, nitrogen and carbon dioxide through normal adult human skin. J Appl Physiol 49:438, 1980

23. Van Duzee BF: Thermal analysis of the human stratum corneum. J Invest Dermatol 65:404, 1975

24. Scheuplein RJ, Blank IH: Permeability of the skin. Physiol Rev 51:702, 1971

25. Tremper KK, Waxman KS: Transcutaneous monitoring of respiratory gases. p. 1. In Nochomovitz ML, Cherniack NS (eds): Noninvasive respiratory monitoring. Churchill Livingstone, New York, 1986

26. Southwood WFW: The thickness of the skin. Plast Reconstr Surg 15:423, 1956

27. Davis MJ, Lawler JC: The capillary circulation of the skin. Arch Dermatol 77:690, 1958

28. Walker A, Phillips L, Powe W, Wood C: A new instrument for the measurement of tissue pO_2 of human fetal scalp. Am J Obstet Gynecol 100:63, 1968

29. Ryan TJ: The blood vessels of the skin. p. 577. In Jarrett A (ed): The physiology and pathphysiology of the skin. Academic Press, New York, 1973

30. Greenfield ADM: The circulation through the skin. p. 1325. In Hamilton WF, Dow P (eds): Handbook of physiology: section circulation. vol 2. American Physiological Society, Washington DC, 1963

31. Edholm OG, Fox RH, MacPherson RK: Effect of body heating on the circulation in skin and muscle. J Physiol (Lond) 134:612, 1956

32. Burnstock G: Autonomic neuroeffector junctions: reflex vasodilation of the skin. J Invest Dermatol 69:47, 1977

33. Levy B, Ghaem M, Verpillat JM, Martineaud J: Antagonistic effects upon cutaneous circulation of muscular exercise and exposure to high ambient temperatures. Pflugers Arch 359:137, 1975

34. Eickhoff JH, Jacobsen E: Correlation of transcutaneous oxygen tension to blood flow in heated skin. Scand J Clin Lab Invest 40:761, 1980

35. Thunstrom AN, Stafford MJ, Severinghaus JW: A two temperature two pO_2 method of estimating the determinants of $tcpO_2$. Birth Defects 15:167, 1979

36. Huch R, Huch A, Lübbers DW: Transcutaneous PO_2. Thieme-Stratton, New York, 1981

37. Lübbers DW: Theoretical basis of transcutaneous blood gas measurements. Crit Care Med 9:721, 1981

38. Al-Siady W, Hill DW: The importance of an elevated skin temperature in transcutaneous oxygen tension measurements. Birth Defects 15:4, 1979

39. Jaszczak P, Poulsen J: Capillary blood temperature in transcutaneous pO$_2$ measurement. Acta Anaesthesiol Scand 25:487, 1981

40. Hensel H: Messkopf zur durchblutungsregisrierung an ohrlappchen. Pflugers Arch 268:604, 1959

41. Friis-Hansen B, Marstrand-Christiansen P, Versterager P: Transcutaneous measurement of arterial blood oxygen tension with a new electrode. Scand J Clin Lab Invest 37Suppl 146:31, 1977

42. Löfgren O: On transcutaneous pO$_2$ measurements in humans: some methodological, physiological and clinical studies. 2nd ed. Radiometer, Malmo, 1978

43. Kimmich HP, Kreuzer F: Catheter pO$_2$ electrode with low flow dependency and fast response. In: Oxygen pressure recording in gases fluids and tissues. Prog Respir Res 3:100, 1969

44. Eberhard P, Mindt W: Reliability of cutaneous oxygen measurement by skin sensors with large-size cathodes. Acta Anaesthesiol Scand Suppl 68:20, 1978

45. Eberhard P, Mindt W, Jann F, Hammacher K: Oxygen monitoring of newborns by skin electrodes: correlation of arterial and cutaneously determined pO$_2$. Adv Exp Med Biol 37:97, 1973

46. Severinghaus JW: Transcutaneous blood gas analysis. Respir Care 27:152, 1982

47. Tolle CD, Beran AV, Johnston WD: Transcutaneous gas monitoring through a dermal window in adults. Respir Care 27:1240, 1982

48. Tremper KK, Waxman K, Shoemaker WC: Effects of hypoxia and shock on transcutaneous pO$_2$ values in dogs. Crit Care Med 7:526, 1979

49. Rithalia SV, Tinker J: Transcutaneous pO$_2$ and tissue pH monitoring during cardiopulmonary bypass. p. 64. In Oberg PE, Odelblad E, Personn J et al (eds): Proceedings of the 5th Nordic Meeting on Medical and Biological Engineering. Linkoping, Sweden, 1981

50. Rooth G, Hedstrand U, Tyden H, Ogren C: The validity of the transcutaneous oxygen tension method in adults. Crit Care Med 4:162, 1976

51. Löfgren O: Transcutaneous oxygen measurement in adult intensive care. Acta Anaesthesiol Scand 23:534, 1979

52. Indyk L: Safe and effective use of transcutaneous blood gas monitors. Acta Anaesthesiol Scand Suppl 68:101, 1978

53. Huch A, Lübbers DW, Huch R: Eine kleine tragbare Elektrode zur Bestimmung des sauerstoffdruckes in kleinen Blutmengen. Klin Wochenschr 52:1021, 1974

54. Fallat R: Getting the blood out of blood gas studies. Respir Ther Sept/Oct:103, 1982

55. Burki NK, Albert RK: Non-invasive monitoring of arterial blood gases: a report of the ACCP section on respiratory pathophysiology. Chest 83:667, 1983

56. Goeckenjan G, Strasser K: Relation of transcutaneous to arterial pO$_2$ in hypoxaemia, normoxaemia and hyperoxaemia. Biotelemetry 7:77, 1977

57. Gray BJ, Heaton RW, Henderson A, Hutchison DCS: In vivo calibration of a transcutaneous oxygen electrode in adult patients. Adv Exp Med Biol 200:75, 1987

58. Spiro SG, Dowdeswell IRG: Arterialised earlobe blood samples for blood gas tensions. Br J Dis Chest 70:263, 1976

59. Gray BJ: Transcutaneous oxygen tension measurements in adult human subjects. MD Thesis. University of Dublin, Dublin, 1989

60. Hughes JA, Gray BJ, Hutchison DCS: Changes in transcutaneous oxygen tension in pulmonary emphysema. Thorax 39:424, 1984

61. Kettler D, Hentze G: Clinical suitability and accuracy of a new combined system for the transcutaneous and intravascular determination of pO$_2$. Biotelemetry Patient Monit 6:66, 1979

62. Lanigan C, Ponte J, Moxham J: Drift in vivo of transcutaneous dual electrodes. Adv Exp Med Biol 220:41, 1987

63. Whitehead MD, Lee BV, Padgin TM, Reynolds EO: Estimation of arterial oxygen and carbon dioxide tensions by a single transcutaneous sensor. Arch Dis Child 60:356, 1985

64. Severinghaus JW, Weiskopf RB, Nishimura M, Bradley AF: Oxygen electrode errors due to polarographic reduction of halothane. J Appl Physiol 31:640, 1971

65. Dent JG, Netter KJ: Errors in oxygen tension measurement caused by halothane. Br J Anaesth 48:195, 1976

66. Tremper KK, Barker SJ, Blatt DH, Wender RH: Effect of anaesthetic agents on the drift of a transcutaneous oxygen tension sensor. J Clin Monit 2:234, 1986

67. Fatt I: An ultra microelectrode. J Appl Physiol 19:326, 1964

68. Kwan M, Fatt I: A non-invasive method of continuous arterial oxygen tension estimation from measured palpebral conjunctival oxygen tension. Anaesthesiology 35:309, 1971

69. Fatt I, Deutsch TA: The relation of conjunctival pO_2 to capillary bed pO_2. Crit Care Med 11:445, 1983

70. Kram HB, Chem B, Lee T et al: Conjunctival oxygen monitoring in postoperative respiratory failure and shock. Circ Shock 19:211, 1986

71. Abraham E, Smith M, Silver L: Continuous monitoring of critically ill patients with transcutaneous oxygen and carbon dioxide and conjunctival oxygen sensors. Ann Emerg Med 11:1021, 1984

72. Yelderman M: Transconjunctival oxygen measurements in critical care medicine. Anaesthesiology 59:266, 1983

73. Podolsky S, Wertheimer J, Harding S: The relationship of conjunctival and arterial blood gas oxygen measurements. Resuscitation 18:31, 1989

74. Abraham E, Fink S: Conjunctival oxygen tension monitoring in emergency department patients. Am J Emerg Med 6:549, 1988

75. Shoemaker WC, Lawler PM: Method for continuous conjunctival oxygen monitoring during carotid artery surgery. Crit Care Med 11:946, 1983

76. Haljamae H, Frid I, Holm J, Holm S: Continuous conjunctival oxygen tension ($pcjO_2$) monitoring for assessment of cerebral oxygenation and metabolism during carotid artery surgery. Acta Anaesthesiol Scand 33:610, 1989

77. Hess D, Evan C, Thomas K et al: The relationship between conjunctival pO_2 and arterial pO_2 in 16 normal persons. Respir Care 31:191, 1986

78. Mahutte CK, Michiels TM, Massell KT, Trueblood DM: Evaluation of a single transcutaneous pO_2/pCO_2 sensor in adult patients. Crit Care Med 12:1063, 1984

79. Larsen J, Linnet N: Solid state transcutaneous combined pO_2/pCO_2 electrode. Radiometer A/S. Copenhagen, 1990

80. Kimmich HP, Spaan JG, Kreuzer F: Transcutaneous measurements of paO_2 at 37°C with a triple electrode system. Acta Anaesthesiol Scand Suppl 68:28, 1978

81. Fallenstein F, Baeckert P, Huch R: Comparison of in vivo response times between pulse oximetry and transcutaneous pO_2 monitoring. Adv Exp Med Biol 220:191, 1987

82. Engel RR, Delpy DT, Parker D: The effect of topical potassium cyanide on transcutaneous gas measurements. Birth Defects 15:117, 1979

83. Ewald U, Huch A, Huch R, Rooth G: Skin reactive hyperemia recorded by a combined $tcpO_2$ and laser Doppler sensor. Adv Exp Med Biol 220:231, 1987

84. Schonfeld T, Sargent CW, Bautista D et al: Transcutaneous oxygen monitoring during exercise stress testing. Am Rev Respir Dis 121:457, 1980

PULSE OXIMETRY

AMAL JUBRAN, MD[†]

The assessment of oxygenation has traditionally involved direct sampling of arterial blood. Although an arterial puncture is relatively easy to perform, arterial blood sampling is invasive and associated with a number of complications, provides intermittent information regarding a patient's status, and is expensive. Recent technologic advances allow the clinician to monitor arterial blood oxygenation noninvasively and continuously. In addition, the new technologies offer promise as a means of decreasing health care costs.[1]

Although noninvasive oximeters have been around since the second World War, it is only in the mid-to-late 1970s, with the development of pulse oximetry, that this technique has become commonplace in the critical care setting.[2] In 1988, 23 manufacturers of pulse oximeters existed, 45 different models were available, and approximately 45,000 units were in use.[3] Indeed, Severinghaus and Astrup considered pulse oximetry to be "the most significant technologic advance ever made in monitoring the well-being and safety of patients during anesthesia, recovery, and critical care."[2]

Severinghaus and Astrup considered pulse oximetry to be "the most significant technologic advance ever made in monitoring the well-being and safety of patients during anesthesia, recovery, and critical care."

HISTORICAL BACKGROUND

The principle of oximetry is based on the spectrophotometric absorption of specific wavelengths of light by a blood specimen. In 1935, Mathes built the first device that continuously measured the oxygen (O_2) saturation of human blood using two wavelengths of light.[2] One wavelength was sensitive to changes in oxygenation, and the second wavelength (which was unaffected by oxygenation) compensated for changes in tissue thickness, hemoglobin content, and light intensity. This device was useful for following trends, but its bulky sensor rendered its use impractical.

Important advances in noninvasive oximetry occurred during World War II, stimulated by the need to monitor oxygenation in pilots flying at high altitude in unpressur-

[†] Staff Physician, Division of Pulmonary and Critical Care Medicine, Edward Hines Jr. Veterans Administration Hospital, Assistant Professor, Loyola University of Chicago Stritch School of Medicine, Hines, Illinois

ized cockpits. A lightweight ear sensor was developed for these aviators, and Millikan referred to this as an "oximeter."[4] In its initial clinical development, the ear oximeter was limited by the laborious two-point calibration that was required—one calibration point was at the bloodless zero to compensate for changes in tissue absorption, and the second point was at a known O_2 saturation. In addition, the earpiece was large, difficult to position, and produced sufficient heat to produce second-degree burns of the pinna.[5] During the 1950s, Wood and colleagues[6] at the Mayo Clinic further improved on Millikan's ear oximeter by incorporating an inflatable balloon that made the earlobe bloodless and consequently enabled the oximeter to obtain a zero reading. In addition, they developed an electronic method for dividing the red signal by the infrared signal to provide a continuous display of O_2 saturation.

In the 1960s, Robert Shaw developed a self-calibrating eight-wavelength ear oximeter that was later marketed by Hewlett-Packard Company.[2] This oximeter identified four species of hemoglobin and compensated for tissue absorbency, but it did not differentiate between venous and arterial blood. As a result, a heater in the probe was used to "arterialize" the capillary blood, thereby bringing the O_2 saturation of venous blood to arterial levels.[7] This device measured arterial O_2 saturation (S_aO_2) with a 95% confidence interval of $\pm 4\%$ for S_aO_2 values above 65%, but it systematically underestimated S_aO_2 values below this level.[8] It was rendered inaccurate in the presence of jaundice, increased carboxyhemoglobin, or darkened skin pigmentation.[9] Despite these limitations, the Hewlett-Packard oximeter quickly became a standard clinical and laboratory tool in pulmonary medicine, especially in sleep laboratories. However, its cumbersome earpiece, delicate fiberoptic cable, and expensive nature prevented its acceptance as a routine monitor in the intensive care unit (ICU).[5]

In the mid 1970s, Takuo Aoyagi, a Japanese bioengineer, made an ingenious discovery regarding oximetry. He found that the variation in tissue arterial blood volume with each pulse could be used to obtain a signal dependent on only the characteristics of arterial blood, and thus could be used to measure arterial O_2 saturation. By focusing on the pulsatile change in light transmission, it was possible to eliminate the absorption of light by venous blood, skin pigment, tissue, and bone. As a result, a self-calibrating device that used a greatly simplified sensor was developed. In 1974, the Japanese firm Nikon Kohden, with the assistance of Aoyagi and his associates, received a Japanese patent for this instrument.[10]

Further development of the pulse oximeter in this coun-

The variation in tissue arterial blood volume with each pulse could be used to obtain a signal dependent on only the characteristics of arterial blood, and thus could be used to measure arterial O_2 saturation.

try was pioneered by the Biox and Nellcor companies in the early 1980s through the application of microprocessor technology to improve oximeter performance.[11,12] Several other companies have now entered the field and improvements in performance continue to be made as new algorithms are developed.

PRINCIPLES OF PULSE OXIMETRY

Oximetry utilizes measurements based on spectrophotometric principles to determine hemoglobin O_2 saturation. The spectrophotometric method is based on the Beer-Lambert law that relates the concentration of a solute to the intensity of light transmitted through a solution:

$$I_{out} = I_{in}^{e-(DC_\epsilon)}$$

where I_{out} is intensity of light coming out of the sample, I_{in} is the light intensity going into the sample, e is the base of the natural algorithm, D is the distance through which light travels, C is the concentration of the substance (hemoglobin), and ϵ is the extinction coefficient of the solute (a constant for a given solute at a specified wavelength). Thus, the concentration of a single substance can be determined by measuring the light absorption at a specific wavelength with a known extinction coefficient through a know path length. In the case of pulse oximetry, two wavelengths have been employed to determine the relative concentration of oxyhemoglobin and reduced hemoglobin.

The noninvasive measurement of S_aO_2 is limited by the presence of many absorbers in the light path other than arterial hemoglobin, such as venous blood, intervening tissues, bone, and skin pigmentation. The early oximeters subtracted the tissue absorbance by compressing and using the absorbance of bloodless tissue as a baseline. In addition, they heated the tissue to obtain a signal related to arterial blood to minimize the absorption interference by venous and capillary blood.[7] In contrast, pulse oximeters correct for absorption characteristics of substances not found in pulsatile blood by separating the pulsatile alternating current (AC) component of the absorption signal from the nonpulsatile direct current (DC) component. The DC component represents the absorbances of the tissue bed, including venous blood, capillary blood, and nonpulsatile arterial blood, while the AC component represents the pulsatile expansion of the arteriolar bed with arterial blood (Fig. 1).

Oximetry utilizes measurements based on spectrophotometric principles to determine hemoglobin O_2 saturation.

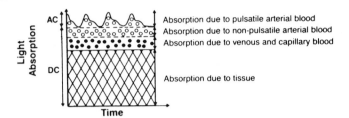

FIGURE 1   Light absorption through living tissue. The alternating current (AC) signal is due to the pulsatile component of the arterial blood while the direct current (DC) signal is comprised of all of the nonpulsatile absorbers in the tissue such as nonpulsatile arterial blood, venous and capillary blood, and all other tissues. From Tremper KK, Barker SJ: Pulse oximetry. Anesthesiology 70:98, 1989. With permission.

The 660 nm and 940 nm wavelengths are used because oxyhemoglobin and reduced hemoglobin have different absorption spectra at these particular wavelengths.

The principle of pulse oximetry is based on the assumption that the only pulsatile absorbance between the light source and the photodetector is that of arterial blood. The light source consists of two light-emitting diodes (LEDs) that emit light at known wavelengths, generally 660 nm (red) and 940 nm (infrared). These two wavelengths are used because oxyhemoglobin and reduced hemoglobin have different absorption spectra at these particular wavelengths. In the red region, oxyhemoglobin absorbs less light than does reduced hemoglobin, while the reverse is true in the infrared region (Fig. 2). The pulse oximeter measures the AC component of light absorbance at each wave-

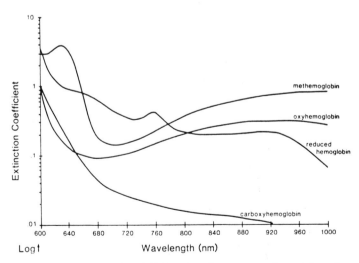

FIGURE 2   Transmitted light absorbance spectra of four hemoglobin species: oxyhemoglobin, reduced hemoglobin, carboxyhemoglobin, and methemoglobin. From Barker SJ, Tremper KK: Pulse oximetry: applications and limitations. Int Anesthesiol Clin 25:155, 1987. With permission.

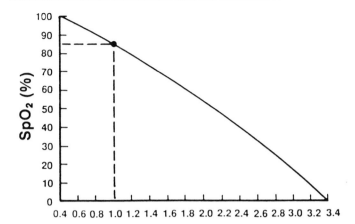

$$R = \frac{AC_{660}/DC_{660}}{AC_{940}/DC_{940}}$$

FIGURE 3   A typical pulse oximeter calibration curve. The S_aO_2 estimate is determined from the ratio (R) of the pulse-added red absorbance at 660 nm to pulse-added infrared absorbance at 940 nm. From Tremper KK, Barker SJ: Pulse oximetry. Anesthesiology 70:98, 1989. With permission.

The S_aO_2 estimate is determined from the ratio of the pulse-added red absorbance at 660 nm to pulse-added infrared absorbance at 940 nm.

length and then divides this by the corresponding DC component; the resulting "pulse-added" absorption is independent of the incident light intensity. By comparing the pulse-added absorption at both wavelengths, a ratio (R) is calculated as follows:

$$R = \frac{AC_{660}/DC_{660}}{AC_{940}/DC_{940}}$$

This ratio is then empirically calibrated against direct arterial blood S_aO_2 measurements obtained in volunteers using a spectrophotometric heme oximeter (CO-oximeter).[5,13] The resulting calibration curve (Fig. 3) is stored in a digital microprocessor within the pulse oximeter. During subsequent use, this calibration curve is used to generate the pulse oximeter's estimate of arterial saturation (S_pO_2).

ACCURACY

Clinical studies have shown large differences in accuracy between different commercial brands of pulse oximeters even though they use similar or identical hardware components. These differences are almost certainly due to the different algorithms used in processing the measured light intensity signals to obtain the S_pO_2 value. These algorithms are limited by the range of O_2 saturations used in generating the calibration curve in volunteers and by the accuracy of the measurement standard, typically a CO-oximeter.[5,14,15]

Numerous studies have evaluated the accuracy of pulse oximeters, but the variation in statistical methods makes it difficult to compare the data. In early studies, linear regression analysis was used to assess accuracy. Such analysis, unfortunately, reports the association between methods rather than the degree of confidence in a new measurement. It is now generally preferred to report the comparison between pulse oximetry and direct CO-oximeter in terms of the mean difference between the two techniques (bias) and the standard deviation of the differences (precision). The bias will show a systematic overestimate or underestimate of one method relative to the other, while the precision will represent the variability or "random error."[16]

NORMAL O$_2$ SATURATION

Most manufacturers claim that the 95% confidence limits of their pulse oximeters are within $\pm 4\%$ when S_aO_2 is above 70%.[17] Indeed, several studies conducted in normal healthy volunteers have shown that pulse oximeters generally have a mean difference of less than 2% and a standard deviation of less than 3% at a $S_aO_2 \geq 90\%$.[18–20] Comparable results have also been obtained in critically ill patients; most oximeters had an absolute bias of less than 1% and precision of less than 2% in patients with good arterial perfusion and S_aO_2 above 90%.[15,21]

LOW O$_2$ SATURATION

The accuracy of pulse oximetry diminishes as S_aO_2 decreases to 80% or less.

The accuracy of pulse oximetry, however, diminishes as S_aO_2 decreases to 80% or less. This is probably due, at least in part, to the difficulty in obtaining reliable human calibration data during extreme hypoxemia.[17,21] An additional factor for the compromised accuracy is the variation in the center wavelength (± 15 nm) of different LEDs that emit light at the 660 nm wavelength—a region in which the concentration of reduced hemoglobin is relatively greater at lower O_2 saturations. Since the absorption spectra for reduced hemoglobin is relatively steep at this region (Fig. 2), a slight shift in the center wavelength of the LED can result in erroneous measurements at lower O_2 saturations.[7]

In a study on normal volunteers, Nickerson et al.[18] used a stepwise reduction in inspired O_2 concentration (F_IO_2) (range, 1.0–0.11) at 5-minute intervals to assess the accuracy of four-pulse oximeters at each hypoxic plateau. They found that the bias ± precision of these oximeters ranged from $-4.9 \pm 2.9\%$ to $3.0 \pm 2\%$ for S_aO_2 values between 65 and 80%. In contrast, Severinghaus et al.[22] tested the accuracy of 14-pulse oximeters during profound hypoxemia by inducing a sudden decrease in S_aO_2 to levels of 55% (range, 40–70%) and maintaining these plateaus for 30 seconds. The mean bias at a S_aO_2 of 55% varied from -15.1 to 5.5, and the precision varied from 14.4 to 2.4. For most oximeters, the mean bias was relatively independent of saturation, although it became more negative in proportion to desaturation with the Nellcor, Ohmeda, and Radiometer oximeters. The accuracy of 14-pulse oximeters was recently examined in 16 healthy adults at 4 20-minute steady-state levels of F_IO_2 (0.21, 0.10, 0.08, and 0.07; range in S_aO_2, 99–55%). The bias and precision were <3% at the two highest F_IO_2 levels (S_aO_2, 99–83%), but at lower F_IO_2 levels (S_aO_2, 78–55%) bias and precision increased to 8% and 5%, respectively.[23]

The reliability of 6-pulse oximeters was recently examined in 17 hypoxemic patients with chronic obstructive pulmonary disease.[24] Unlike most studies where accuracy is examined in the setting of induced hypoxemia, in this study the instruments were tested while the patients were receiving increased levels of F_IO_2, ranging from 0.21 to 0.40 (S_aO_2, 62–100%). The bias and precision were below 1.2% and 3%, respectively, for most of the instruments; however, a systematic instrumental error was noted in which the lower the S_aO_2, the higher the overestimation of S_aO_2 by the pulse oximeter.[24]

The accuracy of pulse oximeters at low O_2 saturations has also been assessed in critically ill patients. In one study, 8 out of the 13 oximeters had a bias $\geq \pm 5\%$ at a $S_aO_2 <$ 80%.[15] In fact, all units were less accurate and most were less precise at these saturations compared with measurements obtained at a $S_aO_2 \geq 80\%$. In patients who had S_aO_2 values as low as 63%, Taylor and Whitman[25] found that agreement between pulse oximetry and a CO-oximeter was poor with a bias of -12% to 18% and pulse oximetry tended to underread at a $S_aO_2 \leq 80\%$. In a study in 54 ventilator-dependent patients, Jubran and Tobin[26] noted that the accuracy of pulse oximetry significantly deteriorated at low S_aO_2 values (Fig. 4). The bias ± precision was $1.7 \pm 1.2\%$ for $S_aO_2 > 90\%$, whereas it increased to $5.1 \pm 2.7\%$ when S_aO_2 was $\leq 90\%$.

In critically ill patients, 8 out of the 13 oximeters had a bias $\geq \pm 5\%$ at a $S_aO_2 < 80\%$.

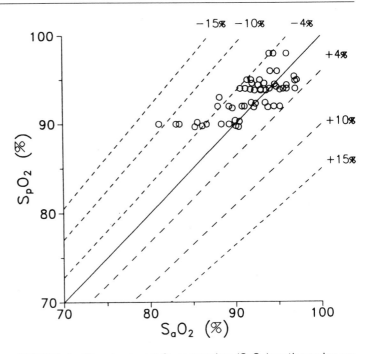

FIGURE 4   Direct arterial O_2 saturation (S_aO_2) vs the pulse ox-imeter O_2 saturation values (S_pO_2) for 55 measurements ob-tained in ventilator-dependent patients. The solid line is the line of identity and the dashed lines are isopleths of different levels of bias. The bias and the precision increased as the S_aO_2 decreased to $\leq 90\%$. From Jubran A, Tobin MJ: Reliability of pulse oximetry in titrating supplemental oxygen therapy in ven-tilator-dependent patients. Chest 97:1420, 1990. With permis-sion.

DYNAMIC RESPONSE

Studies of the accuracy of pulse oximetry have been gen-erally conducted under steady-state conditions, and stud-ies of their accuracy in detecting dynamic or transient changes in S_aO_2 have been limited. Severinghaus and Naifeh[27] examined this problem by inducing a 30–60-sec-ond step hypoxic plateau between an S_aO_2 of 40 and 70% in healthy volunteers. Oximeter probes placed on the ear generally had a much faster response to a sudden decrease in F_IO_2 than did the finger probes. Response times for the ear probes ranged from 9.6 to 19.8 seconds vs 24 to 35.1 seconds for the finger probes (Fig. 5). Likewise, in normal healthy volunteers, Kagle et al.[28] found that the response of a finger probe was 24 seconds slower than an ear probe in measuring rapid resaturation.

West et al.[29] examined the accuracy of the Ohmeda Biox III and Nellcor N-100 oximeters in detecting transient

Oximeter probes placed on the ear generally had a much faster response to a sudden decrease in F_IO_2 than did the finger probes.

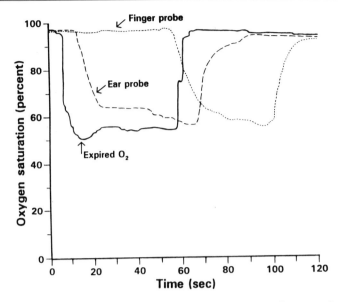

FIGURE 5   Response characteristics of ear and finger pulse oximeter probes in a subject experiencing severe oxygen desaturation. Compared with oxygen saturation calculated from the expired oxygen tension, the ear probe shows a lag of about 50 seconds. From Tobin MJ: Respiratory monitoring. JAMA 264:244, 1990. With permission.

changes in S_aO_2. They used the Hewlett-Packard multi-wavelength transmittance oximeter as a reference, and they studied patients with sleep apnea, since these patients experience rapid and wide fluctuations in S_aO_2. The combined physiologic and instrument response time was calculated as the time from the onset of respiration, immediately following an apnea, to the point at which S_pO_2 changes from the apnea-related desaturation phase to the ventilation-related resaturation phase. This response time was 7 seconds for the Hewlett-Packard ear sensor, with additional delays of 0.1 second for the Biox-Ohmeda ear probe, 20 seconds for the Biox-Ohmeda reusable finger probe, and 7.4 seconds for the Nellcor disposable finger probe. The response time was also dependent on heart rate, and the finger reusable probes displayed longer delays during periods of bradycardia.[29]

LIMITATIONS OF PULSE OXIMETRY

Oximeters have a number of limitations that may lead to inaccurate readings (Table 1).

TABLE 1   Limitations of Pulse Oximetry

Oxygen dissociation curve
Dyshemoglobins
  Carboxyhemoglobin
  Methemoglobin
Anemia
Dyes
  Methylene blue
  Indigo carmine
  Indocyanine green
Nail polish
Ambient light
Motion artifact
Cardiac arrhythmias
Skin pigmentation
Low perfusion state

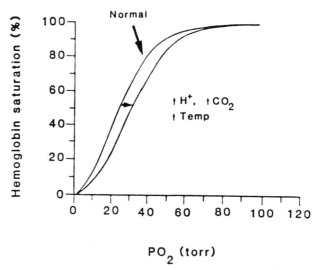

FIGURE 6   Oxygen dissociation curve: arterial saturation plotted against oxygen tension (PO_2). From Tobin MJ: Essentials of critical care medicine. Churchill Livingstone, New York, 1989. With permission.

OXYHEMOGLOBIN DISSOCIATION CURVE

Pulse oximeters measure S_aO_2, which is physiologically related to P_aO_2 according to the oxyhemoglobin dissociation curve (Fig. 6). Factors that shift the oxyhemoglobin dissociation curve, such as temperature, pH, and P_aCO_2, will affect the relationship between S_aO_2 and P_aO_2. However, no evidence shows that these factors affect the accuracy of S_pO_2 measurements.[14] Because of the sigmoid shape of oxyhemoglobin dissociation curve, pulse oximetry is relatively insensitive at detecting significant changes in P_aO_2 at high levels of oxygenation. On the upper horizontal portion of the curve, large changes in P_aO_2 may occur with little changes in S_aO_2.[30,31] Taking the usually stated 95% confidence limits of $\pm 4\%$, an oximeter reading of 95% could represent a P_aO_2 between 60 mmHg ($S_aO_2 = 91\%$) and 160 mmHg ($S_aO_2 = 99\%$).[32]

An oximeter reading of 95% could represent a P_aO_2 between 60 mmHg ($S_aO_2 = 91\%$) and 160 mmHg ($S_aO_2 = 99\%$).

DYSHEMOGLOBINS

Oximeters that use only two wavelengths of light can distinguish between two substances. In the specific case of pulse oximeters, they measure "functional O_2 saturation," which is defined as the percentage of oxyhemoglobin (HbO_2) relative to the total amount of hemoglobin (Hb) available for binding, that is:

$$\text{Functional } S_aO_2 = \frac{HbO_2}{HbO_2 + Hb} \times 100$$

When carboxyhemoglobin (COHb) and methemoglobin (MetHb) are also present, four wavelengths are required to determine the "fractional O_2 saturation," which is defined as percentage of oxyhemoglobin relative to total amount of hemoglobin, that is:

Fractional S_aO_2
$$= \frac{HbO_2}{HbO_2 + Hb + COHb + MetHb} \times 100$$

Currently available pulse oximeters assume that dyshemoglobins (COHb and MetHb) are present only in insignificant concentrations. However, when significant amounts of dyshemoglobins are present, pulse oximetry measurements are likely to be erroneous.

The effect of carbon monoxide inhalation on the accuracy of pulse oximetry has been studied by Barker and Tremper.[33] Dogs were given varying amounts of carbon monoxide to achieve COHb levels between 0 and 75%. Oximetry consistently overestimated the true S_aO_2, with the result that S_pO_2 readings were greater than 90% while the true S_aO_2 was less than 30% (Fig. 7). The two-wavelength oximeter misinterpreted COHb as HbO_2 (since the absorption coefficient of COHb was similar to HbO_2), and thus overestimated the O_2Hb content (Fig. 2). Interestingly, the S_pO_2 readings approximated the sum of COHb and HbO_2.[33] Likewise, in a human study of 149 patients with a mean COHb of 3.9 g%, S_pO_2 readings were consistently higher than corresponding CO-oximeter readings of S_aO_2.[34]

Methemoglobin also interferes with the accurate reporting of HbO_2 by pulse oximetry. Barker and associates[35] examined the performance of pulse oximetry in dogs with MetHb levels of up to 60%. The S_pO_2 readings overestimated the true S_aO_2 values by an amount that was proportional to MetHb until the MetHb reached approximately 35%. At this level, S_pO_2 values reached a plateau of approximately 85% and did not decrease further despite increasing concentrations of MetHb. Methemoglobin has approximately the same absorption coefficient at both the red and infrared wavelengths (Fig. 6), and if enough MetHb is present to dominate all pulsatile absorption, the pulse oximeter will measure a pulse-added absorbance ratio of

Currently available pulse oximeters assume that dyshemoglobins COHb and MetHb are present only in insignificant concentrations.

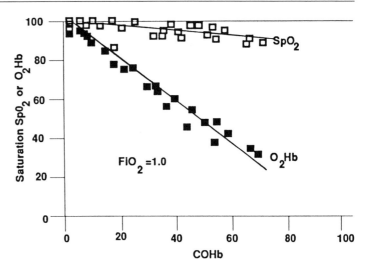

FIGURE 7   Oxygen saturation measured by pulse oximeter (S_pO_2) and CO-oximeter (O_2Hb) versus carboxyhemoglobin (COHb) at a fractional inspired O_2 concentration of 1.0. Pulse oximetry consistently overestimated O_2 saturation in the presence of COHb. At COHb of 70%, S_pO_2 reading is approximately 90%, while directly measured O_2Hb has decreased to 30%. Data from Barker SJ, Tremper KK: The effect of carbon monoxide inhalation on pulse oximeter signal detection. Anesthesiology 67:599, 1987.

these two wavelengths of 1. This ratio of 1 corresponds to an S_pO_2 value near 85% on the pulse oximeter calibration curve.[35,36] Errors have also been reported when pulse oximetry is used in patients with elevated MetHb levels.[37]

ANEMIA

Anemia can affect the accuracy of pulse oximetry since the reading depends on light absorption by hemoglobin. In a study using a Nellcor oximeter mounted on a dog's tongue, Lee et al.[38] noted that at normal levels of S_aO_2, the bias increased from 0.37% at hematocrit values $\geq$ 40% to 5.4% at hematocrit values < 10%, respectively. Recently, Severinghaus et al.[39] retrospectively examined the effect of anemia on the accuracy of pulse oximetry at low S_aO_2 values. In healthy human volunteers, the bias was -6.4% in nonanemic subjects at S_aO_2 level of 54%, whereas the bias was -15% in a subject with Hb of 8 g/dl at the same S_aO_2 value.

Hyperbilirubinemia has little effect on the accuracy of pulse oximetry.

In contrast to the Hewlett-Packard oximeter that underestimates the true O_2 saturation in the presence of jaundice,[40] hyperbilirubinemia has little effect on the accuracy of pulse oximetry. Veyckemans et al.[41] examined the accuracy of a Nellcor pulse oximeter finger probe in patients with jaundice (mean $\pm$ SD bilirubin, 19.2 $\pm$ 18.6 mg/dl) and nonicteric patients (bilirubin, < 1.5 mg/dl). The bias between S_pO_2 and true S_aO_2 was greater in the icteric patients, compared with the control patients, 2.9% and 1.7%, respectively. The icteric patients also had higher COHb levels, and when the S_pO_2 reading was corrected for COHb, the bias between S_pO_2 and S_aO_2 was similar in the two groups of patients. Likewise, Chelluri et al.[42] found no difference between S_pO_2 and S_aO_2 values in patients without jaundice (bilirubin, 1.9 mg/dl) and patients with jaundice (bilirubin, 30.6 mg/dl).

DYES

Intravenous administration of dyes for diagnostic purposes may cause falsely low S_pO_2 readings.[43,44] Scheller et al.[43] showed that in human volunteers, methylene blue, indocyanine green, and, to a lesser extent, indigo carmine, caused falsely low oximeter readings. This effect lasted only a few minutes because of redistribution of the dye. Spurious transient desaturation to S_pO_2 of 65% has also been reported in a patient who was receiving methylene blue for the assessment of ureteral urine flow.[45]

NAIL POLISH

Nail polish also affects the accuracy of pulse oximeters, since many nail polish colors have absorbance at the same wavelengths used by the oximeter sensor (660 and 940 nm) (Fig. 8). Cote et al.[46] found that blue, green, and black nail polish caused artifactually low S_pO_2 readings but red and purple had no effect. It has been suggested that mounting the oximeter probe side-to-side on the finger may alleviate this problem.[47] Indeed, White and Boyle[48] showed that when disposable or nondisposable probes were mounted sideways on the finger, oximetry readings were equally accurate in volunteers with nail polish as in those without.

Nail polish also affects the accuracy of pulse oximeters, since many nail polish colors have absorbance at the same wavelengths used by the oximeter sensor (660 and 940 nm).

AMBIENT LIGHT

In general, pulse oximeters correct for ambient light by adjusting the intensity of LEDs for maximum signal strength.[49] A background signal is generated in the sensor while both the red and infrared LEDs are switched off, and this ambient light signal is then subtracted from the signal generated by switching on the LEDs. However, fluorescent and xenon arc surgical lamps have been shown to cause falsely low S_pO_2 readings.[50] This effect can be minimized

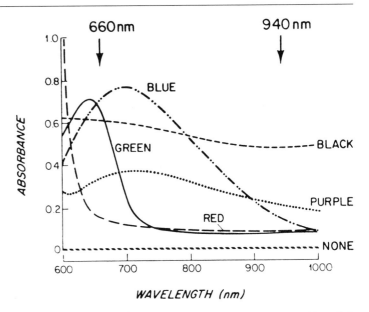

FIGURE 8   Absorption spectra for five different nail polish colors. From Cote CJ, Goldstein EA, Fuchsman WH, Hoaglin DC: The effect of nail polish on pulse oximetry. Anesth Analg 67:683, 1989. With permission.

by isolating the sensor from the interfering signal by wrapping the probe with an opaque shield.

MOTION ARTIFACT

Motion artifact is a significant source of error despite attempts to minimize it.

Motion artifact is a significant source of error despite attempts to minimize it.[7] It has been suggested that these erroneous readings may be decreased if the heart rate signal from the pulse oximeter is synchronized with an electrocardiogram (ECG) signal. However, oximeters that use ECG synchronization have been shown to be no more accurate than unsynchronized oximeters.[22]

CARDIAC ARRHYTHMIAS

The effect of cardiac arrhythmias and pulse deficit on the performance of pulse oximetry was examined in 163 patients in a surgical ICU.[51] When patients who had a discrepancy of >3 beats/min between the ECG and pulse oximeter measurements of heart rate were compared with patients who had no discrepancy between the two measurements of heart rate, no difference in the bias was observed between the two groups; likewise, the bias in the group with normal sinus rhythm and in the group with an irregularly irregular rhythm or >10 ectopic beats per minute were similar.[51]

SKIN PIGMENTATION

Sauders et al.[52] noted that the Hewlett-Packard ear oximeter was equally accurate when used in 5 pigmented subjects compared with 19 nonpigmented healthy volunteers. On the other hand, Ries and colleagues[53] found that the Hewlett-Packard ear oximeter was less accurate in 5 ambulatory patients with moderately dark skin pigmentation than in 18 patients with light pigmentation; interestingly, accuracy of an Ohmeda-Biox IIA ear oximeter was similar in both of these patient groups. Using a Biox and a Nellcor oximeter, Cecil et al.[54] found that the regression lines obtained in a subset of 15 hospitalized black patients were significantly different from those obtained in the total group of 152 hospitalized patients. In a subsequent study, Ries et al.[55] showed that technical problems (inability to obtain a reading, or a warning message indicating poor tissue penetration of the signal) occurred in up to 18% of patients with darkest skin pigmentation, whereas problems occurred in only 1% of patients with lighter pigmentation. In critically ill patients, Jubran and Tobin[26] noted greater bias ± precision in black patients compared with white patients (3.3 ± 2.7 and 2.2 ± 1.8, respectively). In addition, inaccurate readings, that is bias > 4%, occurred more frequently in the black patients (12 of 45, 27%) than in the white patients (6 of 55, 11%).

The reason why pulse oximetry is less accurate in black patients is not known. Darkly pigmented skin may interfere with the absorption of the wavelengths used in pulse oximeters (Fig. 8). Indeed, evidence supporting such a possibility is provided by studies demonstrating that black nail polish[46] and black ink used for fingerprinting[56] produce inaccurate oximeter readings. In addition, the calibration curve programmed into the electronics of oximeters may not be optimally suited to black patients. It is possible that these calibration curves are based predominantly on data derived from white volunteers. As a result, a calibration curve based on data derived from black volunteers may be more accurate when used in black patients.[26]

LOW PERFUSION STATE

All instruments depend on satisfactory arterial perfusion of the skin, thus, low perfusion states such as hypothermia, vasoconstriction, and low cardiac output may impair

Technical problems (inability to obtain a reading or a warning message indicating poor tissue penetration of the signal) occurred in up to 18% of patients with darkest skin pigmentation.

Low perfusion states make it difficult for the sensor to distinguish the true signal from background noise.

peripheral perfusion and make it difficult for the sensor to distinguish the true signal from background noise. Under these conditions, many pulse oximeters will display a message indicating an inadequate pulse signal. Although these clinical situations are frequent, the physiological limits of a pulse oximeter's working conditions are still poorly defined.

Morris et al.[19] examined the accuracy of 15-pulse oximeters in the presence of a pneumatic tourniquet that was used to produce vascular occlusion. Both bias and precision worsened under conditions of poor perfusion. Wilkins et al.[57] studied four-pulse oximeters under conditions of venous engorgement caused by inflation of a sphygmomanometer cuff to 40 mmHg and during vasoconstriction induced by placing the subject's arm in a cold water-filled plastic container. Both experimental conditions significantly increased the time required for detection of induced hypoxemia. The accuracy of pulse oximetry was also examined in patients immediately after open-heart surgery by Palve and Vuori.[58] The lowest cardiac index and temperature at which readings were obtained were 2.4 l/min.m^2 and 26.5°C, respectively. In a subsequent study, the same investigators assessed the accuracy of three-pulse oximeters during low-flow states (cardiac index $\leq$ 2.2 l/min.m^2) and low peripheral temperature (< 28.0°C) as compared with normal cardiac index and peripheral temperature.[59] They found that pulse oximetry was equally reliable in the experimental situation of low cardiac index and low perfusion temperature as in the control situation. In a preliminary study, Tremper et al.[60] examined the effect of temperature and hemodynamics on the accuracy of the Biox III Ohmeda oximeter in 53 critically ill patients. In 57 of the total 383 data sets collected, the pulse oximeter displayed "low perfusion." In the remaining 326 data sets, pulse oximeter was accurate (bias, 1.4%) over a wide range of hemodynamic conditions; that is, cardiac index, 8.7–1.4 l/min/M^2, temperature, 32.8°–39°C, mean arterial pressure, 37–141 mmHg, systemic vascular resistance index, 543–4773 dynes s/M^2/cm^5. In a recent study of 20 pulse oximeters on patients who had undergone cardiac surgery under hypothermic cardiopulmonary bypass (mean rectal temperature, 35.1°C) and had poor perfusion (systolic arterial pressure 114 mmHg, diastolic arterial pressure, 59 mmHg), Clayton et al.[61] found that only 2 pulse oximeters (Criticare CSI 503, Datex Satlite) achieved a combination of accuracy (mean bias) and precision such that 95% of measurements were within ± 4% of the CO-oximeter value. In fact, 4 oximeters (Ohmeda Biox 3700 and 3740, Spectramed pulsat, and Engstrom Eos) had 95% of measurements greater than 6% (range, -15–7%) of the reference. In an accompanying paper by the same investigators, they examined the performances of 10 pulse oximeters under the same conditions of poor peripheral perfusion using finger, ear, nose, or forehead probes. The bias between pulse oximetry and CO-oximetry measurements ranged from 0.2% to 1.7% for finger probes and 0.1% to 8.1% for other probes. Ear probes ranked significantly lower than the finger probes in the number of readings given within 3% of the reference (CO-oximeter) and ranked lower for precision.[62]

CLINICAL USEFULNESS OF PULSE OXIMETRY

Despite their ubiquitous presence in critical care units, it is not clear that pulse oximeters contribute to clinical decision making or alter patient morbidity or mortality. Indeed, most research studies have focused on the accuracy of pulse oximetry and remarkably few studies have examined their clinical usefulness.

In a study examining the effect of information feedback on the incidence of anesthesia complications, Cooper et al.[63] found that pulse oximetry did not increase the number of reports of hypoxemic events in the recovery room. They pointed out, however, that oximetry may provide a warning that is sufficiently early to permit correction of clinical problems and decrease the need to report them to the recovery room staff. The introduction of pulse oximetry resulted in a significant decrease in recovery room impact events (ie, events that affected recovery room care) although a cause-and-effect relationship could not be clearly established. This study was weakened by the lack of concurrent controls (ie, a matched group without feedback or without pulse oximetry). Cote et al.[64] undertook a more carefully designed study to examine the frequency of hypoxemic episodes (arbitrarily defined as a $S_pO_2 < 85\%$ for at least 30 s) in 152 pediatric surgical patients undergoing general anesthesia. They found that 32% of patients whose anesthesiologists did not have oximetry data immediately available to them experienced major hypoxemia compared with only 14% of the patients whose anesthesiologists had continuous oximetry data available. The investigators concluded that oximetry helped to guide anesthesia management, although no morbidity was documented in any patient who experienced a hypoxemic episode.[64]

Pulse oximetry is commonly employed to assist with titration of F_IO_2 in ventilator-dependent patients. Jubran

It is not clear that pulse oximeters contribute to clinical decision making or alter patient morbidity or mortality.

Physicians employ a wide scatter of target S_pO_2 values when titrating F_1O_2.

and Tobin[26] found that physicians employ a wide scatter of target S_pO_2 values when titrating F_1O_2 (Fig. 9). Even though a target S_pO_2 value of 90% or less was commonly used by physicians, this could result in dangerously low P_aO_2 values (41 mmHg). These investigators found that pulse oximetry was reliable when assessing the response to adjustments of F_1O_2, but the optimal S_pO_2 target value depended on the patient's skin color. In white patients, a S_pO_2 target value of 92% was reliable in predicting a satisfactory level of oxygenation. In black patients, however, such a S_pO_2 reading was commonly associated with significant hypoxemia and a higher target S_pO_2 value (95%) was required (Fig. 10).

Relatively few investigators have examined the cost-effectiveness of pulse oximetry. In 24 patients being weaned from mechanical ventilation following elective cardiac surgery,[65] those patients monitored by oximetry had fewer arterial blood gas determinations than a control group that were monitored with periodic arterial blood gas sampling, 5.9 ± 2.7 (SD) and 10.5 ± 1.8 samples per patient, respectively. However, no difference in the length of intubation in the two groups was found. Alford et al.[66] found that the number of arterial blood gas measurements obtained from patients receiving mechanical ventilation de-

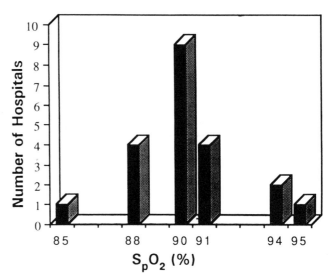

FIGURE 9   Target oxygen saturation values (S_pO_2) used by physicians. When titrating fractional inspired O_2 concentration, a wide scatter of target S_pO_2 values is apparent. From Jubran A, Tobin MJ: Reliability of pulse oximetry in titrating supplemental oxygen therapy in ventilator-dependent patients. Chest 97:1420, 1990. With permission.

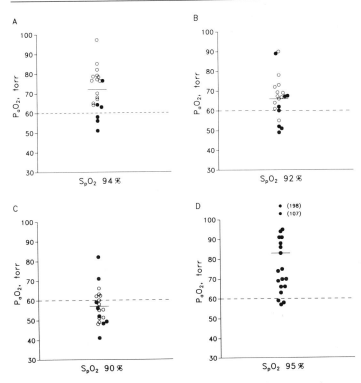

FIGURE 10   Arterial oxygen tension (P_aO_2) values at pulse oximetry O_2 saturation (S_pO_2) value of 94%, 92%, 90%, and 95%. The inspired O_2 concentration (F_IO_2) was adjusted until the desired steady-state S_pO_2 value was achieved. The solid horizontal line represents the mean P_aO_2 value obtained for each S_pO_2 target. The closed and open circles represent values obtained in black and white patients, respectively. In white patients, a S_pO_2 target of 92% resulted in a satisfactory level of oxygenation, whereas a higher S_pO_2 target (95%) was required in black patients. From Jubran A, Tobin MJ: Reliability of pulse oximetry in titrating supplemental oxygen therapy in ventilator-dependent patients. Chest 97:1420, 1990. With permission.

creased by 3% in the year that pulse oximeters were installed in their ICU. Studies of a similar nature are sorely needed to determine the cost-effectiveness of oximetry in the management of critically ill patients.

In conclusion, pulse oximetry is probably one of the most important advances in noninvasive monitoring. Oximeters are accurate and easy to operate. Although numerous studies have examined their accuracy, especially during steady-state conditions in healthy subjects, a relative paucity of information regarding the clinical usefulness and cost-effectiveness of pulse oximetry in the critical care setting remains.

ACKNOWLEDGMENT

Supported in part by the Chicago Lung Association.

References

1. Bone RC, Balk RA: Noninvasive respiratory care unit: a cost effective solution for the future. Chest 93:1988, 1988

2. Severinghaus JW, Astrup PB: History of blood gas analysis. VI. Oximetry. J Clin Monit 2:270, 1986

3. Berlin SL, Branson PS, Capps JS et al: Pulse oximetry: a technology that needs direction. Respir Care 33:243, 1988

4. Millikan GA: An oximeter: an instrument for measuring continuously oxygen saturation of arterial blood in man. Rev Sci Instrum 13:434, 1942

5. Tremper KK, Barker SJ: Pulse oximetry. Anesthesiology 70:98, 1989

6. Wood E, Geraci JE: Photoelectric determination of arterial oxygen saturation in man. J Lab Clin Med 34:387, 1949

7. Pologe JA: Pulse oximetry: technical aspects. Int Anesthiol Clin 25(3):137, 1987

8. Tobin MJ: State of the art: respiratory monitoring in the intensive care unit. Am Rev Respir Dis 138:1625, 1988

9. Wukitisch MW, Peterson MT, Tobler DR, Pologe JA: Pulse oximetry: analysis of theory, technology, and practice. J Clin Monit 4:290, 1988

10. Aoyagi T, Kishi M, Yamaguchi K, Watanabe S: Improvement of the earpiece oximeter. Abstracts of the 13th annual meeting of the Japanese Society of Medical Electronics and Biological Engineering 90, 1974

11. Severinghaus JW, Honda Y: History of blood gas analysis. VII. Pulse oximetry. J Clin Monit 3:135, 1987

12. Welch JP, De Cesari R, Hess D: Pulse oximetry: instrumentation and clinical applications. Respir Care 35:584, 1990

13. Kelleher JF: Pulse oximetry. J Clin Monit 5:37, 1989

14. Ralston AC, Webb RK, Runciman WB. Potential errors in pulse oximetry. I. Pulse oximeter evaluation. Anaesthesia 46:202, 1991

15. Emergency Care Research Institute: Pulse oximeters. Health Devices 18:185, 1989

16. Altman DG, Bland JM: Measurement in medicine: the analysis of method comparison studies. Statistician 32:307, 1983

17. Tobin MJ: Respiratory monitoring. JAMA 264:244, 1990

18. Nickerson BG, Sarkisian C, Tremper KK: Bias and precision of pulse oximeters and arterial oximeters. Chest 93:515, 1988

19. Morris RW, Nairn M, Torda TA: A comparison of fifteen pulse oximeters. Part I: A clinical comparison; Part II: A test of performance under conditions of poor perfusion. Anaesthesia and Intensive Care 17:62, 1989

20. Choe H, Tashiro C, Fukumitsu K et al: Comparison of recorded values from six pulse oximeters. Crit Care Med 17:678, 1989

21. Webb RK, Ralston AC, Runciman WB: Potential errors in pulse oximetry. II. Effects of changes in saturation and signal quality. Anaesthesia 96:207, 1991

22. Severinghaus JW, Naifeh KH, Koh SO: Errors in 14 pulse oximeters during profound hypoxemia. J Clin Monit 5:72, 1989

23. Hannhart B, Haberer JP, Saunier C, Laxenaire MC: Accuracy and precision of fourteen pulse oximeters. Eur Respir J 4:115, 1991

24. Hannhart B, Michalski H, Delorme N et al: Reliability of six pulse oximeters in chronic obstructive pulmonary disease. Chest 99:842, 1991

25. Taylor MB, Whitman JG: The accuracy of pulse oximeters: a comparative clinical evaluation of five pulse oximeters. Anaesthesia 43:229, 1988

26. Jubran A, Tobin MJ: Reliability of pulse oximetry in titrating supplemental oxygen therapy in ventilator-dependent patients. Chest 97:1420, 1990

27. Severinghaus JW, Naifeh KH: Accuracy of response of six pulse oximeters to profound hypoxia. Anesthesiology 67:551, 1987

28. Kagle DM, Alexander CM, Berko RS, et al: Evaluation of the Ohmeda 3700 pulse oximeter: steady-state and transient response characteristics. Anesthesiology 66:376, 1987

29. West P, George CF, Kryger MH: Dynamic in vivo response characteristics of three oximeters. Hewlett Packard 47201 A, Biox III, and Nellcor N-100. Sleep 10:263, 1987

30. Severinghaus JW: Simple, accurate equations for human blood O_2 dissociation computations. J Appl Physiol 46:599, 1979

31. Roughton FJW, Severinghaus JW: Accurate determination of O_2 dissociation curve of human blood above 98.7% saturation with data on O_2 solubility in unmodified human blood from 0° to 37°C. J Appl Physiol 6:861, 1973

32. Ries AL: Oximetry: know thy limits (editorial). Chest 91:316, 1987

33. Barker SJ, Tremper KK: The effect of carbon monoxide inhalation on pulse oximeter signal detection. Anesthesiology 67:599, 1987

34. Tawaklna MT, Greville HW: The effect of carboxyhemoglobin on the accuracy of pulse oximetry in ambulatory care patients. Chest 143:A72, 1991

35. Barker SJ, Tremper KK, Hyatt J: Effects of methemoglobinemia on pulse oximetry and mixed-venous oximetry. Anesthesiology 70:112, 1989

36. Barker SJ, Tremper KK: Pulse oximetry: applications and limitations. Int Anesthesiol Clin 25:155, 1987

37. Eisenkraft JB: Pulse oximeter desaturation due to methemoglobinemia. Anesthesiology 68:279, 1988

38. Lee SE, Tremper KK, Barker SJ: Effects of anemia on pulse oximetry and continuous mixed venous oxygen saturation monitoring in dogs. Anesth Analg 67:S130, 1988

39. Severinghaus JW, Koh SO: Effect of anemia on pulse oximeter accuracy at low saturation. J Clin Monit 6:85, 1990

40. Chaudhary BA, Burki NK: Ear oximetry in clinical practice. Am Rev Respir Dis 117:173, 1978

41. Veyckemans F, Baele P, Guillaume JE et al: Hyperbilirubinemia does not interfere with hemoglobin saturation measured by pulse oximetry. Anesthesiology 70:118, 1989

42. Chelluri L, Snyder JV, Bird JR: Comparison of pulse oximetry with CO-oximeter in patients with hyperbilirubinemia. Chest 96:288S, 1989

43. Scheller MS, Unger RJ, Kelner MJ: Effects of intravenously administered dyes on pulse oximetry readings. Anesthesiology 65:550, 1986

44. Sidi A, Paulus DA, Rush W et al: Methylene blue and indocyanine green artifactually lower pulse oximetry reading of oxygen saturation: studies in dogs. J Clin Monit 3:249, 1987

45. Kessler MR, Eide T, Humanyun B, Poppers PJ: Spurious pulse oximeter desaturations with methylene blue injection. Anesthesiology 65:435, 1986

46. Cote CJ, Goldstein EA, Fuchsman WH, Hoaglin DC: The effect of nail polish on pulse oximetry. Anesth Analg 67:683, 1989

47. Ralston AC, Webb RK, Runciman WB: Potential errors in pulse oximetry. III: Effects of interference, dyes, dyshemoglobins and other pigments. Anaesthesia 46:291, 1991

48. White PF, Boyle WA: Nail polish and oximetry. Anesth Analg 68:546, 1989

49. Hanowell L, Eisele JH, Donns D: Ambient light affects pulse oximeters. Anesthesiology 67:864, 1987

50. Amar D, Neidzwski J, Wald A, Finck AD: Fluorescent light interferes with pulse oximetry. J Clin Monit 5:135, 1989

51. Wong DH, Tremper KK, Davidson J et al: Pulse oximetry is accurate in patients with dysrhythmias and a pulse deficit. Anesthesiology 70:1024, 1989

52. Saunders NA, Powles ACP, Rebuck AS: Ear oximetry: accuracy and practicability in the assessment of arterial oxygenation. Am Rev Respir Dis 113:745, 1976

53. Ries AL, Farrow JT, Clausen JL: Accuracy of two ear oximeters at rest and during exercise in pulmonary patients. Am Rev Respir Dis 132:685, 1985

54. Cecil WT, Thorpe KJ, Fibuch EE, Tuohy GF: A clinical evaluation of the accuracy of the Nellcor N-100 and Ohmeda 3700 pulse oximeters. J Clin Monit 4:31, 1988

55. Ries Al, Prewitt LM, Johnson JJ: Skin color and ear oximetry. Chest 96:287, 1989

56. Battito MF: The effect of fingerprinting ink on pulse oximetry (letter). Anesth Analg 69:265, 1989

57. Wilkins CJ, Moores M, Hanning CD: Comparison of pulse oximeters: effects of vasoconstriction and venous engorgement. Br J Anaesth 62:439, 1989

58. Palve H, Vuori A: Pulse oximetry during low cardiac output and hypothermia states immediately after open heart surgery. Crit Care Med 17:66, 1989

59. Palve H, Vuori A: Accuracy of three pulse oximeters at low cardiac index, and peripheral temperature. Crit Care Med 19:560, 1991

60. Tremper KK, Hufstedler SM, Barker SJ et al: Accuracy of a pulse oximeter in the critically ill adult: effect of temperature and hemodynamics (Abstr). Anesthesiology 63:175, 1985

61. Clayton D, Webb RK, Ralston AC et al: A comparison of the performance of 20 pulse oximeters under conditions of poor perfusion. Anaesthesia 46:3, 1991

62. Clayton D, Webb RK, Ralston AC et al: Pulse oximeter probes: a comparison between finger, nose, ear, and forehead probes under conditions of poor perfusion. Anesthesia 46:260, 1991

63. Cooper JB, Cullen DJ, Nemeskal R et al: Effects of information feedback and pulse oximetry on the incidence of anesthesia complications. Anesthesiology 67:686, 1987

64. Cote JB, Goldstein EA, Cote MA et al: A single blind study of pulse oximetry in children. Anesthesiology 68:184, 1988

65. Niehoff J, DelGuercio C, LaMorte W et al: Efficacy of pulse oximetry and capnometry in postoperative ventilatory weaning. Crit Care Med 16:701, 1988

66. Alford PT, Hawkins P, Sherrill TR et al: Impact of pulse oximetry on demand for arterial blood gases in an ICU. Chest 96:288S 1989

CLINICAL AND PHYSIOLOGIC RATIONALE FOR CONTINUOUS MEASUREMENT OF MIXED VENOUS OXYGEN SATURATION

PATRICK J. FAHEY, MD[†]

Patients are admitted to intensive care units (ICU) primarily because of potential or actual threats to the adequacy of tissue oxygenation. This premise is often forgotten in the myriad of therapeutic interventions, including central access lines, antibiotics, nutritional interventions, nasogastric suction tubes, and the other assorted routine medical therapeutic measures instituted in these patients. Nevertheless, the foundation of ICU care is the assurance of sustaining adequate oxygen (O_2) delivery relative to tissue O_2 needs. In a post-myocardial infarction patient who is alert and stable, the ICU therapeutic measures are poised to immediately intervene if tissue O_2 is threatened by a sudden change in cardiovascular function. In this setting, the ICU is used to ensure continued ongoing adequate tissue oxygenation. In contrast, a patient with adult respiratory distress syndrome (ARDS) and sepsis with hypotension who requires high levels of positive end-expiratory pressure (PEEP) requires specific and aggressive interventions in order to return O_2 delivery levels to normal and to continue adequate O_2 consumption by tissues. While O_2 delivery can be assumed to be adequate for tissue O_2 needs in the alert post-myocardial infarction patient with stable vital signs and normal laboratory values, the clinician is more challenged in assessing the adequacy of tissue oxygenation in the unstable patient receiving multiple thera-

The foundation of ICU care is the assurance of sustaining adequate oxygen delivery relative to tissue O_2 needs.

[†] Chief, Pulmonary and Critical Care Medicine, Loyola University Medical Center, Maywood, Illinois

peutic interventions. In this setting, studies have shown that experienced physicians are incorrect in gauging cardiac output ranges and pulmonary capillary wedge pressures in over 50% of such patients. It is in this setting that other methods of assessing tissue oxygenation must be employed. This chapter will focus on the role of continuous measurement of mixed venous O_2 saturation (S_vO_2) in helping the clinician assess the adequacy of tissue O_2 needs relative to O_2 delivery in a variety of clinical disorders.

PHYSIOLOGIC RATIONALE

The continued interest of critical care physicians in the levels of O_2 in venous blood stems from its use as an index of the adequacy of tissue oxygenation. Early in the twentieth century, Krogh proposed a model of tissue oxygenation in which a tissue consisted of cells encircling a capillary.[16] Oxygen diffuses out of the capillary from the arterial end to the venous end and into the surrounding cells. Tenney has adapted this theory as depicted in Figure 1. In this model of tissue oxygenation, the cells that are most vulnerable to decreased O_2 levels are those that are situated at the most downstream portion of the capillary and those that are furthest in radial distance from the capillary. Tenney describes these cells as residing in the "lethal corner," that is, as O_2 enters the capillary bed, the capillary O_2 level decreases as more and more O_2 is unloaded from hemoglobin as the red blood cell traverses the capillary. Sufficient decreases in the amount of O_2 reaching the capillary

The cells that are most vulnerable to decreased O_2 levels are those that are situated at the most downstream portion of the capillary and those that are furthest in radial distance from the capillary.

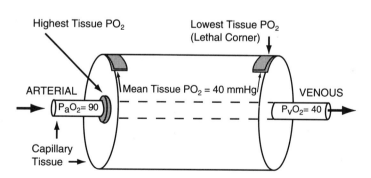

FIGURE 1   Traditional mode of tissue oxygenation where O_2 enters the tissue cylinder at arterial end, diffuses from capillary into surrounding cells, and exits at venous end. Cells at the venous end and furthest from the capillary are said to reside in the "lethal corner." From Prof. S. M. Tenney, Dartmouth Medical School, Hanover, New Hampshire. With permission.

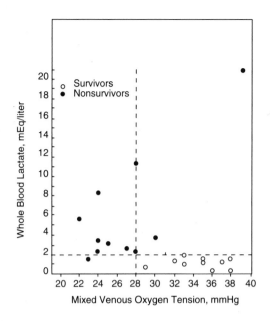

FIGURE 2   Relation between mixed venous O$_2$ tension and blood lactate concentration. Horizontal dashed line at 2 mEq/l is the upper limit of normal lactate concentration. Vertical dashed line at venous O$_2$ 28 mmHg is arbitrary "critical level" of venous O$_2$. From Krasnitz P et al: Mixed venous O$_2$ tension and hyperlactemia. JAMA 236:570, 1976. With permission.

or increased cellular extraction can result in O$_2$ levels in the distal end of the capillary that are reduced to the point of an inadequate partial pressure for O$_2$ to diffuse O$_2$ to those cells lying in the lethal corner. Tenney has calculated that the oxygen pressure (PO$_2$) of venous blood is equal to or a very close index of the PO$_2$ at the end capillary.[25] An important clinical question is determining the level at which the driving pressure of O$_2$ at the end capillary is inadequate to provide adequate O$_2$ to the cells residing in the lethal corner.

Krasnitz et al.[15] approached this problem by studying the mixed venous O$_2$ level, a reflection of the average venous level of all tissue beds, of patients brought to the Emergency Room at various stages of acute hemodynamic distress and correlating these venous O$_2$ levels with simultaneously obtained measurements of lactic acid, the classic indicator of tissue hypoxia. Results of this study indicate that when the mixed venous PO$_2$ (P$_v$O$_2$) fell below 28 mmHg the incidence of tissue hypoxia as measured by lactic acid substantially increased (Fig. 2). Elevated lactate

Studies have indicated that in most acute clinical conditions when venous O_2 levels fall below 28 mmHg (corresponding to venous O_2 saturation of 50%), the likelihood of inadequate tissue oxygenation and lactic acid formation is high.

levels also identified all of the subjects who expired. This study and others have indicated that in most acute clinical conditions when venous O_2 levels fall below 28 mmHg (corresponding to venous O_2 saturation of 50%), the likelihood of inadequate tissue oxygenation and lactic acid formation is high.

VARIATIONS IN VENOUS O_2 LEVELS

The amount of O_2 remaining in blood at the end of the tissue capillary and in venous blood is dependent on the amount of O_2 transported to the tissue (O_2 delivery) and the amount of O_2 consumed in the tissue (VO_2). The determinants of O_2 delivery are:

1. Hemoglobin (Hgb) concentration. Each gram of Hgb is capable of combining with 1.34 ml of O_2.

2. The saturation percentage (Sat%) of Hgb. This is directly dependent on the PO_2 dissolved in plasma, and this relationship is described by the O_2 Hgb dissociation curve.

3. Cardiac output.

The O_2 content of blood is described by the following equation:

$$O_2 \text{ content (ml } O_2/100 \text{ ml blood)}$$

$$= O_2 \text{ dissolved}$$

$$+ O_2 \text{ combined with Hgb}$$

$$O_2 \text{ dissolved} = 0.003 \text{ (ml/dl/mmHg)}$$

$$\times PO_2 \text{ (mmHg)}$$

$$O_2 \text{ Hgb} = 1.34 \text{ (ml } O_2/g)$$

$$\times \text{ Hgb (g/dl)} \times \text{ sat\%}$$

Example

Hgb = 15 g%, PO_2 = 100 mmHg, sat% = 98

O_2 content = (0.003 × 100) + (1.34 × 15 × 0.98)

0.3 ml O_2 + 20.0 ml O_2

20.3 ml/dl

O_2 delivery (DO_2) is defined as the amount of O_2 that leaves the heart and is delivered to the tissues in 1 minute. O_2D is calculated as:

O_2D = cardiac output (CO) × arterial O_2 content (C_aO_2)

Example

When   CO = 5.0 l/min and C_aO_2 = 20 volume %

Then O_2 = 5.0 l/min × 20 ml/100 ml

$\qquad$ = 1000 ml/min

VO_2 is defined as the volume of O_2 consumed by the body's tissues in 1 minute and is calculated by using the Fick equation:

$$O_2 \ VO_2 = CO \times (C_aO_2 - C_vO_2 \times 10)$$

When $\qquad$ CO = 5.0 l/min,

$\qquad$ C_aO_2 = 20 volume %, and C_vO_2

$\qquad$ = 15 volume %

Then $\qquad$ VO_2 = 250 ml/min

Where $\qquad$ C_vO_2 = mixed venous O_2 content.

When the terms of the Fick equation are rearranged, it is apparent that the determinants of venous O_2 levels are the components of DO_2 and VO_2

$$VO_2/(CO \times 10) = C_aO_2 - C_vO_2$$

$$VO_2 \ (CO \times 10) - C_aO_2 = - C_vO_2$$

$$C_vO_2 = C_aO_2 - [VO_2/(CO \times 10)]$$

$$C_vO_2/C_aO_2 = 1 - [VO_2/(CO \times 10 \times C_aO_2)]$$

(if S_aO_2 = 1.0 then S_vO_2 = 1.0,

then $S_vO_2 = C_vO_2 \times C_aO_2$)

$$S_vO_2 = 1 - [VO_2/CO \times 10 \times C_aO_2]$$

$$S_vO_2 = 1 - VO_2/DO_2$$

An increase in VO_2 or decrease in cardiac output, Hgb concentration, or arterial O_2 saturation (S_aO_2) will produce a decrease in S_vO_2, provided there is no change in other components of the equations.

PRINCIPLES OF SPECTROPHOTOMETRIC BLOOD O₂ MEASUREMENTS

Present laboratory techniques for determining the amount or percentage of O_2 bound to Hgb rely on spectrophotometric methods to determine the relative amounts of deoxygenated and oxygenated Hgb. Typically, light of precisely determined wavelengths is transmitted through a cuvette containing the blood sample. The wavelengths of light are chosen to maximize the difference in light absorption by the Hgb molecule when it is oxygenated and deoxygenated. Frequently used wavelengths are 660 nm and 805 nm. The amount of light of each of these wavelengths that is transmitted through the blood samples varies depending on the relative concentration of oxyhemoglobin and deoxygenated Hgb. By analyzing these differences at various wavelengths, the ratio of Hgb to oxyhemoglobin can be accurately determined.

Attempts to determine oxyhemoglobin saturation *in vivo*, for instance in the pulmonary artery, rely on the same principles of measurement, but the measurement is complicated by the necessity of the transmitted light being reflected and refracted off the moving red blood cells and back to the catheter tip for analysis (Fig. 3).

Initial attempts at *in vivo* reflective measurements relied on stiff fiberglass bundles transmitting light of two wave-

Fiberoptic catheter oximetry (*in vivo*)

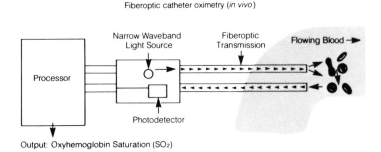

FIGURE 3   Schematic of principles of reflection spectrophotometry with wavelengths of light being transmitted down catheter, reflected off blood cells back into photo detection for analysis.

lengths through flowing blood.[8] The amount of each wavelength of reflected light was detected and the ratio computed. Besides their considerable stiffness, these early catheters that attempted to measure *in vivo* oxyhemoglobin saturation suffered from inaccuracies due to calibration assumptions and artifactual measurements resulting from vessel wall reflectance. In addition, the catheters were stiff and relatively large, and the glass fibers broke easily, making the instruments impractical for routine clinical care. The introduction of plastic optical fibers that could be bundled together allowed the production of flexible, small, and less-breakable fiber optic catheters beginning in 1979.

In addition to the technological improvements in catheter design, the new generation of catheters incorporated a third wavelength of light that improved accuracy compared to two-wavelength systems. The three-wavelength system also reduced the system's sensitivity to physiological factors such as changes in Hgb concentration and pulsatile flow. In addition, changes in the light scattering from red blood cell surfaces and blood vessel walls that could artifactually increase the measured oxyhemoglobin saturation were eliminated.

At present, two fiberoptic pulmonary catheters are marketed in the United States: the Opticath (Oximetrix, Sunnyvale, CA), a three-wavelength system, and the Swan-Ganz Oximetry TD Catheter (Edwards Labs, Santa Ana, CA), a two-wavelength system. The catheter systems appear comparable in terms of flexibility, ease of insertion, and initial calibration. The two-wavelength system requires input of the Hgb concentration and must be updated with changes in Hgb concentration as they occur. In addition, the two-wavelength system is unable to reliably distinguish reflectance of the optical signal from the vessel wall, which can falsely elevate the measured Hgb saturation. Differences in accuracy of the two systems has been reported by Gettinger et al.[9] In this study, 5 two-wavelength and 5 three-wavelength catheters were placed in 10 dogs. Mixed venous saturation was recorded by the fiberoptic catheters and compared to simultaneously obtained samples of mixed venous blood measured with a co-oximeter. A wide range of S_vO_2 was obtained by changing the inspired O_2 concentration, lowering Hgb, and decreasing cardiac output. The measured venous O_2 achieved with these techniques was between 10% and 90%. This study found significantly greater accuracy with the three-wavelength system. The two-wavelength system was found to drift during the experiments, resulting in deviation from the measured S_vO_2 between 5% and 31% at the end of the experiment.

Gettinger et al. found significantly greater accuracy with the three-wavelength system.

RELATIONSHIP OF O_2 SUPPLY AND O_2 CONSUMPTION

VO₂ declines with further decreases in DO₂, that is, VO₂ becomes dependent on DO₂—a condition referred to as pathologic supply dependency of VO₂.

The clinical utility of continuously measured S_vO_2 relies on the independence of tissue VO_2 from DO_2. Decreases in DO_2 are reliably detected by decreased venous O_2 levels only if VO_2 remains constant and unaffected by changes in delivery. The result of this independent relationship is that when DO_2 decreases, VO_2 remains unchanged until a critical level of DO_2 is reached. At that point, VO_2 declines with further decreases in DO_2, that is, VO_2 becomes *dependent* on DO_2—a condition referred to as pathologic supply dependency of VO_2. Venous O_2 levels do not change when VO_2 declines in concert with decreases in DO_2.

A number of studies have investigated the "critical" level of DO_2, that point on the curve at which further changes in DO_2 decrease VO_2. Shibutani et al. studied 58 patients undergoing cardiovascular surgery who were anesthetized and paralyzed and found that VO_2 remained constant until DO_2 was decreased to 325 ml/m^2/min.[24] This level of DO_2 corresponds to approximately a 50% decrease from normal (recall that a 70 kg normal person delivers 1,000 ml O_2 per minute or close to 15 ml/O_2/kg/min). This study also found increased production of lactic acid at this level of reduction in DO_2. Rashkin studied 44 critically ill patients and also found increased lactic acid levels when DO_2 declined to below 8 ml O_2/kg/min.[21] Fallat and Eberhart studied patients with ARDS receiving extracorporeal membrane oxygenation, and, with this mechanical set-up, they could mechanically alter DO_2 by varying pump speed.[7] In this setting, CO_2 production, which is directly related to VO_2 by the respiratory quotient, could be measured continuously. This study found that CO_2 production remained constant in patients with ARDS until DO_2 was reduced to 7 ml O_2/kg/min. Krasnitz et al. also found that the production of lactic acid was strongly correlated with mixed venous O_2 levels below 27 mmHg, which would correlate with a 50% reduction in DO_2.[15]

These studies support the concept that in a wide variety of clinical disorders, the critical point of DO_2 that results in threatened adequacy of tissue oxygenation occurs near where DO_2 falls to levels below 50% of normal. This would correspond to an DO_2 of approximately 500 ml/min (50% of normal); with VO_2 constant at 250 ml/min, this would result in a S_vO_2 of 50% and a mixed venous PO_2 of approximately 27 mmHg. This value of S_vO_2 corresponds well to our clinical observations that patients are generally stable with S_vO_2 between 60% and 75%, in moderate hemodynamic stress with levels between 50% and 60%, and often in severe hemodynamic stress with levels below 50%.

Other studies have found evidence of VO_2 being dependent on DO_2 at much higher levels of delivery compared to normal.[3,14,18] In particular, this has been reported in patients with ARDS. These studies suggested that a pathologic supply dependency of O_2 uptake may play a role in the high incidence of multiple organ failure that frequently accompanies ARDS. Controversy continues over the existence of pathologic O_2 supply dependency and, if it does exist, its clinical significance.

Villar et al. performed a prospective study in 28 critically ill patients in order to document changes in VO_2 and O_2 transport that occurred spontaneously, without any experimental interventions aimed at altering DO_2.[26] They measured cardiac output and blood gases three to five times in a given patient with the interval between any two measurements of 20–60 minutes. Spontaneous variation in VO_2 within each study was between 7% and 147% (mean, 38%), and the variation of DO_2 was between 9% and 189% (mean, 42%). These authors concluded that changes in VO_2 and DO_2 occur spontaneously in patients with normal blood lactate levels, even in the absence of therapeutic interventions. These spontaneous changes make it extremely difficult to interpret studies that find VO_2 to be supply-limited. This study found that an apparent relationship between O_2 supply and VO_2 consumption was usually the result of increased tissue O_2 demand resulting in a physiologically appropriate increase in DO_2. In no instance, when blood lactate levels were normal, could VO_2 be called pathologically dependent on DO_2.

Changes in VO_2 and DO_2 occur spontaneously in patients with normal blood lactate levels, even in the absence of therapeutic interventions.

In some studies that reported that VO_2 was O_2 supply-dependent, vasodilators were used to increase cardiac output. In this setting, drug-induced vasodilatation may well interfere with peripheral vasoregulatory compensatory mechanisms and, in addition, could generate a sympathetic response themselves and thereby increase VO_2. In a study by Gilbert et al., the relationship between DO_2 and consumption was analyzed in 54 patients with sepsis and septic shock before and after fluid loading, blood transfusion, or catecholamine administration.[10] This study found that in patients receiving fluid and blood to increase DO_2, VO_2 increased only in the subgroup with an elevated blood lactate concentration. In the group with a normal blood lactate, VO_2 did not change. By contrast, all patients receiving catecholamines to increase DO_2 showed increases in VO_2 irrespective of the presence or absence of lactic acidosis.

In the setting of pathologic supply dependency of VO_2, venous O_2 levels do not accurately reflect the adequacy of tissue oxygenation. In the study by Danek et al., patients with ARDS experienced large decreases in DO_2 through decreases in cardiac output, yet venous O_2 levels did not change.[3] These results raised serious questions regarding the value of monitoring venous O_2 levels in patients with ARDS. In a recent review of the subject of DO_2 versus VO_2, Dantzker (one of the authors of the original Danek paper) et al. concluded that with a given set of DO_2 and consumption points obtained at random time intervals, the most likely relationship will be a linear one.[4] This linear relationship follows a *normal* interaction between the two variables, making them physiologically rather than pathologically linked. Analysis of the accumulated data in this area indicates that the dependence of O_2 uptake on DO_2 is primarily a statistical coupling and has not been shown to be of physiologic or clinical significance.

The dependence of O_2 uptake on DO_2 is primarily a statistical coupling and has not been shown to be of physiologic or clinical significance.

CLINICAL UTILITY OF CONTINUOUS MEASUREMENTS OF S_vO_2

The normal value for S_vO_2 is near 75%, reflecting normal DO_2 of 1,000 ml/min and normal O_2 extraction of 250 ml/min. The range of S_vO_2 values that have been measured in hemodynamically stable patients varies between 68% and 77%. Values above this range reflect increased DO_2 relative to VO_2 or decreased extraction of O_2 relative to delivery. Clinical conditions that have been associated with elevated S_vO_2 include the hyperdynamic phase of sepsis and cirrhosis of the liver with systemic arterial venous malformations, as well as peripheral arteriovenous fistulas. In addition, technologic problems with monitoring of S_vO_2 can cause falsely elevated venous O_2 measurements resulting from either inaccurate calibration or distal migration of the pulmonary artery catheter tip with increased reflectance of the transmitted light signal from the vessel wall.

It should be recalled that a normal value of between 68% and 77% for S_vO_2 does not guarantee that all capillary beds are equally well oxygenated. As shown in Table 1, there exists a wide variation in venous O_2 levels from the tissue beds in the body reflecting local differences in tissue blood flow and VO_2. The measured mixed venous O_2 level reflects the "flow-weighted" mixture of all contributions of end-capillary tissue O_2 levels from all body organs. The average measurement may be not sensitive to a change in

TABLE 1   Variations in Tissue Oxygenation

	P_vO_2 (mmHg)	S_vO_2 (%)	AVO_2 (m/O_2/dl)
Brain	36	70	6.0
Heart	20	45	11.0
Liver	40	75	5.0
Kidney	70	93	1.5
Skin	65	90	2.0
Mean	40	75	4.5

O_2 status in a particular tissue bed, unless the magnitude of the change or the amount of flow to that tissue bed is a substantial portion of the total O_2 extraction or blood flow. Attempts at more specific analysis of tissue O_2 levels by measuring specific-organ venous blood, such as the renal vein or jugular vein, have been of limited value in extrapolating their values to other tissue beds.[11] Normal venous O_2 level in the jugular vein cannot give the clinician assurance that myocardial or diaphragmatic blood flow is adequate.

Venous O_2 levels that fall below 0.68 are potentially due to either a decrease in the Hgb concentration, arterial PO_2 (P_aO_2), or cardiac output or an increase in O_2 extraction as occurs with increased muscle activity, agitation, and fever. Under most circumstances, declines in Hgb and P_aO_2 do not lead to similar declines in venous O_2 levels because of the corresponding increase in cardiac output. Thus, in the usual clinical setting, the two major determinants of a decreased S_vO_2 are VO_2 and cardiac output. In normal subjects, the arteriovenous O_2 content is protected and remains more constant than either cardiac output or VO_2.[22] If VO_2 should increase, an increase in cardiac output would result. If some pathologic process prevented an increase in cardiac output, tissue oxygenation would be sustained by an increase in O_2 extraction and a widened arteriovenous O_2 difference with a corresponding decrease in venous O_2.

As discussed previously, O_2 extraction under normal circumstances can double before venous O_2 levels approach the critical level, that is, S_vO_2 of about 50% or P_vO_2 of 27 mmHg. Under special conditions, such as chronic congestive heart failure, tissues may adapt to chronic tissue hypoxia by increasing their O_2 extraction capabilities as shown by Schlichtig et al.[23] In this report, three patients with long-standing congestive heart failure were shown to tolerate levels of S_vO_2 as low as 25% for over 24 hours without evidence of elevated tissue lactate production. The authors concluded that the level of S_vO_2 associated with inadequate VO_2 is highly variable and depends on the body's ability to employ vasoconstrictor mechanisms that appropriately match O_2D to VO_2. In patients with chronic low cardiac output states, very low S_vO_2 did not imply diminished VO_2 but rather an increased ability of a number of organs to extract O_2. Chronic or recurrent episodes of tissue hypoxia as occur with congestive heart failure, living at high altitude, or physical training appear to allow tissues to become more efficient at extracting O_2 and able to tolerate levels of venous O_2 that would result in lactic acid production in other individuals.

CLINICAL EXAMPLES

The value of continuously measured S_vO_2 in the clinical management of critically ill patients has been demonstrated by many investigators.[1,2,5,11,14,20,28,30] Examples listed below are taken from my own clinical experience and are representative of patients cared for in the ICU with continuous S_vO_2 monitoring.

> **Case 1** A 25-year-old factory worker complained of the sudden onset of severe headache at work followed by collapse to the floor. When evaluated in the Emergency Room, he was in severe respiratory distress and required endotracheal intubation. While breathing fractional inspired oxygen (F_IO_2) of 1.0, the measured P_aO_2 was only 47 mmHg and 15 cm H_2O of PEEP was required to raise the PO_2 to 84 mmHg. A chest radiograph revealed fluffy bilateral infiltrates, and a computerized axial tomography scan of the head showed evidence of intracerebral hemorrhage. Neurogenic pulmonary edema was suspected, and intravenous mannitol and dexamethasone were given in an attempt to decrease cerebral edema. Vital signs remained stable except for tachycardia of 115 beats per minute. A pulmonary artery catheter was inserted and revealed slightly elevated pressure in the pulmonary artery (35/15 mmHg; mean, 21 mmHg) with a normal pulmonary capillary wedge pressure (12 mmHg). Continuous measurement of S_vO_2 initially showed a value of 0.38 (Fig. 4). The amount of PEEP was reduced to 5 cm H_2O and resulted in a prompt increase in the s_vO_2 to near 0.60. The P_aO_2 however, declined to 51 mmHg following the decrease in PEEP.

This case presents a seeming paradox in that tissue oxygenation improved, as measured by the impressive rise in

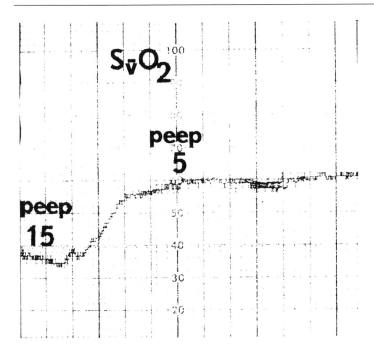

FIGURE 4   Continuous measurement of S_vO_2 during reduction in PEEP from 15 to 5 cm H_2O in a patient with neurogenic pulmonary edema. From Fahey PJ et al: Clinical experience with continuous monitoring of mixed venous O_2 saturation in respiratory failure. Chest 86:748, 1982. With permission.

S_vO_2, yet arterial O_2 levels decreased following the decrease in PEEP. Since mixed venous O_2 levels reflect the balance between arterial O_2 content, blood flow, and tissue O_2 extraction, a decrease in arterial O_2 content can result in an increased venous O_2 level only if a simultaneous increase in blood flow or decrease in VO_2 occurs. It is suspected that a decrease in cardiac output occurred in this case as PEEP of 15 cm H_2O is likely to have decreased cardiac output. The patient had diuresed 4 liters during the mannitol infusion and was intravascularly depleted, making the vascular system more susceptible to the adverse effects of PEEP. The reduction of PEEP to 5 cm H_2O not unexpectedly resulted in a decrease in P_aO_2, but the rise in S_vO_2 indicates that the increase in cardiac output more than compensated for the small change in P_aO_2.

In a subsequent study of 13 patients with hypoxemic respiratory failure, PEEP was varied between 5 and 20 cm H_2O and the corresponding arterial O_2 content, VO_2, and O_2D was measured.[6] Increasing PEEP from 5 to 20 cm H_2O decreased S_vO_2 steadily from 72% to 62%, with a corresponding decrease in cardiac output. Also, strong intra-subject correlation between DO_2 and S_vO_2 was noted (Fig.

A decrease in arterial O_2 content can result in an increased venous O_2 level only if a simultaneous increase in blood flow or decrease in VO_2 occurs.

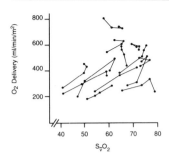

FIGURE 5 Correlation of changes in O_2 with S_vO_2 in 13 patients with ARDS. Changes in O_2 were accomplished by altering PEEP between 5 and 20 cm H_2O. From Fahey PJ et al: Clinical experience with continuous monitoring of mixed venous O_2 saturation in respiratory failure. Chest 86:748, 1982. With permission.

Detection of unexpected changes in VO_2 has been one of the most useful aspects of continuous S_vO_2 monitoring in the ICU.

5), while VO_2 remained constant. Despite the reports of others,[3,14,18] I have found S_vO_2 to be a reliable monitor of the balance of DO_2 and consumption in patients with ARDS.

Case 2 A 70-year-old retired man came to the hospital with long-standing idiopathic cardiomyopathy and suspected amiodarone hydrochloride-induced pulmonary and neurologic toxicity. He was admitted to the hospital for evaluation of increasing shortness of breath. The patient had requested that no extraordinary means be undertaken to prolong his life and he specifically refused endotracheal intubation. While breathing with a high-flow face mask delivering F_IO_2 of 1.0, the S_aO_2 was 75%, corresponding to an P_aO_2 of near 40 mmHg. Figure 6 shows the continuous measurement of S_vO_2 that was 38% at the time the S_aO_2 was 75%. A tight-fitting mask providing continuous positive airway pressure (CPAP) set at 10 cm H_2O cwp was applied and resulted in a prompt increase in S_aO_2 to 90%, but more importantly the S_vO_2 rose from 38% to 67%.

The Fick equation predicts that a 15% increase in S_aO_2, as occurred in this case, would result in a similar increase in S_vO_2 if other variables remained constant. The increase in S_vO_2 in this case exceeded that associated with the increase in S_aO_2 and must be a result of either a corresponding increase in cardiac output or decrease in VO_2. We had no reason to believe that the application of CPAP would increase cardiac output, but CPAP is known to decrease the O_2 cost of breathing in patients with reduced lung compliance. Indeed, in the present case, the measured VO_2 following application of CPAP mask decreased from 342 ml/min to 256 ml/min. Detection of unexpected changes in VO_2 has been one of the most useful aspects of continuous S_vO_2 monitoring in the ICU.

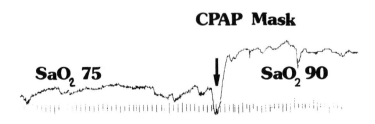

FIGURE 6 Continuous measurement of S_vO_2 in a patient with pulmonary edema. When the CPAP mask is in place, S_aO_2 rose from 75% to 90%, while S_vO_2 increased from 38% to 67%.

Case 3 Figure 7 shows acute decreases in S_vO_2 during endotracheal suctioning in a 60-year-old patient with ARDS secondary to aspiration pneumonia. Decreases in S_vO_2 in this setting could be due to a decrease in S_aO_2 associated with detachment from the ventilator tubing during suctioning with corresponding reduction of F_IO_2 and S_aO_2, a decrease in cardiac output, or increase in VO_2. Significant morbidity has been associated with endotracheal suctioning, including development of hypotension, arrhythmias, and even death. Declines in S_aO_2 have been thought to account for most of this morbidity. My colleagues and I suspected that declines in S_vO_2 could also explain some of the morbidity associated with endotracheal suctioning, and we therefore systematically investigated the etiology of declines in S_vO_2 during suctioning in 10 patients.[28] In this study, we found that declines in S_vO_2 regularly accompany endotracheal suctioning and are usually due to increases in VO_2 associated with coughing and muscular straining that frequently occur during the procedure. Declines in S_aO_2 were quite modest and were insensitive indicators of alteration in S_vO_2.

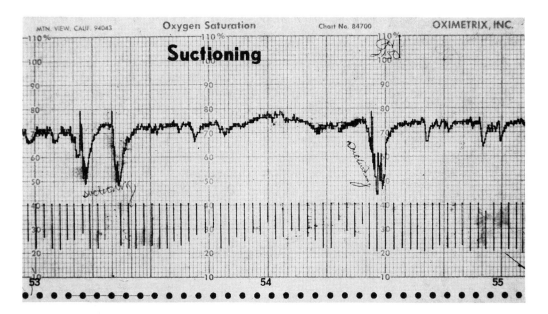

FIGURE 7   Continuous measurement of S_vO_2 during endotracheal suctioning in a patient with ARDS. Note the sharp increases in S_vO_2 immediately preceding each suctioning event. This corresponds to the brief period of lung hyperinflation with F_IO_2 of 1.0 prior to suctioning. From Walsh JM et al: Unsuspected hemodynamic alterations during endotracheal suctioning. Chest 95:162, 1989. With permission.

COST–BENEFIT ANALYSIS OF S_vO_2 MONITORING

To this date, no randomized and controlled study has documented an improved clinical outcome attributable to continuous measurement of S_vO_2. Most studies have been limited in size and too small to detect a clinical significant difference if one existed. Indeed, most studies have found that S_vO_2 has had no significant impact on ICU days, hospital days, or mortality, and variable results have been reported on the frequency of blood gas analysis, cardiac output determinations, and other assessments of hemodynamic status.[12,19,20] These findings may not be surprising given the variable patient populations studied and the lack of standardized protocols for addressing the steps to be taken in the evaluation of a change in S_vO_2. In addition, probability analysis indicates that for a study to be able to detect a 10% reduction in expected mortality in patients with a 90% chance of survival, a minimum of 200 patients well matched and randomized in each group is required. No study has approached this number.

In our experience with continuous monitoring of S_vO_2, patients can reasonably be divided into three groups based on the severity of illness and probability of outcome. In the first group are patients who are stable and do not require frequent assessment of hemodynamic status or experience unexpected changes in cardiac output or VO_2. Typical patients in this group are routine cardiovascular surgery patients and patients who had a pulmonary artery catheter placed during the initial phase of pulmonary edema but are currently improving. In this setting of stable hemodynamics, S_vO_2 changes are likely to be infrequent and the patients' clinical course stable and improving independent of ongoing monitoring. Studies that include large numbers of these type of patients will most likely not show significant differences in outcome or resource utilization when compared to standard monitoring. Another group of patients that is challenging to cost–benefit and outcome studies includes those whose severity of illness is so great that the chances for survival are minimal, making any type of monitoring unlikely to have an impact on outcome. Examples of this type of patient are those with cardiogenic shock and lactic acid production or sepsis with hypotension and increased lactic acid concentration. Because the chances of death are high in this group, it is unreasonable to expect that a measurement of one variable could alter the expected outcome significantly. Our experience has found continuous monitoring of S_vO_2 most helpful in the group of patients whose hemodynamic status lies between the two previous groups. That is, those patients who are more unstable than the "routine" monitoring groups, but not so hemodynamically unstable that survival is unlikely. In this intermediate illness group are patients with shock of any type but without increased lactic acid production. It is in this group of patients that S_vO_2 monitoring is of most value in initiating therapies and detecting early changes in tissue oxygenation.

In order to reliably perform studies evaluating the cost-effectiveness and impact on clinical outcome of continuous S_vO_2, the following factors must be considered: (1) the patient population being studied, (2) the number of patients studied and the power of the study to detect a significant difference, (3) the standard of practice within the ICU and in particular the protocol adapted for assessing changes in S_vO_2, and (4) the cost and charge figures for the individual hospital.

In the final assessment, the real value of S_vO_2 may be to decrease the number of unnecessary blood gas and hemodynamic measurements in stable patients and to serve as an early warning to the ICU team of the need for additional measurements if an imbalance develops between DO_2 and VO_2.

References

1. Baele P, McMichan J, Marsh H et al: Continuous monitoring of mixed venous O_2 saturation in critically ill patients. Anesth Analg 61:513, 1982

2. Divertie M, McMichan J: Continuous monitoring of mixed venous O_2 saturation. Chest 85:423, 1984

3. Danek SJ, Lynch JP, Weg JG, Dantzke DR: The dependence of O_2 uptake on O_2 delivery in the adult respiratory distress syndrome. Am Rev Respir Dis 122:387, 1980

4. Dantzker, DK, Forseman B, Gutierrez G: O_2 supply and utilization relationships. Am Rev Respir Dis 143:675, 1991

5. Fahey PJ: An overall assessment of the role of continuous S_vO_2 measurement in hemodynamic monitoring in the ICU. p. 113. In Schweis JE (ed): Continuous measurement of blood O_2 saturation in the high risk patient. Vol. 1. Beach International, San Diego, 1983

6. Fahey PJ, Harris K, Vanderwarf C: Clinical experience with continuous monitoring of mixed venous O_2 saturation in respiratory failure. Chest 86:748, 1984

7. Fallat RJ, Eberhart R: Independence of CO_2 production and systemic O_2 delivery in severe adult respiratory distress syndrome. Am Rev Respir Dis 129:96, 1984

8. Gamble WJ: The use of fiber optics in clinical cardiac catheterization. 1. Intracardiac oximetry. Circulation 31:328, 1965

9. Gettinger A, DeTraglia MC, Glass D: In vivo compression of two mixed venous saturation catheters. Anaesthesia 66:373, 1987

10. Gilbert EM, Haupt MT, Mandennas RY et al: The effect of fluid loading, blood transfusion and catecholamine infusion on O_2 delivery and consumption in patients with sepsis. Am Rev Respir Dis 134:873, 1989

11. Haljamae H, Frid I, Holm J: Continuous conjunctional O_2 tension ($PcjO_2$) monitoring for assessment of cerebral oxygenation and metabolism during cardiac artery surgery. Acta Anaesthesiol Scand 33:610, 1989

12. Jastremski MS, Chelluri L, Beney KM: Analysis of the effects of continuous on line monitoring of mixed venous O_2 saturation on patient outcome and cost effectiveness. Crit Care Med 17:148, 1989

13. Kandel G, Aberman A: Mixed venous O_2 saturation: its' role in the assessment of the critically ill patient. Arch Intern Med 143:1400, 1983

14. Kariman K, Burns S: Regulation of tissue O_2 extraction is disturbed in adult respiratory distress syndrome. Am Rev Respir Dis 132:109, 1985

15. Krasnitz P, Druger GL, Yorra F, Simmons DH: Mixed venous O_2 tension and hyperlactemia: survival in severe cardiopulmonary disease. JAMA 236:570, 1976

16. Krogh A: The number and distribution of capillaries in muscles with calculations of the O_2 pressure head necessary for supplying the tissue. J Physiol (Lond) 52:409, 1919

17. McMichan JC, Baele PL, Wignes MW: Insertion of pulmonary artery catheters: a comparison of fiberoptic and nonfiberoptic catherters. Crit Care Med 12:517, 1984

18. Mohsenifar Z, Goldbach P, Tashkin DP et al: Relationship between O_2 delivery and O_2 consumption in the adult respiratory distress syndrome. Chest 84:267, 1983

19. Orlando R: Continuous mixed venous oximetry in critically ill surgical patients. Arch Surg 121:470, 1986

20. Pearson KS, Gomez MN, Moyers JR et al: A cost/benefit analysis of randomized invasive monitoring for patients undergoing cardiac surgery. Anesth Analg 69:336, 1989

21. Rashkin MC, Bosken C, Boughman RP: O_2 delivery in critically ill patients: relationship to blood lactate and survival. Chest 87:580, 1985

22. Reeves T, Graver RF, Felley GF et al: Cardiac output in resting man. J Appl Physiol 16:276, 1961

23. Schlichtig R, Cowden WL, Chaitman BR: Tolerance of unusually low mixed venous O_2 saturation: adaption in the chronic low cardiac output syndrome. Am J Med 80:813, 1986

24. Shibutani K, Komatsu T, Kubal K et al: Critical level of O_2 delivery in anesthetized man. Crit Care Med 11:640, 1983

25. Tenney SM: A theoretical analysis of the relationship between venous blood and mean tissue O_2 pressures. Respir Physiol 20:283, 1974

26. Villar J, Slutsky A, Hew E, Aberman A: O_2 transport and O_2 consumption in critically ill patients. Chest 98:687, 1990

27. Waller JL, Bauman DL, Craver JM: Clinical evaluation of a new fiber optic catheter oximeter during cardiac surgery. Anesth Analg 61:676, 1982

28. Walsh JM, Vanderwaarf C, Hoscheidt D, Fahey PJ: Unsuspected hemodynamic alterations during endotracheal suctioning. Chest 95:162, 1989

29. Watsons CB: The PA catheter as an early warning system. Anesth Rev 10:34, 1983

CAPNOMETRY AND TRANSCUTANEOUS CARBON DIOXIDE MONITORING

STEVEN KESTEN, MD, FRCPC[†]
KENNETH R. CHAPMAN, MD, FRCPC[††]

CO_2 PRODUCTION AND ELIMINATION

When dissolved in water, carbon dioxide is present almost entirely as unhydrated CO_2 with a solubility coefficient close to 1. The relationship among carbonic acid (H_2CO_3), carbon dioxide (CO_2), water (H_2O) and the bicarbonate (HCO_3^-) and hydrogen (H^+) ions may be represented as[1]:

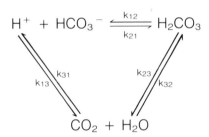

The rate constants k_{21} and k_{12} are significantly greater than the others shown. Thus, the equilibrium of the reaction $CO_2 + H_2O \rightleftharpoons H_2CO_3$ in plasma is so far to the left that the concentration of dissolved CO_2 is about 1,000 times greater than the concentration of H_2O_3.[2] Measured at body temperature, 0.0301 mM/l (067 volume percent) of CO_2 is dis-

[†] Assistant Professor of Medicine, University of Toronto, Division of Respiratory Medicine, The Toronto Hospital, Toronto, Ontario, Canada

[††] Acting Director, Asthma Centre of the Toronto Hospital, Assistant Professor of Medicine, University of Toronto, Toronto, Ontario, Canada

solved in plasma for each mmHg partial pressure of CO_2. Thus, arterial blood in the normocapnic individual contains 1.2 mM/l of dissolved CO_2.

With only minute quantities of carbonic acid present in plasma, this compound is responsible for the manufacture of only small amounts of bound CO_2 in the form of HCO_3^-. Of greater importance, the erythrocyte enzyme carbonic anhydrase promotes the formation of HCO_3^- from tissue CO_2, contributing OH^- to CO_2 in the direction of hydration and withdrawing OH^- from HCO_3^- in the dehydration reaction. Within the red cell, hemoglobin provides the basic groups that neutralize H^+ ions formed by H_2CO_3 dissociation, hence promoting the formation of HCO_3^-. Hypoxic conditions intensify hemoglobin's efficacy as a buffer since reduced hemoglobin is a better H^+ ion acceptor than oxyhemoglobin.

In humans, the physically dissolved carbon dioxide produced by the tissues is transported between the systemic and pulmonary capillaries both in plasma and erythrocytes. In the lungs, the blood gives up its excess CO_2 to the alveoli—a process aided by oxygen's displacement of CO_2 from hemoglobin. The gases are highly soluble in aqueous media and diffuse rapidly. As a result, a steady-state between the CO_2 tension in mixed venous blood (PCO_2 = 46 mmHg), alveolar air, and pulmonary capillary blood (PCO_2 = 40 mmHg) occurs swiftly.

A steady-state between the CO_2 tension in mixed venous blood (PCO_2 = 46 mmHg), alveolar air, and pulmonary capillary blood (PCO_2 = 40 mmHg) occurs swiftly.

METHODS FOR MEASURING CO_2 IN GAS MIXTURES

Physiologists and clinicians have been interested in the measurement of expired CO_2 since Brown-Sequard and d'Arsonval[3] and Haldane and Lorrain Smith[4] made formal studies of "poisonous organic substances given off in expired air." Using a 70-cubic-foot chamber, Haldane observed the process of partial asphyxiation, noting that when air was rebreathed the resulting tachypnea was the consequence of CO_2 excess. To estimate CO_2 tensions in alveolar gas, Haldane collected expired gas samples using a 4-foot length of 1-inch rubber hose. He relied upon his subjects to provide the necessary valving by opening and closing the open end of the hose with their tongues. Gas analysis was performed with a portable apparatus that he transported to coal mines, factories, railway tunnels, and to the lodging houses of dyspneic workers. The principle of Haldane's method was to draw a sample of gas into a graduated burette over mercury, recording its volume. The

CO_2 was then absorbed by exposure of the gas to potassium hydroxide (KOH), after which the measurement of volume was repeated. The volume of CO_2 in the original sample was the difference. (An analagous method allowed early investigators to quantify O_2 using pyrogallol or anthraquinone and sodium hydrosulphite as absorbents). Many chemical and physical methods for CO_2 analysis in expired gas have since been developed and are summarized below.

CHEMICAL METHODS

Haldane's apparatus was simplified and applied to clinical studies by Campbell[5] who used a burette holding 10 ml of gas within an absorbent chamber and reservoir filled with 10–20% KOH solution. The gas was moved chamber to chamber by a syringe-driven mercury column. The method, although simplified from Haldane's original, still required considerable technical skill to obtain reliable results. In the hands of an experienced operator, CO_2 tensions could be estimated to within $+0.1\%$ CO_2.

The most accurate of chemical absorption methods is Lloyd's modification of the Haldane apparatus.[6] Lloyd and Cormack paid strict attention to temperature stabilization and dryness of the compensating chamber, achieving, even in the hands of a technician new to the instrument an accuracy of $\pm0.01\%$. For gas samples as small as 0.5 ml, the micro-Scholander[7] apparatus can be used, although it is far less accurate.

The PCO_2 of any gas or liquid may also be determined directly by the use of a PCO_2-sensitive electrode,[8] which allows a film of HCO_3^- solution to come into contact with the sample across a membrane permeable to CO_2. The pH of the HCO_3^- solution is monitored, and the PCO_2 is inversely proportional to the recorded pH. The pH-sensitive electrode has a 95% limit of error on the order of ±0.5 kPa when operated correctly.

The PCO_2 of any gas or liquid may also be determined directly by the use of a PCO_2-sensitive electrode, which allows a film of HCO_3^- solution to come into contact with the sample across a membrane permeable to CO_2.

PHYSICAL METHODS

Several rapid, continuous, and simple to operate physical methods for measuring CO_2 in gas mixtures are available. Instruments employing physical methods are usually calibrated against gas mixtures analyzed previously by chemical absorption methods. Like many of the gases and vapors of interest in respiratory and anesthetic practice, CO_2 has an absorption band in the infrared spectrum allowing its continuous and rapid measurement.[9] Due to a process known as collision broadening, other gases influence the response of the infrared instrument that varies according to the CO_2 concentrations.[10] Hence, such instruments must be calibrated with known concentrations of CO_2 in a diluent gas mixture similar to that of the gas sample intended for analysis. The major value of infrared analyzers is that they can respond within less than a quarter of a second and will thus show the changes in CO_2 concentration during a single respiratory cycle, assuming sufficiently high sampling flow rates.[11]

Mass spectrometry is the most sophisticated of the physical methods for CO_2 analysis in expired gas.

Mass spectrometry is the most sophisticated of the physical methods for CO_2 analysis in expired gas.[12] Respiratory mass spectrometers ionize a sample stream of gas with an electrical discharge. The ions accelerated in an electric field by an amount directly proportional to their charge and inversely proportional to their mass. A magnetic field at right angles to the accelerating electric fields deflects the ions by an amount dependent upon their charge and speed. Detectors are placed so as to be in the known trajectories of the ions characteristic of each gas to be measured. The electric charge that accumulates is proportional to the concentration of each gas in the sample. Mass spectrometers are both more versatile and more rapid than infrared analyzers, sampling up to four low molecular weight gases simultaneously and responding in as little as 0.1 second. Such versatility and speed is costly and spectrometers may be difficult to operate and maintain. In the clinical setting, one of their more troublesome traits is their susceptibility to condensation in the sampling tube.[13]

In summary, the chemical analysis of CO_2 concentration in expired gas yields great accuracy in competent technical hands, but is applicable only to single samples. For continuous monitoring of expired gas, the most appropriate clinical method is by physical means, using infrared absorption. The method is technically simple and virtually immediate but requires calibration with test gases in a similar range of concentration.

NONINVASIVE MEASUREMENT OF PCO₂

TRANSCUTANEOUS CO₂ MONITORING

An electrochemical sensor to measure PCO_2 was initially developed by Severinghaus in 1958.[14] The sensor, composed of a pH-sensing glass electrode, actually measures the concentration of H^+ ions in a solution. Carbon dioxide released from the skin diffuses through a permeable membrane and combines with water, resulting in the production of H_2CO_3. The pH sensor within the transcutaneous electrode then measures the H^+ ion concentration in the solution. The results are referenced to a silver/silver chloride electrode and calibrated to the CO_2 tension.[15]

Transcutaneous carbon dioxide tensions ($tcPCO_2$) are invariably higher than the corresponding arterial tensions.[16,17] This difference is the consequence of, or is influenced by (1) the higher temperature at which the electrodes operate, typically 44°C in adults; (2) local metabolic production of carbon dioxide; (3) capillary blood flow; and (4) cardiac output.[15] The elevated temperature is necessary to increase gas permeability across the cutaneous barrier, but increases local production of CO_2 and requires a site change every 4 hours to avoid burns. Reduced tissue perfusion results in an increase in $tcPCO_2$.

It is important at this point to emphasize that $tcPO_2$ values estimate no other physiologic parameter in common clinical usage. That is, the $tcCO_2$ approximates, if anything, a tissue CO_2 tension, not an arterial tension, and is measured in no other way. One important implication is that the transcutaneous value cannot be validated. By contrast, oximetry readings of S_aO_2 can be verified by testing in arterial blood samples; end-tidal CO_2 values can be verified against arterial CO_2 tensions. Moreover, no normal physiologic range for $tcCO_2$ has been defined and each subject acts as his or her own control. Initial readings immediately following application to the skin have little meaning; the device is best viewed as a trend monitor.

While earlier designs required fastidious skin preparation to insure a certain degree of accuracy,[18] later models, several of which combine a Clark-type O_2 electrode and a Severinghaus-type CO_2 electrode in a single unit, are simple to apply without the need to abrade the skin. The major disadvantages of $tcPCO_2$ monitoring are relatively lengthy response times (3–7 minutes) and lag times (15–56 seconds).[19,21] Calibration times of at least 5–10 minutes limit the usefulness of transcutaneous monitoring during cardiorespiratory resuscitation. To such instrument response times we must also add the time for the care giver to recognize a significant change in trend. This is not a simple task given the absence of a defined physiologic range for $tcPCO_2$ or critical levels at which alarms might be set. Response will also be influenced by each patient's moment-to-moment variability in $tcPCO_2$. The $tcPCO_2$ value must exceed by a subjective degree the normal excursion of $tcCO_2$ baseline. Finally, additional time may be lost while the monitor signal is verified, a task more rapidly and sensibly done by cross-checking other monitored variables

Transcutaneous carbon dioxide tensions are invariably higher than the corresponding arterial tensions.

The most extensive clinical experience in transcutaneous monitoring is in subjects with thin skin (neonates) where studies have demonstrated a high degree of accuracy with little variability.

than by the time-consuming process of reapplying and re-calibrating the instrument.

The most extensive clinical experience in transcutaneous monitoring is in subjects with thin skin (neonates) where studies have demonstrated a high degree of accuracy with little variability.[22,23] Although several studies have shown a significant correlation between transcutaneous and arterial PCO_2 in stable adults[18,20,24] (Fig. 1), the relationship in the acute care setting in the presence of pulmonary disease is less well documented. While $tcPCO_2$ generally increases proportionally to P_aCO_2, in states of extremely low perfusion (ie, shock) a disproportionate increase in $tcPCO_2$ occurs.[25] When transcutaneous devices are used as trend monitors in the critical care setting, a rise or fall in $tcCO_2$ values hints at a significant change in the cardiopulmonary system as a unit, leaving the clinician to determine the cause of the trend more specifically. For example, a rise in transcutaneous CO_2 may imply worsened alveolar ventilation from a variety of causes, ranging from ventilator malfunction to worsened $\dot{V}/Q$ mismatch, but may just as plausibly imply decreased tissue perfusion either globally or locally.

There appears to be a role for $tcPCO_2$ monitoring in neonatal intensive care units; the devices are most accurate in this age group and allow monitoring where vascular access is problematic. The role of $tcPCO_2$ monitoring in adult critical care is as yet to be defined; the long response and lag times and the less than ideal relationship to arterial values

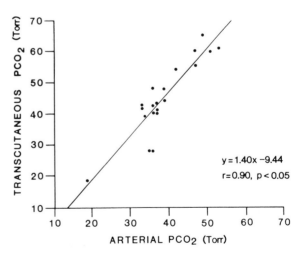

FIGURE 1   Relationship between $tcPCO_2$ (dashed line) and P_aCO_2 (solid line) in 20 patients with stable respiratory disease. From Kesten S, Chapman KR, Rebuck AS: Response characteristics of a dual transcutaneous oxygen/carbon dioxide monitoring system. Chest 99:1211, 1991. With permission.

fail to offer the characteristics necessary for useful monitoring in a rapidly changing clinical situation. Viewed as trend monitors, transcutaneous monitors offer little additional information not already provided by other means. Significant changes in cardiopulmonary status sufficient to perturb the transcutaneous record are likely to have been manifest minutes earlier as changes in heart rate, blood pressure, respiratory rate, tidal volume, mean airway pressure, or other continuously recorded variable. When nursing care approximates a one-to-one ratio and the critically ill patient is instrumented for continuous hemodynamic monitoring, transcutaneous devices are most often sluggish and redundant. Their merit is more obvious in the setting of the step-down unit where nurse-to-patient ratios are lower and invasive forms of monitoring are absent.

ALVEOLAR GAS SAMPLING

Arterial PCO_2 can be estimated rapidly and noninvasively by the analysis of gas sampled continuously at the mouth or by the use of end-tidal sampling. A capnogram is the displayed CO_2 concentration of the gas sample (Fig. 2). Expired gas consists of four components: apparatus dead space, anatomical dead space, "ideal" alveolar gas, and alveolar dead space gas. Apparatus and anatomical dead space gases are exhaled in series, contain almost no CO_2, and are seen as an initial flat portion of the capnogram (phase 1). An elevated phase 1 suggests rebreathing or a stuck inspiratory or expiratory valve. Dead space gas mixed with alveolar gas causes a rapid rise in the capnogram tracing (phase 2). During a single expiration, after exhalation of the instrument and anatomical dead space gas, the tension of CO_2 attains a fairly constant level, called the alveolar plateau. It is probably more accurate to refer to this

Expired gas consists of four components: apparatus dead space, anatomical dead space, "ideal" alveolar gas, and alveolar dead space gas.

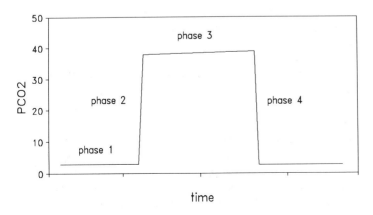

FIGURE 2   Shape of a normal capnogram.

so-called plateau as phase 3 because this expiratory "plateau" continues to rise slightly. In healthy subjects, phase 3 most closely approximates a plateau with any slight upward slope being attributed to gas exchange continuing during expiration.[26] The end of the alveolar plateau represents end-tidal CO_2. Any factor that influences the rate of gas exchange will by necessity influence the slope of phase 3, these factors being composition of inspired gas, alveolar volume, composition of mixed venous blood, and the flow rate at which it enters the lungs. As the flow rate of mixed venous blood plays an inspired role in determining the slope of phase 3, measurement of the slope can be used as the basis of a noninvasive method for estimating cardiac output.[27] Alveolar gas and alveolar dead space are exhaled in parallel.[28] In the presence of any appreciable alveolar dead space, it is therefore impossible to sample or analyze ideal alveolar gas. Furthermore, the PCO_2 of end-expiratory gas will invariably be less than that of "ideal" alveolar gas since it is diluted with alveolar dead space. Finally, inspiration follows phase 3 with a rapid fall in CO_2 (phase 4) and the cycle begins again.

The most important factor that influences the slope of the expired CO_2 trace is uneven lung function. Alveoli with lower ventilation/perfusion ratios empty late in expiration. By contrast, alveoli that are well ventilated with respect to their perfusion empty earlier. Since no gas exchange takes place in the conducting airways, all of the CO_2 eliminated by the lungs must be contained in the alveolar gas. In a steady-state, the volume of CO_2 being eliminated must equal that being produced by the tissues. Although a single value can be calculated from the CO_2 production and alveolar ventilation, there is no single value for alveolar PCO_2 in a lung in which inequalities between ventilation and perfusion exist. In alveoli that are ventilated but not perfused, the alveolar gas approaches that of inspired gas. In the alveoli that are perfused but not ventilated, the CO_2 tension is equal to that of mixed venous blood. Analysis of alveolar gas thus becomes a better method for evaluating $\dot{V}/Q$ characteristics of the lung[29] than for estimating arterial PCO_2. Mean arterial PCO_2 tends to be higher than mean alveolar gas PCO_2, thereby creating an arterial-to-end-tidal CO_2 tension difference. The single expiration may be displayed at high chart or monitor speeds, but more commonly capnograms are displayed at slower speeds to show trends over many breaths. Inspection of the single breath tracing offers a crude graphic estimate of $\dot{V}/Q$ mismatch evident as the steepness of phase 3. However, the presence of significant $\dot{V}/Q$ mismatch in critical care settings is seldom a mystery and the capnogram simply confirms clinical information already at hand. Nonetheless, this inspection step should not be omitted before long-term monitoring is commenced. A nonphysiologic appearance to the expired capnogram suggests technical problems such as a partially clogged sampling tube. The capnogram should be reviewed periodically for such artifacts during prolonged monitoring. The shape of the capnogram at slower display speeds may also provide useful information. An abrupt exponential decay in end-tidal CO_2 levels may be seen in cardiac arrest. A gradual rise in end-tidal levels may reflect worsening pulmonary status or increased metabolic production of CO_2 such as during fever. A progressive rise in both end-tidal and baseline (end-inspiratory) CO_2 levels alerts the caregiver to ventilator malfunction or misuse with consequent rebreathing. In mechanically ventilated subjects, a low alveolar PCO_2 may indicate a disturbance in the ventilator circuit, an ineffectual endotracheal tube, cardiac arrest or pulmonary embolism. End-tidal sampling can be employed as a method for prolonged monitoring of respiratory rate or, with suitable electronic manipulation, as an apnea alarm. Alveolar or end-tidal PCO_2 most closely approximates arterial PCO_2 in subjects with normal lungs. The presence of an arterial-to-alveolar PCO_2 difference renders the method inaccurate when lung disease is present unless the patient has stable cardiorespiratory function and a consistent breathing pattern; nevertheless, in the latter scenario an increase in end-tidal CO_2 may represent hypoventilation due to pulmonary or extra pulmonary (ie, respiratory depression) causes, an obstructed airway, or increased CO_2 production (ie, fever, malignant hyperthermia).

It has been demonstrated in animals that the arterial-to-end tidal CO_2 difference may be used to find the optimal level of positive end-expiratory pressure (PEEP) for mechanical ventilation, the smallest gradient presumably being associated with the best $\dot{V}/Q$ matching.[30] However, this has not proven reliable in clinical contexts.[31]

In summary, a rapid estimate of the arterial PCO_2 can be obtained by determining alveolar PCO_2, either by continuous sampling at the mouth or by use of end-tidal sampling. Although alveolar PCO_2 approximates closely the arterial PCO_2 in subjects with normal lungs, the existence of the arterial-to-alveolar PCO_2 difference renders the estimate inaccurate when lung disease is present; its value is therefore in trend monitoring when applied in the critical care setting.[32] Expired PCO_2 can be used to measure physiological dead space.

A progressive rise in both end-tidal and baseline (end-inspiratory) CO_2 levels alerts the caregiver to ventilator malfunction or misuse with consequent rebreathing.

Although alveolar PCO_2 approximates closely the arterial PCO_2 in subjects with normal lungs, the existence of the arterial-to-alveolar PCO_2 difference renders the estimate inaccurate when lung disease is present.

MIXED EXPIRED PCO$_2$ AND THE CALCULATION OF VD/VT RATIO

The alveolar dead space is assumed to be the difference between the anatomical and physiological dead spaces, determined separately but simultaneously. One simply measures the arterial and end-expiratory PCO$_2$ simultaneously, and the difference becomes an estimate of alveolar dead space.[33] Although the arterial-to-end-expiratory difference is stable in healthy anesthetized subjects,[34] in patients with respiratory disease the difference is so large and variable as to be of little value. It is, after all, impossible to sample or analyze "ideal" alveolar gas.

The determination of physiological dead space is of greater clinical utility. Physiological dead space may simply be defined as that part of tidal volume that does not participate in gas exchange. Its measurement has been generally accepted as being useful in patients who have required assisted ventilation for prolonged periods. To measure physiological dead space, arterial blood and expired air are collected simultaneously over a period of 2 or 3 minutes. Carbon dioxide gas tensions of each are then determined. Tidal volume is measured during the expired gas collection with apparatus as simple as a Wright spirometer. The results are expressed as the ratio of the physiological dead space to tidal volume (V_D/V_T), which is calculated as follows:

$$\frac{\text{Physiological dead space}}{\text{Tidal volume}} = \frac{\text{arterial PCO}_2 - \text{mixed expired PCO}_2}{\text{arterial PCO}_2}$$

or by using the Bohr equation:

$$\frac{V_D}{V_T} = \frac{P_aCO_2 - P_ECO_2}{P_aCO_2}$$

The functional concept of physiological dead space is of clinical value to physicians caring for patients on mechanical ventilation. A V_D/V_T of 0.6 is considered as the upper limit at which weaning from mechanical ventilation is feasible.[35] The V_D/V_T ratio increases with age, body size, and a change from erect to the supine posture.[36] For healthy nonsmoking males, values for V_D/V_T between 33 and 45% can be expected, with lower values for women. The monitoring of V_D/V_T levels provides a useful method for evaluating changes in the level of PEEP in patients undergoing assisted ventilation.[37]

The monitoring of V_D/V_T levels provides a useful method for evaluating changes in the level of PEEP in patients undergoing assisted ventilation.

MIXED VENOUS PCO_2
Rebreathing

The PCO_2 in mixed venous blood may be obtained by a rebreathing method in which the lung is used as a tonometer. Gas is rebreathed from a small bag until complete equilibration is obtained with mixed venous PCO_2. The method, which was developed for clinical use by Campbell and Howell,[38] requires a bag of about 2 liters capacity, a mask or mouthpiece by which the bag is connected to the subject, and a three-way valve to permit switching the subject from bag rebreathing to room air breathing. The bag is fitted with a small-bore side connection from which gas can be sampled. As first developed by Campbell and Howell, the procedure was designed in such a way that an estimate of P_VCO_2 could be made from analysis of a single gas sample, drawn at the conclusion of the maneuver, and taken away for chemical analysis by the Haldane method. The procedure entailed two separate but essentially related stages: the first comprised preparation by the subject of a bag of gas mixture that roughly approximated his or her P_VCO_2, the second stage refined the bag mixture and created a bag-lung-blood equilibrium. Starting with 1.0–1.5 l O_2, the subject rebreathed for 90 seconds or until the ventilation had started to rise. The bag was then sealed and the subject allowed to breathe air for 3 minutes. This allowed correction of the CO_2 retention that had inevitably occurred during the 90-second rebreathing period. After the 3-minute rest period, the subject then rebreathed from the bag mixture he/she had created for a further 20 seconds, or five breaths. This procedure raised the tension of CO_2 in the bag to the level of the mixed venous blood when it is fully saturated with oxygen.

Campbell and Howell's refinement of Collier's[39] concept of a rebreathing method for estimating P_VCO_2 provided a widely accepted method of noninvasive CO_2 measurement. With the advent of rapid physical methods for CO_2 analysis, the rebreathing events could be observed continuously, ensuring that a true CO_2 equilibrium occurred (Fig. 3). Powles and Campbell[40] later used a single-stage procedure, obviating the need for initial rebreathe by starting with a gas mixture of 7% CO_2 balance oxygen. Using their approach in 102 subjects, Sealey et al.[41] showed that P_VCO_2 is relatively constant within individuals. It tends to be lower in premenopausal women (mean = 46.0 ± 2.48 mmHg) than men (mean = 51.0 ± 2.9 mmHg). Values in women fluctuate throughout the menstrual cycle and are influenced by taking oral contraceptives.

The rebreathing method for measuring mixed venous

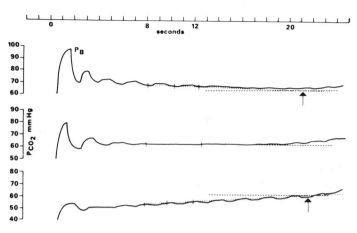

FIGURE 3   Three representative tracings of tidal PCO_2 during rebreathing different CO_2 concentrations. The middle trace shows an ideal equilibrium, the upper is too high, and the lower is too low. Extrapolation of the lines joining the end-expiratory values between 8 and 12 seconds intersect at the sample point, at 20–22 seconds (indicated by arrows) in each example. From Jones NL, Rebuck AS: Rebreathing equilibration of CO_2 during exercise. J Appl Physiol 35:538, 1973. With permission.

The rebreathing method for measuring mixed venous PCO_2 has been modified for use in children, but its main value to respiratory physiologists has been during exercise studies, in which it can be used to estimate cardiac output by the indirect Fick method.

PCO_2 has been modified for use in children,[42] but its main value to respiratory physiologists has been during exercise studies, in which it can be used to estimate cardiac output by the indirect Fick method.[43] If the mixed venous and arterial PCO_2 are known, the venoarterial CO_2 content difference may be derived using a standard CO_2 dissociation curve.[44] Even if an ideal equilibration plateau is not obtained, accurate equilibration values for P_VCO_2 within ± 2 mmHg of true equilibrium can be calculated from "too high" and "too low" test results by extrapolation (Fig. 3).[45]

The collection of a gas sample that has been equilibrated with mixed venous blood provides an opportunity for measurement of PCO_2 where no facilities are available for analysis of blood samples. The best approximation to arterial PCO_2 is obtained by multiplying the oxygenated, rebreathing PCO_2 by a factor of 0.8.[46] This method is inaccurate, however, in patients with markedly reduced cardiac output, or in those with large intracardiac shunts. It is also reasonable to suggest that the method should be feasible in the unconscious or anesthetized patient, yet the method has not been reported in these clinical situations, nor has it found a place in many routine laboratories. Reasons for this general lack of popularity may include difficulties sometimes encountered in obtaining acceptable equilibration PCO_2 plateaus and the now widespread use of arterial puncture. The volume of the rebreathing bag must be adjusted carefully for each subject to twice the tidal volume,[47] and the initial bag PCO_2 must be adjusted for each patient to a PCO_2 that is approximately 10 mmHg higher than yet unknown P_VCO_2. Equilibration plateaus must appear after gas mixing is completed and before recirculation occurs. If a plateau is short (ie, lasts for less than 10 seconds), the result is invalid because the initial PCO_2 has been too low, and the PCO_2 in the bag will continue to increase as mixed venous blood adds CO_2 to the bag and the lungs. Delayed plateaus also give unacceptable values for P_VCO_2 because initial bag CO_2 has been too high or the bag volume too large, such that CO_2 is added to mixed venous blood and the plateau appears when recirculation has occurred.[48] Thus, the PCO_2 of a delayed plateau will be higher than the P_VCO_2. In the light of these difficulties inherent in rebreathing techniques, other methods such as breathholding have been developed in the search for noninvasive measurement of the PCO_2 in the mixed venous blood.

Breath Holding

Haldane[49] observed that mixed venous PCO_2 could be estimated by having subjects inspire various mixtures of CO_2. The inspired gas was held in inspiration and then exhaled in two stages 10 seconds apart. After trying a wide range of inspired CO_2 mixtures, eventually one would be found in which the two expiratory samples had identical PCO_2 values. This value must be equal to mixed venous PCO_2. Defares[50] made a detailed analysis of these events and showed that only two gas mixtures need to be inhaled to produce the same result. He took a high CO_2 mixture, which produced gradually decreasing PCO_2 levels in the expirate, and a low CO_2 mixture, which, of course, produced gradually increasing levels as the breath was held and then exhaled. He then determined P_VCO_2 by estimating visually the common asymptote of the two curves. Dubois et al.[51] made a mathematical analysis of the breath-holding PCO_2 curve and concluded that, unless more than one inspirate was used, the final result was likely to underestimate the true P_VCO_2. If multiple data points are collected during expiration, a differential equation can be used to calculate P_VCO_2,[52] but a high coefficient of a variance results from using this method.[53]

Frankel et al.[54] evaluated these breath-holding methods and developed a clinical method that they tested in healthy volunteers, conscious subjects with lung diseases, and unconscious patients undergoing mechanical ventilation. They then demonstrated the feasibility of using their method in anesthetized patients.[55] Frankel et al. used two

Haldane observed that mixed venous PCO_2 could be estimated by having subjects inspire various mixtures of CO_2.

standard gas mixtures (0% and 12% CO_2 in O_2), allowed or delivered a full inspiration of the first gas mixture, and then the subject held his/her breath. After 5 seconds, 500 ml of gas was exhaled into a collection bag and, after a total of 10 seconds, a further 500 ml was collected, the subject then resuming normal breathing pattern. The procedure was then repeated with the second gas mixture. The four data points (two during expiration of a breath-held sample of 0% CO_2 and two following 12% CO_2) were used to calculate P_VCO_2 using two simultaneous equations (Fig. 4). The results correlated well with the rebreathing PCO_2 and with values obtained directly by drawing blood from the pulmonary artery. The method has the advantage of using only two standard gas mixtures, the inspired volume does not have to be related to tidal volume, and the low coefficient of the variance suggested that a single test would yield acceptable results in patients of chronic lung disease. The breath-holding method can be used to estimate cardiac output, with the P_VCO_2 obtained substituting for the right heart catheter,[56] and has now been simplified to the use of three expiratory samples obtained from a single breath hold of 100% oxygen.[57]

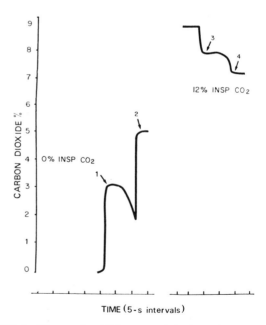

FIGURE 4   The expired CO_2 record during a breath-hold measurement of mixed venous PCO_2. The four data points define two exponential curves, each approaching the true mixed venous PCO_2 asymptomatically. From Frankel DZN, Sandham G, Rebuck AS: A new method for measuring PCO_2 during anesthesia. Br J Anaesth 215:51, 1979. With permission.

Neither the breath-hold method or rebreathing method for estimating P_VCO_2 has found widespread application in the critical care arena. This is regrettable; such measurements could obviate the need for more invasive forms of monitoring. For example, when coupled with arterial puncture, one of these noninvasive methods of estimating P_VCO_2 could be used to estimate cardiac output with accuracy sufficient for clinical purposes. Such low-cost methodology might find a useful role in step-down units where care needs are less intensive.

Neither the breath-hold method or rebreathing method for estimating P_VCO_2 has found widespread application in the critical care arena.

SUMMARY

The tension and content of CO_2 and the concentration of H ions in the blood plasma are related through the Henderson-Hasselbalch equation. The PCO_2 in arterial blood is readily measured by drawing a small blood sample and analyzing it with pH-sensitive CO_2 electrodes. Clinically used noninvasive methods for analyzing blood CO_2 include: (1) expired gas analysis, which is continuous and accurate, but highly influenced by V/Q inequalities; (2) transcutaneous monitoring, which is continuous and slow and reflects tissue PCO_2, a variable influenced by local metabolic processes and tissue perfusion; and (3) estimation of mixed venous PCO_2 by rebreathing or breath holding.

References

1. Eigen M, Kustin K, Maass G: Die geschwindigkeit der hydration von SO_2 in wasseriges losung. Z Physik Chem 30:130, 1961

2. Cherniack RM, Cherniack L, Naimark A: Respiration in Health and Disease. 2nd ed. WB Saunders, Philadelphia, 1971

3. Brown-Sequard CE, d'Arsonval A: Untitled discussion. CR Soc Biol 4:814, 1887

4. Haldane JS, Smith JL: The physiological effects of air vitiated by respiration. J Pathol Bactiol 1:168, 1893

5. Campbell EJM: Simplification of Haldane's apparatus for measuring CO_2 concentration in respired gases in clinical practice. Br Med J 1:457, 1960

6. Cormack RS: Eliminating two sources of error in the Lloyd-Haldane apparatus. Resp Physiol 14:382, 1972

7. Scholander PF: Analyzer in the accurate estimation of respiratory gases in one-half cubic centimeter samples. J Biol Chem 167:235, 1947

8. Severinghaus JW: Blood gas concentrations. p. 1475. In Fenn WO, Rahn H (eds): Handbook of physiology. Section 3. Waverly Press, Baltimore, 1965

9. DuBois AB, Fowler RC, Soffer A et al: Alveolar CO_2 measured by expiration into the rapid infrared gas analyzer. J Appl Physiol 4:526, 1952

10. Cooper EQ: Infrared analysis of the estimation of carbon dioxide in the presence of nitrous oxide. Br J Med Soc 30:486, 1957

11. Cormack RS, Powell JN: Improving the performance of the infrared carbon dioxide meter. Br J Med 34:131, 1972

12. Fowler KT, Hugh-Jones P: Mass spectrometry applied to clinical practice and research. Br Med J 1:1205, 1957

13. Davies CTM, Shirling DS: The rapid sampling, storage and analysis of expired air. Ergonomics 10:349, 1967

14. Severinghaus JS, Bradley FA: Electrodes for blood PO_2 and PCO_2 determination. J Appl Physiol 13:515, 1958

15. Tremper KK, Waxman KS: Transcutaneous monitoring of respiratory gases. p. 1. In Nochomovitz ML, Cherniack NS (eds): Noninvasive respiratory monitoring. Churchill Livingstone, New York, 1986

16. Hansen TN, Tooley WH: Skin surface carbon dioxide tension in sick infants. Pediatrics 64:942, 1979

17. Severinghaus JS, Stafford M, Bradley AF: $tcPCO_2$ electrode design, calibration and temperature gradient problems. Acta Anaesthesiol Scand 68:118, 1978

18. McClellan PA, Goldstein RS, Ramcharan V, Rebuck AS: Transcutaneous carbon dioxide monitoring. Am Rev Respir Dis 124:199, 1981

19. Lanigan C, Ponte J, Moxham J: Performance of transcutaneous PO_2 and PCO_2 dual electrodes in adults. Br J Anaesth 60:736, 1988

20. Kesten S, Chapman KR, Rebuck AS: Response characteristics of a dual transcutaneous oxygen/carbon dioxide system. Chest 99:1211, 1991

21. Stradling JR, Cover ND, Hughes JMB: Speed of response and accuracy of two transcutaneous carbon dioxide monitors. Bull Eur Physiopathol Respir 19:407, 1983

22. Martin RJ, Beoglos A, Miller MJ et al: Increasing arterial carbon dioxide tension: influence on transcutaneous carbon dioxide tension measurements. Pediatrics 81:684, 1988

23. Bucher HU, Fanconi S, Fallenstein F, Duc G: Transcutaneous carbon dioxide tension in newborn infants: reliability and safety of continuous 24 hour measurement at 42°C. Pediatrics 78:531, 1986

24. Goldman MD, Gribbin HR, Martin RJ, Loh L: Transcutaneous PCO_2 in adults. Anaesthesia 37:944, 1982

25. Tremper KK, Menteles RA, Shoemaker WC: Effects of hypercarbia and shock on transcutaneous carbon dioxide at different electrode temperatures. Crit Care Med 8:608, 1980

26. Cotes JE: Distribution of ventilation and perfusion. p. 131. In: Lung function assessment and application in medicine. 4th ed. Blackwell Scientific Publications, Oxford, 1979

27. Kim TS, Rahn H, Farhi LE: Estimation of true venous and arterial PCO_2 by gas analysis of a single breath. J Appl Physiol 81:1338, 1966

28. Nunn JF: Respiratory dead space and distribution of the inspired gas. p. 213. In Nunn JF (ed): Applied respiratory physiology. 2nd ed. Butterworths, London, 1977

29. West JB: Ventilation/blood flow and gas exchange. 2nd ed. Blackwell Scientific Publications, Oxford, 1970

30. Murray IP, Modell JH, Gallagher TJ, Banner MJ: Titration of PEEP by arterial minus end-tidal carbon dioxide gradient. Chest 85:100, 1984

31. Jardin F, Genevray B, Pazin M, Margairaz A: Inability to titrate PEEP in patients with acute respiratory failure using end-tidal carbon dioxide measurements. Anesthesiology 62:530, 1985

32. Sykes MK, McNicol MW, Campbell EJM: Gas and blood gas analysis. p. 378. In: Respiratory Failure. 2nd ed. Blackwell Scientific Publications, Oxford, 1976

33. Rahn H, Mohney J, Otis AB et al: A method for the continuous analysis of alveolar air. Aviat Med 17:173, 1946

34. Nunn JF, Hill DW: Respiratory dead space and arterial to end tidal CO_2 tension difference in anesthetized man. J Appl Physiol 15:383, 1960

35. Skillman JJ, Malhotra IV, Pallota JA et al: Determinants of weaning from controlled ventilation. Surg Forum 22:198, 1971

36. Craig DB, Wahba WM, Don HF et al: Closing volume and its relationship to gas exchange in seated and supine positions. J Appl Physiol 31:717, 1971

37. Suter PM, Fairley HB, Isenberg MD: Optimum end expiratory airway pressure in patients with acute pulmonary failure. N Engl J Med 292:284, 1975

38. Campbell EJ, Howell JBL: Rebreathing method for measurement of mixed venous PCO_2. Br Med J 2:630, 1962

39. Collier CR: Determination of mixed venous CO_2 tensions by rebreathing. J Appl Physiol 9:25, 1956

40. Powles ACP, Campbell EJM: An improved rebreathing method for measuring mixed venous carbon dioxide tensions and its clinical applications. Can Med Assoc J 118:501, 1978

41. Sealey KG, Rebuck AS, Campbell EJM: Oxygenated mixed venous PCO_2 in healthy subjects. Can Med Assoc J 113:1047, 1976

42. Sykes MK: Observations on a rebreathing technique for the determination of arterial PCO_2 in the apneic patient. Br J Anesth 32:256, 1960

43. Jones NL, Campbell EJM, McHardy GJR et al: The estimation of carbon dioxide pressure of mixed venous blood during exercise. Clin Sci 32:311, 1967

44. Jones NL, Campbell EJM, Edwards RHT et al: Alveolar blood PCO_2 difference during rebreathing in exercise. J Appl Physiol 27:356, 1969

45. Jones NL, Rebuck AS: Rebreathing equilibration of CO_2 during exercise. J Appl Physiol 35:538, 1973

46. McEvoy JDS, Jones NL, Campbell EJM: Mixed venous and arterial PCO_2. Br Med J 4:687, 1974

47. McEvoy JDS, Jones NL, Campbell EJM: Alveolar-arterial PCO_2 difference during rebreathing in patients with chronic hypercapnia. J Appl Physiol 35:542, 1973

48. Douglas CG, Haldane JS: The regulation of the general circulation rate in man. J Physiol (Lond) 56:69, 1922

49. Haldane JS: Respiration. Yale University Press, New Haven, Connecticut, 1922

50. Defares JG: A study of the carbon dioxide time course during rebreathing. p. 124. PhD Thesis, Utrecht, The Netherlands, 1956

51. DuBois AB, Britt AG, Fenn WO: Alveolar CO_2 during the respiratory cycle. J Appl Physiol 4:535, 1952

52. Knowles JH, Newman W, Fenn WO: Determination of oxygenated mixed venous CO_2 tension by a breath hold method. J Appl Physiol 15:225, 1960

53. Godfrey S, Wolf E: An evaluation of rebreathing methods for measuring mixed venous PCO_2 during exercise. Clin Sci 42:345, 1972

54. Frankel DZN, Mahutte CK, Rebuck AS: A noninvasive method for measuring the PCO_2 of mixed venous blood. Am Rev Respir Dis 117:63, 1978

55. Frankel DZN, Sandham G, Rebuck AS: A new method for measuring PCO_2 during anesthesia. Br J Anaesth 215:51, 1979

56. Hoffstein V, Rebuck AS: Determination of cardiac output based on breath holding. Crit Care Med 8:671, 1980

57. Hoffstein V, Rebuck AS: A simplified breath holding method for measurement mixed venous PCO_2. J Lab Clin Med 98:437, 1981

RESPIRATORY NEUROMUSCULAR FUNCTION

MARTIN J. TOBIN, MD[†]
JOHN M. WALSH, MD, MS[††] [*]

An elevated arterial carbon dioxide tension (P_aCO_2) is a common finding in critically ill patients, and, by definition, indicates the presence of alveolar hypoventilation.[1] Accordingly, ventilatory depression resulting from reduced respiratory neural drive or respiratory muscle dysfunction should be suspected. While the level of respiratory drive is inadequate to maintain normocapnia in such patients, it is not necessarily subnormal and formal measurements may be required to achieve a clearer diagnosis. Such testing should always be preceded by more simple tests of pulmonary mechanics, in order to distinguish patients who "won't breathe" from those who "can't breathe" because of severe mechanical abnormalities. In general, an abnormality in the respiratory control system should be suspected when hypercapnia is observed in the following settings: (1) a relatively well maintained forced expiratory volume in 1 second (FEV_1), that is, >1.3 l[2,3]; (2) a normal alveolar-arterial oxygen (O_2) gradient; (3) ability to achieve normocapnia during voluntary hyperventilation; and (4) ability to generate a negative inspiratory pressure of at least −30 cm H_2O (which eliminates respiratory muscle weakness as a cause).

An elevated arterial carbon dioxide tension is a common finding in critically ill patients, and, by definition, indicates the presence of alveolar hypoventilation.

RESPIRATORY CENTER FUNCTION

A number of techniques have been used to evaluate respiratory center output, typically in response to hyper-

[†] Professor of Medicine, Division of Pulmonary and Critical Care Medicine, Stritch School of Medicine, Loyola University of Chicago, Chicago, Illinois

[††] Assistant Professor of Medicine and Physiology, Division of Pulmonary and Critical Care Medicine, Loyola University Medical Center, Maywood, Illinois

[*] Recipient of a Parker B. Francis Research Fellowship award

capnic or hypoxic stimulation. These include measurements of minute ventilation, diaphragmatic electromyogram (EMG) activity, airway occlusion pressure, and breathing pattern. Since increased respiratory resistance or decreased compliance cause a reduction in the ventilatory response to hypercapnia or hypoxia (independent of changes in the central control function),[4,5] the ventilatory response to chemical stimulation is not an accurate way of assessing respiratory control in patients with underlying lung disease. Measurement of diaphragmatic EMG activity has never gained popularity as a method of studying respiratory motor output, although it has proved useful in studying respiratory muscle function (*vide infra*). The airway occlusion pressure technique will be discussed immediately below, and breathing pattern analysis will be discussed separately at the end of this chapter.

The ventilatory response to chemical stimulation is not an accurate way of assessing respiratory control in patients with underlying lung disease.

AIRWAY OCCLUSION PRESSURE

The negative pressure generated by an isometric contraction of the inspiratory muscles against an occluded airway is directly related to its neural stimulus, as reflected by the diaphragmatic EMG.[3,6] Whitelaw et al.[7] showed that a useful index of respiratory center motor output can be obtained by performing inspiratory occlusions without warning at irregular intervals and by measuring the change in airway pressure at a point (typically 0.1 s) before the subject recognizes the occlusion and reacts to it, that is, $P_{0.1}$.

A useful index of respiratory center motor output can be obtained by performing inspiratory occlusions without warning at irregular intervals and by measuring the change in airway pressure at a point (typically 0.1 s).

$P_{0.1}$ measurements have several attractive features. They are relatively independent of respiratory resistance and compliance since there is no airflow during the inspiratory occlusion.[7] The force-velocity relationships of the respiratory muscles have a relatively small influence since the muscles can be expected to shorten much less during an occluded inspiration compared with unobstructed breathing.[7] They are not influenced by vagal lung volume-related reflexes.[7] Although an increase in functional residual capacity (FRC) can cause a reduction in $P_{0.1}$,[8] the effect is usually slight,[9] and making the measurements in a supine position further decreases this likelihood.[10]

The typical circuit used to measure $P_{0.1}$ has the following features. An airway adaptor or mouthpiece is attached to a one-way valve to facilitate independent control over the inspiratory and expiratory limbs of the circuit. During expiration, a shutter or valve is activated (manually or electronically) in the inspiratory limb; this has no effect on expiratory flow because of the one-way circuit. The occlusion is maintained during the subsequent inspiration for less than 0.25–0.30 seconds and the airway pressure generated at 0.1 second is calculated (Fig. 1). A pneumotach-ograph is usually included in the circuit to provide a si-multaneous measure of airflow. To permit accurate cal-culations from a strip-chart recorder, the paper speed needs to be run at 25–100 mm/s.[11,12] Methods of making the measurements using computerized techniques have been also described.[12,13] At least 6 measurements should be obtained at irregular intervals, and at least 5–8 regular breaths are usually permitted between each occlusion.[11] Measurements may be made while breathing room air, during hypercapnic or hypoxic stimulation, or while re-ceiving supplemental O_2.

Although $P_{0.1}$ values represent negative pressures, it is customary to report them in positive units. During resting breathing in normal subjects, $P_{0.1}$ is about 0.93 ± 0.48 (SD) cm H_2O.[9,14,15] The coefficient of variation within individual subjects is about 50%.[9,15] Between subjects, the coefficient of variation is about 20–33% during a single set of mea-surements,[9,15] but on repeated measurements (during CO_2 rebreathing trials) it is about 60%.[16]

Measurements of $P_{0.1}$ have been recently examined as a means to predict the outcome of a trial of weaning from mechanical ventilation. Herrera et al.[17] noted unsuccessful weaning attempts on 89% of the occasions when $P_{0.1}$ values were > 4.2 cm H_2O, and Sassoon et al.[18] found that every patient with a $P_{0.1}$ value of > 6 cm H_2O failed a trial of weaning. However, Montgomery and co-workers[19] found that $P_{0.1}$ values were similar in patients who were suc-cessfully weaned and those who failed a weaning trial. In addition, they found that $P_{0.1}$ measurements during a hy-percapnic challenge were similar in the weaning success and weaning failure groups. However, hypercapnic aug-mentation of $P_{0.1}$, expressed as the ratio of the CO_2-stim-ulated $P_{0.1}$ to the baseline $P_{0.1}$, was greater in the patients who were successfully weaned, 2.04 ± 0.25, than in the failure group, 1.17 ± 0.03.

RESPIRATORY MUSCLE FUNCTION

The respiratory muscles consist primarily of the dia-phragm, intercostal/accessory muscles, and abdominal muscles.[20] They are unique in that they are the only skeletal muscles that are essential for life, since breathing is de-pendent upon their repetitive contraction. Considerable in-formation regarding muscle performance can be gleaned from careful clinical assessment, radiological examination, and routine pulmonary function testing, in addition to that

During resting breathing in normal subjects, $P_{0.1}$ is about 0.93 ± 0.48 (SD) cm H_2O.

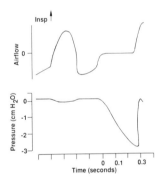

FIGURE 1 Measurement of airway occlusion pres-sure. The airway pres-sure at 0.1 s ($P_{0.1}$) after commencing inspiration against an occluded airway provides a useful measure of respiratory drive. During the period of occlusion, the speed of the tracing was in-creased 10-fold.

The respiratory muscles are the only skeletal muscles that are essential for life.

obtained by formal evaluation of respiratory muscle strength and endurance.[21]

CLINICAL ASSESSMENT

The symptoms of respiratory muscle dysfunction are subtle and the condition frequently goes undetected until late in its natural evolution. Coexisting impairment of other skeletal muscles may prevent patients from exceeding their limited ventilatory capacity and as a result they may not develop dyspnea.[22] The development of orthopnea immediately on lying supine should arouse suspicion of paralysis or severe weakness of the diaphragm; this contrasts with more gradual development of orthopnea in patients with congestive heart failure. In general, orthopnea tends to occur when maximal transdiaphragmatic pressure (P_{di}-max) is less than 30 cm H_2O.[23] Cough may be impaired due to the inability to take a deep inspiration and also because of poor expulsive forces as a consequence of expiratory muscle weakness. The hazards of impaired cough are multiplied by coexisting neuromuscular weakness, and these patients commonly have problems with swallowing, which predisposes to aspiration and asphyxiation of food particles. Many patients display a further decrease in ventilation during sleep, which leads to morning headaches and daytime somnolence.[24] This has been considered a characteristic feature of patients with bilateral diaphragmatic paralysis, who by necessity are dependent on their intercostal and accessory muscles. These muscles are less active during rapid eye movement (REM) sleep, and this leads to profound hypoventilation.

Physical examination may reveal deformity of the chest wall, as in kyphoscoliosis, or evidence of generalized neuromuscular disease such as wasting and fasciculation.[23] Evidence of increased patient effort is reflected by increased activity of the sternomastoid and scalene muscles, recession of the suprasternal, supraclavicular and intercostal spaces, nasal flaring, diaphoresis, and tracheal tug.[25] The pattern of breathing can give very helpful clues to the presence of severe respiratory muscle weakness and increased loads (*vide infra*). Finally, cor pulmonale may be present.

RADIOLOGICAL ASSESSMENT

Unilateral phrenic nerve paralysis is associated with an elevated hemidiaphragm, but this is a nonspecific finding since it can also occur with pneumonia, atelectasis, and other conditions. In patients with bilateral diaphragmatic

The development of orthopnea immediately on lying supine should arouse suspicion of paralysis or severe weakness of the diaphragm.

Evidence of increased patient effort is reflected by increased activity of the sternomastoid and scalene muscles, recession of the suprasternal, supraclavicular and intercostal spaces, nasal flaring, diaphoresis, and tracheal tug.

paralysis, it may be difficult to note any abnormality on the chest radiograph and the availability of previous films for comparison is important.[26] Fluoroscopy is a time-honored method of diagnosing diaphragmatic paralysis. During inspiration or a sniff, the diaphragm normally descends. With unilateral diaphragmatic paralysis, the entire leaf shows at least 2 cm of paradoxic motion. Unfortunately, paradoxic motion is also observed in 6% of healthy people.[27] In patients with bilateral diaphragmatic paralysis, fluoroscopy is commonly misleading. For example, Newsom-David et al.[28] observed paradoxic motion in only 17% ($\frac{1}{6}$) of patients with this disorder. This appears to be due to the fact that some patients with paralyzed diaphragms contract their abdominal muscles during expiration, displacing the abdomen inwards and the diaphragm into the rib cage. At the onset of inspiration, relaxation of the abdominal muscles causes outward recoil of the abdominal wall and diaphragmatic descent. Measurement of transdiaphragmatic pressure (*vide infra*) is a more reliable method of diagnosing diaphragmatic paralysis.

In patients with bilateral diaphragmatic paralysis, fluoroscopy is commonly misleading.

PULMONARY FUNCTION TESTS

Routine pulmonary function tests can provide a clue to the presence of respiratory muscle dysfunction. If evidence of severe airway obstruction is present, this implies that the muscles have to contract against a high load. Severe weakness of the respiratory muscles produces a restrictive pattern with a decrease in vital capacity (VC), total lung capacity (TLC) and FRC, while FEV_1/VC ratio, residual volume (RV), and diffusing capacity (D_LCO) remain relatively normal. Based on the shape of the normal pressure-volume curve, one would expect a considerable loss of respiratory muscle strength before seeing a fall in VC and other lung volumes.[21,26,29] This is the case in many patients with acute respiratory muscle weakness. However, in patients with chronic muscle weakness, the loss in VC is greater than expected because of an associated decrease in lung compliance, probably due to the presence of diffuse microatelectasis, and a decrease in chest wall compliance, probably due to stiffening of the rib cage tendons and ligaments, and ankylosis of the costovertebral and thoracovertebral joints.[29]

If diaphragmatic paralysis is suspected, it is helpful to check the fall in forced vital capacity (FVC) that occurs when a patient switches from an erect to a supine position. Normally, there is an average fall of 8%, and the upper limit of normal is 19%.[30] A greater fall is commonly seen in patients with diaphragmatic paralysis.

If diaphragmatic paralysis is suspected, it is helpful to check the fall in forced vital capacity that occurs when a patient switches from an erect to a supine position.

RESPIRATORY MUSCLE STRENGTH

Airway Pressures

Like other skeletal muscles, the maximum force that can be generated by the respiratory muscles is related to their degree of stretching, and thus, it is important to control the lung volume at which the measurements are made.

Respiratory muscle strength is assessed by measuring the maximum inspiratory and maximum expiratory pressure ($P_I$max and $P_E$max, respectively) generated against an occluded airway. In the ICU setting, these measurements can be readily obtained with an inexpensive aneroid manometer.[25] Like other skeletal muscles, the maximum force that can be generated by the respiratory muscles is related to their degree of stretching, and thus, it is important to control the lung volume at which the measurements are made. $P_I$max is usually measured after expiration to RV.[25] Some physicians prefer to make the measurement at FRC, because this reflects the pressure available for inspiratory efforts made from end-expiratory lung volume, and, also, because respiratory system recoil has little or no effect on the pressure measured.[31] $P_E$max should be measured after inspiration to TLC, because the expiratory muscles are maximally stretched in this position.

Published normal values of $P_I$max and $P_E$max show considerable variation between reports. This variation may depend on the cohorts employed to establish the normal range and on the method used to make the measurement. For example, $P_I$max and $P_E$max values are 9% and 20% higher, respectively, if a simple rubber tube (4.5 cm length, 4 cm internal diameter) rather than a typical scuba-type (ie, semirigid plastic flanged) mouthpiece is used when making the measurements.[32] In general, when a flanged mouthpiece is employed, $P_I$max and $P_E$max values are approximately 111 ± 34 (SD) and 151 ± 68 cm H_2O, respectively, in healthy men.[32–35] Values are lower in women: $P_I$max 72 ± 26 and $P_E$max 93 ± 30 cm H_2O. Strength tends to decrease with age: $P_I$max values are reported to be 6%, 25%, and 32% lower in men who are 31–35, 40–60, and 61–75 years old, respectively, compared with those who are 16–30 years old.[36]

$P_I$max is one of the standard measurements employed to determine the need for the institution or continuation of mechanical ventilation.

$P_I$max is one of the standard measurements employed to determine the need for the institution or continuation of mechanical ventilation. The team of Bendixin and Bunker[37] was one of the first investigators to suggest that $P_I$max might provide a useful reflection of respiratory reserve; this conclusion was based on pressure measurements in dogs that had their airways occluded for 50 seconds. In a companion study in human subjects recovering from neuromuscular blockade, they shortened the period of occlusion to 30 seconds and concluded that a $P_I$max of -20 cm H_2O indicated sufficient reserve to transfer a patient to the recovery room (provided that there was no underlying lung disease).[38] In subsequent studies in which $P_I$max was examined as a predictor of weaning outcome, the period of occlusion was not standardized during the measurement. Sahn and Lakshminarayan[39] found that $P_I$max values that were more negative than -30 cm H_2O predicted weaning success, whereas values that were no lower than -20 cm H_2O predicted weaning failure. However, a high rate of false positive and false negative results has been reported with these criteria.[40] Recently, attention has again been turned to standardizing the method of measuring $P_I$max in critically ill patients. Using a valve attached to the airway to ensure that inspiration begins at a low volume, and standardizing the period of occlusion to 20 seconds, Marini and associates[41] obtained $P_I$max values that were approximately one-third more negative than nonstandardized measurements. Multz et al.[42] recently examined the reproducibility of this method of measuring $P_I$max. Triplicate measurements were obtained by 5 experienced investigators in 14 ventilator-dependent patients. Measurements of $P_I$max obtained at a single sitting by a single investigator showed good reproducibility: coefficient of variation, $12 \pm 1\%$. However, there was significant variation among $P_I$max measurements obtained by different investigators studying the same patient on the same day: coefficient of variation, $32 \pm 4\%$. Since true inspiratory muscle strength must be equal to or greater than the highest recorded $P_I$max, the variation in values by different investigators indicates that $P_I$max values, even when obtained in a standardized manner, commonly underestimate true strength.

Sahn and Lakshminarayan found that $P_I$max values that were more negative than -30 cm H_2O predicted weaning success, whereas values that were no lower than -20 cm H_2O predicted weaning failure.

Recently, attention has again been turned to standardizing the method of measuring $P_I$max in critically ill patients.

Transdiaphragmatic Pressure

While $P_I$max and $P_E$max measured at the airway reflect the global strength of the respiratory muscles, these pressures do not directly assess diaphragmatic function. The diaphragm is the single most important respiratory muscle, being responsible for about two thirds of tidal volume during breathing. Transdiaphragmatic pressure provides the most direct method of assessing diaphragmatic strength. This requires passage of two balloon catheters, one to measure esophageal pressure (P_{es}) and the other to measure gastric pressure (P_{ga}); P_{di} is calculated as $P_{ga} - P_{es}$ (Fig. 2). The highest and most reproducible measurements of maximal P_{di} are obtained if the patient can see the P_{es} and P_{ga} tracings while combining a maximal static inspiratory effort against an occluded airway (Mueller maneuver) with an abdominal expulsive maneuver.[43] However, many patients find it difficult to perform this maneuver. In contrast,

The diaphragm is the single most important respiratory muscle, being responsible for about two thirds of tidal volume during breathing.

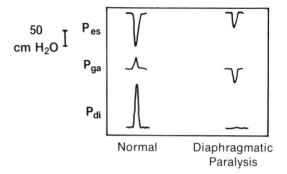

Normal   Diaphragmatic
Paralysis

P_{di} is measured by inserting balloon catheters into the esophagus and stomach, and P_{di} is electrically calculated by subtracting esophageal pressure from gastric pressure.

FIGURE 2   Measurement of transdiaphragmatic pressure (P_{di}) in a normal subject and in a patient with bilateral diaphragmatic paralysis. P_{di} is measured by inserting balloon catheters into the esophagus and stomach, and P_{di} is electrically calculated by subtracting esophageal pressure (P_{es}) from gastric pressure (P_{ga}). When a patient with diaphragmatic paralysis makes a maximal inspiratory effort, the negative P_{es} generated by the other inspiratory muscles pulls the flaccid diaphragm cephalad, thereby resulting in a fall in P_{ga}. From Tobin MJ: Essentials of critical care medicine. Churchill Livingstone, New York, 1989. With permission.

most patients are able to perform a sniff, that is, a short, sharp, voluntary effort through the nostrils with the mouth closed. The values of P_{di} during a sniff are higher and more reproducible than those achieved during a Mueller maneuver, with the result that the normal range is narrower: men—mean 148, range 112–204 cm H_2O; women—mean 122, range 82–182 cm H_2O.[44] In patients with bilateral diaphragmatic paralysis, P_{di} values are close to zero.[23,28]

RESPIRATORY MUSCLE ENDURANCE

Endurance is the capacity of a muscle to sustain a contractile force. It is related to muscle capillary and mitochondrial density and overall oxidative enzyme capacity.[45] The converse of endurance is fatigue, which can be defined in operational terms as the inability of a muscle to generate and sustain a required contractile force.[46] Respiratory muscle fatigue can be divided into central, transmission, and contractile fatigue (Table 1).[46,47] *Central fatigue* is considered present when a voluntary contraction generates less force than does electrical stimulation. In a well-motivated subject, the force generated by voluntary contraction should be the same as that resulting from electrical stimulation.[46,47] Although central fatigue has been demonstrated

Respiratory muscle fatigue can be divided into central, transmission, and contractile fatigue.

TABLE 1   Diagnostic Features of Diaphragmatic Fatigue

Type of Fatigue	Voluntary Effort		Phrenic Nerve Stimulation		Direct Muscle Stimulation (animal)
	EMG Response	P_{di} Response	EMG Response	P_{di} Response	
Central	Decreased	Decreased	Normal	Normal	Normal
Transmission	Decreased	Decreased	Decreased	Decreased	Normal
Contractile	Normal	Decreased	Normal	Decreased	Decreased

EMG = electromyogram; P_{di} = transdiaphragmatic pressure. From Tobin MJ: Respiratory monitoring during mechanical ventilation. p. 691. In Tobin MJ (ed): Mechanical ventilation. WB Saunders, Philadelphia, 1990. With permission.

in some healthy subjects breathing against high respiratory loads,[48] it remains unclear as to whether central fatigue has any relevance to ventilatory failure.[47] *Transmission fatigue* is thought to be due to impaired neuromuscular transmission; its pathognomonic feature is a decrease in the EMG response to phrenic nerve stimulation. The clinical significance of transmission fatigue has yet to be resolved. *Contractile fatigue* is characterized by a decrease in the contractile response to neural stimulation (see Fig. 3). A number of techniques have been employed to detect the presence or development of respiratory muscle fatigue. These include the transdiaphragmatic pressure response to phrenic nerve stimulation, the ratio of the diaphragmatic electromyogram signal to transdiaphragmatic pressure, power spectral analysis of the electromyogram, calculation of the pressure-time product, and the relaxation rate of respiratory pressures.

It remains unclear as to whether central fatigue has any relevance to ventilatory failure.

Contractile fatigue is characterized by a decrease in the contractile response to neural stimulation.

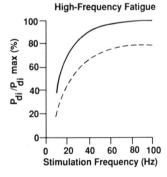 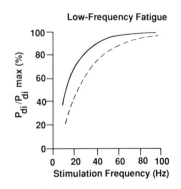

FIGURE 3   Force-frequency curves of the diaphragm. The phrenic nerve is stimulated transcutaneously at increasing frequencies (abscissa), and diaphragmatic contractility is quantitated by using transdiaphragmatic pressure (P_{di}) measurements (ordinate). The development of fatigue causes the curve to shift to the right.

Phrenic Nerve Stimulation

The most sophisticated way of studying respiratory muscle contractility is to generate a force-frequency or pressure-frequency curve.

Low-frequency fatigue may be due to structural alterations within the muscle and up to 24 hours may be required for recovery.

Phrenic nerve conduction time is measured as the time from stimulus artifact to the onset of the diaphragm action potential.

Probably the most sophisticated way of studying respiratory muscle contractility is to generate a force-frequency or pressure-frequency curve by stimulating the phrenic nerve at various frequencies (10, 20, 50, and 100 Hz) and recording the resulting increase in P_{di} (Fig. 3). Supramaximal impulses of 50–160 V and 0.1 ms duration are applied transcutaneously to one or both phrenic nerves in the neck.[49,50] The diaphragmatic EMG is recorded to determine optimal electrode position and ensure constant phrenic stimulation.[50] A decrease in the contractile response to phrenic nerve stimulation (ie, a shift in the force-frequency curve to the right) indicates the development of contractile fatigue. Contractile fatigue is subdivided into two types: *high-frequency fatigue*, which is manifested by a decrease in the contractile response at high stimulation frequencies (50–100 Hz), and *low-frequency fatigue*, which occurs at nerve firing frequencies of normal daily activities (10–20 Hz).[47] High-frequency fatigue is thought to be due to accumulation of toxic metabolites and it has a rapid recovery phase (within minutes). Low-frequency fatigue may be due to structural alterations within the muscle and up to 24 hours may be required for recovery.

In addition to assessing diaphragmatic contractility, this technique can be used to determine phrenic nerve conduction time (Fig. 4). This is measured as the time from stimulus artifact to the onset of the diaphragm action potential.[50] The normal phrenic nerve conduction time is less

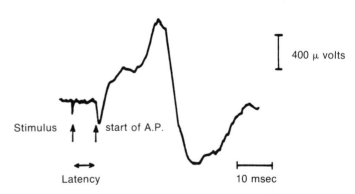

FIGURE 4 Measurement of phrenic nerve conduction time. Surface electrodes placed in the 7th intercostal space record the diaphragmatic action potential (AP) following a single twitch stimulation of the phrenic nerve in the neck. The conduction time (latency) is measured as the time from stimulus artifact to the onset of AP. From Laroche CM, Moxham J, Green M: Respiratory muscle weakness and fatigue. Q J Med 71:373, 1989. With permission.

than 9.25 ms. A prolonged conduction time is seen with phrenic nerve damage due to the use of chilled cardioplegic solutions during cardiac surgery,[21] phrenic neuritis, mediastinal tumors, and peripheral neuropathy. A normal conduction time in the presence of diaphragmatic paralysis suggests the presence of an upper motor neuron lesion (eg, infarct or tumor in medulla), brainstem encephalitis, or a high spinal cord lesion. In patients being considered for phrenic nerve pacing, phrenic nerve conduction time should be normal, as this indicates that the diaphragm can be adequately excited.

In patients being considered for phrenic nerve pacing, phrenic nerve conduction time should be normal, as this indicates that the diaphragm can be adequately excited.

Electromyogram

The EMG is the electrical signal emanating from an active muscle. It can be detected by various electrodes, and the signal can be amplified, recorded, and analyzed in numerous ways. The EMG signal represents the temporal and spatial summation of individual action potentials of activated motor units as detected at the site of the recording electrodes. In practice, the presence and magnitude of the EMG signal identifies and quantifies muscle activation, and more detailed analysis of the EMG signal can predict and identify muscle fatigue. While EMGs of numerous respiratory muscles have been examined, the inspiratory muscles (especially the diaphragm) are most often studied. EMG recordings are obtained with surface or intramuscular (needle or fine wire) electrodes. While surface electrodes are the simplest, the resulting EMG may be contaminated by the activity of adjacent muscles.

The presence and magnitude of the EMG signal identifies and quantifies muscle activation, and more detailed analysis of the EMG signal can predict and identify muscle fatigue.

Quantification of the EMG signal provides information on the degree of muscle activation. Quantification is commonly done by rectifying (ie, inverting negative components of the raw EMG) and then averaging the EMG (referred to as a "moving time average"). The quantity (or magnitude) of an EMG signal normally correlates with force generation of a muscle. The relationship between the magnitude of the diaphragmatic EMG signal (E_{di}) and P_{di} is useful for studying the development of contractile fatigue.[51] Commonly, the E_{di}/P_{di} ratio is examined over time, and an increasing ratio represents reduced force generation for a given level of muscle activation and indicates the development of contractile fatigue of the diaphragm.

The relationship between the magnitude of the diaphragmatic EMG signal and P_{di} is useful for studying the development of contractile fatigue.

The frequency components of the EMG signal can also be employed to detect muscle fatigue. Contractile fatigue is preceded by a shift in the EMG signal consisting of an increase in the low-frequency and a decrease in the high-frequency components. It should be emphasized that this is not related to the frequency of nerve stimulation (see

The H/L ratio is somewhat crude, and current methods of characterizing the frequency components of the EMG signal are more sophisticated.

The power spectrum is typically described by its mean or median frequency.

Fig. 3), but instead refers to specific frequency components that constitute the complex raw EMG signal. In early studies, fatigue-related alterations in the EMG signal were detected by a fall in the ratio of high-frequency EMG power (typically 150–350 Hz) to low-frequency EMG power (typically 20–47 Hz), referred to as the high-low (H/L) ratio. The H/L ratio is somewhat crude, and current methods of characterizing the frequency components of the EMG signal are more sophisticated. Fourier transform is used to generate a frequency-power spectrum[52]; this is a plot of frequency versus power (ie, magnitude) and it reveals the entire spectrum of frequencies within the raw EMG. The power spectrum is typically described by its mean or median frequency.[53] The mean frequency represents the average frequency of the power spectrum, and the median frequency represents the frequency that divides the power spectrum into two halves of equal power. The EMG of a fresh (nonfatigued) muscle and the change in frequency-power spec-

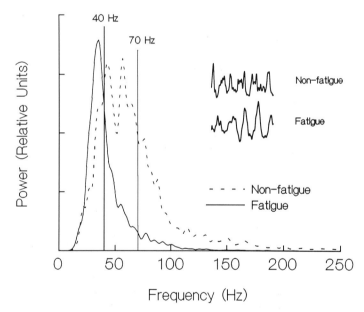

FIGURE 5   The raw EMG (inset) and the associated power spectra of a nonfatigued and fatigued muscle. Fatigue was induced by maintaining a constant increased load. Note the generalized slowing of the raw EMG that occurs with fatigue. Secondly, there is a leftward shift of the power spectrum representing an increase in low frequency and a decrease in high frequency components. Thirdly, the spectrum itself is characterized by its mean frequency (fm), which decreases with fatigue. The mean frequency (represented by the vertical line) of nonfatigued muscle is 70 Hz, whereas it is only 40 Hz in the fatigued muscle.

trum that occurs with the development of fatigue are shown in Fig. 5. These changes in the EMG power spectrum occur before the development of mechanical fatigue, that is, inability to sustain constant force.

Fatigue-related changes in the diaphragmatic EMG were first described by Gross et al.,[54] who imposed an inspiratory resistance to increase the swings in P_{di} being generated with each breath. Resistances that resulted in the generation of 50% and 75% of maximum P_{di} with each breath (which is known to result in mechanical fatigue) produced a decrease in the H/L ratio over time. In contrast, inspiratory pressures of 25% maximum P_{di} (which do not produce mechanical failure) produced no change in the H/L ratio. Detection of fatigue by EMG analysis has been used in studying quadraplegic patients, assessing respiratory muscle training,[55] and in studying other respiratory muscles such as the parasternal intercostal muscles.[56]

The use of EMG analysis to detect respiratory muscle fatigue has a number of limitations: (1) a baseline, non-fatigued, reference state is required for comparison; (2) proper placement of electrodes and signal analysis require a considerable level of technical skill; and (3) the frequency-power spectrum is affected by factors other than fatigue per se, such as change in muscle length (Fig. 6).[57] The effect of muscle length on the power spectrum is particularly worrisome, since length of the inspiratory muscles inevitably changes with each breath. If greater control can be

Changes in the EMG power spectrum occur before the development of mechanical fatigue, that is, inability to sustain constant force.

The effect of muscle length on the power spectrum is particularly worrisome.

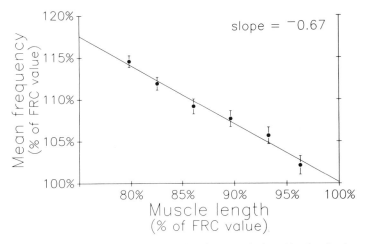

FIGURE 6 The effect of alteration in muscle length of a dog's diaphragm on the mean frequency of the EMG power spectrum. A 20% decrease in muscle length from that at functional residual capacity (FRC) produced a 15% increase in the median frequency. From Walsh JM, Ito T, Grassino A: The effect of diaphragm length on the EMG power spectrum. Clin Res 38:847A, 1990. With permission.

achieved over this and other confounding variables,[58,59] EMG analysis may prove to be a very useful means of monitoring respiratory muscle fatigue in critically ill patients.

Pressure–Time Product

Tension–time index of the diaphragm has been reported to be a better predictor of the O_2 cost of breathing than measurements of the mechanical work of breathing.

The tension developed and the duration of respiratory muscle contraction are important determinants of the energy consumption and fatigability of the respiratory muscles.[60,61] Indeed, a tension–time index of the diaphragm has been reported to be a better predictor of the O_2 cost of breathing ($\dot{V}O_2$ resp) than measurements of the mechanical work of breathing. A variety of different methods have been used to combine tension and time into a single index. Collett et al.[62] derived a pressure–time product by electrically integrating negative mouth pressure (P_{mo}) with respect to time ($\int P_{mo}dt$), which is equivalent to the product of mean P_{mo} and inspiratory time (T_I). Another approach has been popularized by Bellemare and Grassino[63] based on the fact that the diaphragm contracts mainly during inspiration. They reasoned that the relative duration of T_I to the duration of a total respiratory cycle (T_{TOT}) should be an important determinant of diaphragmatic fatigue. In healthy subjects breathing against resistive loads, they found that mean P_{di} during each inspiration as a fraction of P_{di}max and T_I/T_{TOT} were equally important as determinants of diaphragmatic fatigue. They combined these factors into a tension time index of the diaphragm (TT_{di}), calculated as

P_{di}max and T_I/T_{TOT} are equally important as determinants of diaphragmatic fatigue.

$$TT_{di} = \text{mean } P_{di}/P_{di}\text{max} \times T_I/T_{TOT}$$

Evidence of respiratory muscle fatigue was observed when TT_{di} exceeded 0.15. Normal subjects breathing at rest have a TT_{di} value of 0.02, indicating approximately an eight-fold reserve.[63] Although TT_{di} is a major determinant of $\dot{V}O_2$ resp, it is not the only factor. Other factors that influence $\dot{V}O_2$ resp include respiratory work rate,[64] lung volume,[62] and possibly mean inspiratory flow rate.[64–66]

Pressure Relaxation Rate

Quantitative assessment of the rate of decay of various respiratory pressure swings has aroused considerable interest as a method of diagnosing respiratory muscle fatigue. Two indices have been developed. The *maximum relaxation rate* (MRR) is calculated as the slope of a tangent drawn to the steepest portion of the pressure decay.[67,68] Since MRR increases linearly with increase in the peak pressure of a contraction, it should be normalized by dividing by peak pressure. The *time constant* (tau) is calculated by replotting the pressure signal on a semilog scale and taking the reciprocal of the slope of the lower portion of this line.[67,68] These indices have been calculated from P_{di}, P_{es}, P_{np}, and P_{mo} tracings during a voluntary sniff (with or without an occluded airway) and during phrenic nerve stimulation. In healthy subjects, the MRR/P_{peak} is typically about 9% ± 1% (SD) pressure loss over 10 msec, and the time constant is about 50–55 msec. A 15–30% decrease in MRR and a 30–45% increase in the time constant are typically observed with the development of respiratory muscle fatigue.

A 15–30% decrease in MRR and a 30–45% increase in the time constant are typically observed with the development of respiratory muscle fatigue.

BREATHING PATTERN ANALYSIS

In recent years, it has been increasingly recognized that detailed analysis of breathing pattern can provide valuable information regarding the respiratory system.[69–71] In addition, improvements have occurred in the instrumentation used to record ventilation, especially in the nonintubated patient.[72]

TECHNIQUE OF MEASUREMENT

Direct Measurement

In the intubated patient, ventilation can be easily measured by attaching a spirometer or pneumotachograph to the patient's endotracheal tube. The prototype pneumotachograph, the Fleisch instrument, presents a problem in this setting because condensation of moist gases and mucus can easily clog the narrow metal tubes within the instrument, and thus alter resistance and produce inaccurate results. The development of newer variable-orifice pneumotachographs will hopefully diminish this problem. In the nonintubated patient, problems arise in attempting to measure ventilation with a spirometer or pneumotachograph because critically ill patients have a low tolerance of devices that require a direct connection to the patient's airway. In addition, the use of a mouthpiece produces spurious alterations in breathing pattern, causing tidal volume to increase and respiratory frequency to decrease.[73] Consequently, several devices have been developed to measure ventilation indirectly.

The use of a mouthpiece produces spurious alterations in breathing pattern, causing tidal volume to increase and respiratory frequency to decrease.

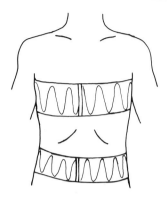

FIGURE 7 Transducer bands of the respiratory inductive plethysmography placed around the rib cage and abdomen. From Tobin MJ: Noninvasive evaluation of respiratory movement. p. 37. In Nochomovitz ML, Cherniack NS (eds): Noninvasive respiratory monitoring. Churchill Livingstone, New York, 1986. With permission.

Indirect Measurement

The respiratory inductive plethysmography (RIP) is the most widely accepted method of obtaining quantitative and noninvasive measurements of ventilation.[72,74] The transducers consist of two coils of insulated wire sewn onto bands placed around the rib cage and abdomen (Fig. 7). The coils are connected to a small oscillator module that puts out frequency-modulated signals that are proportional to alterations in the self-inductance of the coil. The self-inductance of the coil, and so the frequencies of its oscillator, is proportional to the cross-sectional area enclosed by the coil. These signals are sent to a demodulator/calibrator unit that converts the signal into a proportional voltage that can be amplified and recorded. Calibration of the RIP is based on the assumption that the respiratory system can be considered as a simple physical system with two moving parts, the rib cage and abdomen. Consequently, volume measured at the mouth is equivalent to the sum of volume changes of the rib cage and abdomen. This concept of two degrees of freedom forms the basis of the various techniques that can be used to calibrate the RIP. While the least squares technique is probably the most robust technique of calibration,[75,76] it can be tedious, especially in critically ill patients. Recently, Sackner et al.[77] reported an innovative technique of calibrating the RIP that is independent of the need for a spirometer or pneumotachograph and thus particularly suited to clinical monitoring in critically ill patients. This new calibration technique can provide accurate quantitative measurements of respiratory timing and rib cage–abdominal coordination, and an accurate measurement of relative changes in tidal volume.

ANALYSIS

Volume and Time Components

In resting healthy subjects, minute ventilation ($\dot{V}_E$) is about 6 l/min.[70] A $\dot{V}_E$ of less than 10 l/min is commonly used as a predictor of weaning outcome,[39] but this criterion is associated with a high rate of false positive and false negative results.[40,78] In healthy subjects, respiratory frequency (f) is approximately 17 breaths/min and tidal volume is approximately 0.40 l.[70] Rapid shallow breathing is a common finding in patients who fail a trial of weaning from mechanical ventilation,[79] and this can be quantitated in terms of the f/V_T ratio (Table 2)—a value above 100 breaths/min/l suggests that a weaning trial is likely to be unsuccessful.[78] An elevated respiratory frequency is often the earliest sign of an impending respiratory disaster,[80,81] and the degree of

TABLE 2   Rapid Shallow Breathing Index

RSB index

$$= \frac{\text{Respiratory frequency (breaths per min)}}{\text{Tidal volume (l)}}$$

RSB if $f/V_T > 100$ breaths per min/l, eg, f of ≥ 30 breaths/min and V_T of ≤ 0.3 l

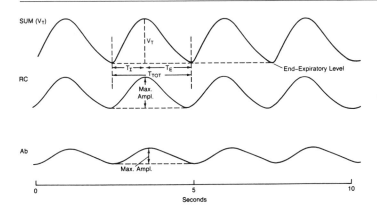

FIGURE 8   Schematic recording of the respiratory cycle that depicts the points of reference for computation of the various breathing pattern parameters. The signals have been obtained with a respiratory inductive plethysmography; thus SUM (V_T) indicates tidal volume, which has been calibrated to spirometry and represents the algebraic sum of the rib cage (RC) and abdominal (Ab) excursions. T_I = inspiratory time; T_E = expiratory time; T_{TOT} = time of a total breath; V_T/T_I = mean inspiratory flow rate. Alterations in the end-expiratory level represent changes in functional residual capacity, provided movement artifact is absent. Maximal amplitude is the trough-to-peak amplitude of the rib cage and abdominal excursions, irrespective of their phase relationship to the SUM (V_T) signal; their arithmetic sum, designated maximal compartmental amplitude (MCA), is equivalent to the algebraic SUM (V_T) signal when the rib cage and abdomen move in phase. From Tobin MJ: State of the art: respiratory monitoring in the intensive care unit. Am Rev Respir Dis 138:1625, 1988. With permission.

Alterations in the end-expiratory level represent changes in functional residual capacity, provided movement artifact is absent.

The arithmetic sum of the rib cage and abdomen signals, designated maximal compartmental amplitude, is equivalent to the algebraic SUM (V_T) signal when the rib cage and abdomen move in phase.

elevation is proportional to the severity of the underlying disease.[82]

More detailed analysis of the breathing pattern can provide additional helpful information (Fig. 8). Minute ventilation ($\dot{V}_E$) has been traditionally analyzed in terms of tidal volume (V_T) and respiratory frequency (f)

$$\dot{V}_E = V_T \times f \qquad (1)$$

This equation can be rearranged, as respiratory frequency is equal to 60 divided by T_{TOT} or time of a single breath.

$$\dot{V}_E = V_T \times 60/T_{TOT} \qquad (2)$$

Conceptually, 60 can be deleted and the equation reduced to

$$\dot{V}_E = V_T \times 1/T_{TOT} \qquad (3)$$

Dividing V_T by T_I while multiplying $1/T_{TOT}$ by T_I gives

$$\dot{V}_E = V_T/T_I \times T_I/T_{TOT} \qquad (4)$$

The first parameter, V_T/T_I, has been termed mean inspiratory flow rate, and the second parameter, T_I/T_{TOT}, has been called fractional inspiratory time.

V_T/T_I has been widely employed as a measure of respiratory drive, and the neurogenic basis of doing so has been demonstrated by a number of investigators.[83,84] Once inspiration has begun, changes in pulmonary afferent activity produce no appreciable change in the slope of integrated phrenic nerve activity.[83–87] V_T/T_I, which is the mechanical transformation of this neural activity, has been shown to be related to standard indices of respiratory center output, such as $P_{0.1}$ and the ventilatory response to hypercapnia.[12,16,87] An inherent disadvantage of V_T/T_I is that it may underestimate respiratory drive in the presence of marked abnormalities in pulmonary mechanics. However, an elevated V_T/T_I in this situation reflects elevated respiratory drive, albeit it may be underestimated.

Fractional inspiratory time, T_I/T_{TOT}, indicates the relationship between inspiration and expiration, and it provides a crude measure of the degree of airway obstruction.[71] Since the respiratory muscles are normally active only during inspiration, T_I/T_{TOT} has also been termed the duty cycle of the respiratory system, and it is an important determinant of the amount of stress being placed on the respiratory muscles.[63]

The reproducibility of breathing pattern measurements is very appealing compared with traditional methods of assessing the respiratory control system. The ventilatory and mouth occlusion pressure responses to hypercapnia and hypoxia display enormous inter- and intraindividual variability.[88,89] The greater reproducibility of breathing pattern components[90] permits the construction of a relatively narrow normal range, permitting the detection of abnormalities in individual patients. For example, although V_T/T_I is commonly considered an insensitive index of respiratory drive in patients with abnormal lung mechanics, it was elevated above the normal 95% confidence limits in 71% of 28 patients with COPD (Fig. 9).[21,71]

Rib Cage–Abdominal Motion

Additional information about the amount of stress being placed on the respiratory system can be obtained from examination of the pattern of rib cage–abdominal motion— an added attraction of employing an indirect method of

V_T/T_I has been widely employed as a measure of respiratory drive, and the neurogenic basis of doing so has been demonstrated by a number of investigators.

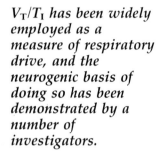

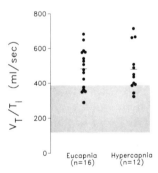

FIGURE 9 Mean inspiratory flow (V_T/T_I), an index of respiratory drive, during resting breathing in patients with chronic obstructive pulmonary disease. The shaded area represents the 95% confidence limits of V_T/T_I in healthy subjects. From Tobin MJ: Respiratory muscles in disease. Clinics Chest Med 9:263, 1988. With permission.

measuring ventilation (Fig. 10). Normally, the rib cage and abdomen inflate in unison with each other during inspiration and simultaneously deflate during expiration. There are three major types of abnormal rib cage–abdominal motion[91,92]: (1) asynchronous motion is characterized by a time lag between motion of the rib cage and abdominal compartments; (2) paradoxic motion is characterized by one compartment moving in an opposite direction to the other; and (3) the third type of abnormal motion is characterized by an increase in the breath-to-breath variability of relative contribution of the rib cage and abdomen to tidal

There are three major types of abnormal rib cage–abdominal motion: asynchrony, paradox, and increased breath-to-breath variability in compartmental contribution.

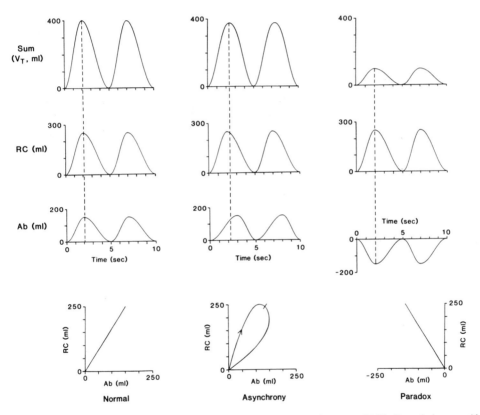

FIGURE 10   Schematic representation of the motion of the rib cage (RC), the abdomen (Ab), and their sum signal, representing tidal volume (V_T) during (A) normal breathing, (B) asynchronous breathing, and (C) abdominal paradox. It should be noted that the pattern of rib cage motion is identical in each panel; the vertical dashed lines represent maximal inspiration of the sum signal. The respective X-Y (Konno-Mead) plot for each type of motion is shown below the time tracings. Normal, synchronous breathing results in a straight line (actually a closed loop) with a positive slope. Asynchronous breathing produces an open loop (the direction of inspiration is indicated by the arrow, and the point of end inspiration is represented by the tick mark). Paradoxical motion of the abdomen (ie, movement in a direction opposite of the sum signal) results in a straight line (or closed loop) with a negative slope. From Tobin MJ: State of the art: respiratory monitoring in the intensive care unit. Am Rev Respir Dis 138:1625, 1988. With permission.

Fatigue is neither a sufficient nor a necessary condition for the development of abdominal paradox.

Although abdominal paradox has been considered a useful predictor of an unsuccessful weaning outcome, this belief has been based on nonquantitative measurements obtained in a nonstandardized manner.

volume; this has sometimes been termed "respiratory alternans."[93]

In the past, paradoxic motion of the abdomen was thought to reflect the presence of diaphragmatic fatigue.[93] In recent studies, however, fatigue was shown to be neither a sufficient nor a necessary condition for its development, and instead, abnormal motion was shown to reflect increased respiratory load.[92] Although abdominal paradox has been considered a useful predictor of an unsuccessful weaning outcome,[93] this belief has been based on nonquantitative measurements obtained in a nonstandardized manner. In a study where precise quantitative measurements of rib cage–abdominal motion were obtained over fixed intervals, no significant difference was noted in the degree of abdominal paradox in weaning success and weaning failure patients.[91] The lack of difference in abdominal paradox between the two groups of patients was due, at least in part, to the considerable breath-to-breath fluctuation in the relative contribution of the rib cage and abdomen to tidal volume, and the fact that the extent of paradoxic motion tended to be divided between the two compartments. Instead, weaning outcome was better predicted by an index that combines asynchrony *and* paradox of *both* the rib cage and abdomen (the ratio of maximum

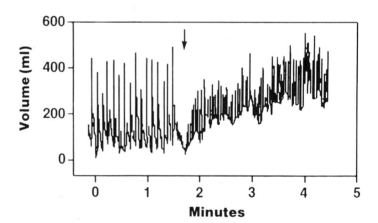

FIGURE 11 A compressed microprocessor plot of breathing pattern in a patient who failed a weaning trial. Each vertical line represents the volume of a single breath, and alterations in the baseline or end-expiratory level are equivalent to changes in functional residual capacity (FRC). The arrow indicates the point of resuming spontaneous breathing after discontinuation of ventilator support—note the development of tachypnea and dynamic hyperinflation. From Tobin MJ, Perez W, Guenther SM et al: The pattern of breathing during successful and unsuccessful trials of weaning from mechanical ventilation. Am Rev Respir Dis 134:111, 1986. With permission.

compartmental amplitude to tidal volume, MCA/V_T) (see Fig. 8) and an index that quantitates the breath-to-breath variability in the contribution of the rib cage and abdomen to tidal volume.[91]

Change in End-expiratory Level

Alterations in the end-expiratory level of a RIP signal provide a measure of the change in functional residual capacity, provided that motion artifact is absent (Fig. 11).[94,95] If inductive plethysmography is employed for this purpose, it is important to use thermally stable oscillators and the direct current (DC) coupling mode. It is also important to note that this device measures the change in FRC rather than absolute FRC. Recently, Hoffman and colleagues[96] reported the use of RIP to estimate auto-PEEP. By noting the level of external PEEP at which a patient's end-expiratory lung volume increased, they obtained a remarkably close estimate of the patient's original level of auto-PEEP.

Alterations in the end-expiratory level of a RIP signal provide a measure of the change in functional residual capacity, provided that motion artifact is absent.

SUMMARY

In recent years, significant advances have occurred in our ability to monitor respiratory neuromuscular function. Respiratory drive can be monitored by measuring airway occlusion pressure ($P_{0.1}$) or mean inspiratory flow (V_T/T_I). Careful clinical examination, radiological examination, and routine pulmonary function testing can provide helpful information regarding respiratory muscle function. More formal testing includes measurement of maximum respiratory pressures, force-frequency curves in response to phrenic nerve stimulation, phrenic nerve conduction time, electromyography, pressure–time product, and pressure relaxation rates. Advances in noninvasive monitoring make it possible to monitor ventilation without a physical connection to the airway. Quantification of the volume and time components of the respiratory cycle and rib cage–abdominal motion provide valuable information regarding respiratory system performance.

Advances in noninvasive monitoring make it possible to monitor ventilation without a physical connection to the airway.

References

1. Madias NE, Adrogué HJ: Respiratory acidosis and alkalosis. Contemp Management Crit Care 1(2):37, 1990

2. Gilbert R, Keighley J, Auchincloss JH: Mechanisms of chronic carbon dioxide retention in patients with obstructive pulmonary disease. Am J Med 38:217, 1965

3. Lopata M, Lourenco RV: Evaluation of respiratory control. Clinics Chest Med 1:33, 1980

4. Cherniack RM, Snidal DP: The effect of obstruction to breathing on the ventilatory respone to CO_2. J Clin Invest 35:1286, 1956

5. Lourenco RV, Cherniack NS, Malm JR et al: Nervous output from the respiratory center during obstructed breathing. J Appl Physiol 21:527, 1966

6. Evanich MJ, Franco MJ, Lourenco RV: Force output of the diaphragm as a function of phrenic nerve firing rate and lung volume. J Appl Physiol 35:208, 1973

7. Whitelaw WA, Derenne JP, Milic-Emili J: Occlusion pressure as a measure of respiratory center output in conscious man. Respir Physiol 23:181, 1975

8. Eldridge FL, Vaugn KZ: Relationship of thoracic volume and airway occlusion pressure: muscular effects. J Appl Physiol 43:312, 1977

9. Burki NK: The effects of changes in functional residual capacity with posture on mouth occlusion pressure and ventilatory pattern. Am Rev Respir Dis 16:895, 1977

10. Grassino AE, Derenne JP, Almirall J et al: Configuration of the chest wall and occlusion pressures in awake humans. J Appl Physiol 50:134, 1981

11. Burki NK: Measurements of ventilatory regulation. Clinics Chest Medicine 10:215, 1989

12. Lind FG, Truve AB, Lindborg BPO: Microcomputer-assisted on-line measurement of breathing pattern and occlusion pressure. J Appl Physiol 56:235, 1984

13. Brenner M, Mukai DS, Russell JE et al: A new method for measurement of airway occlusion pressure. Chest 98:421, 1990

14. Sorli J, Grassino A, Lorange G, Milic-Emili J: Control of breathing in patients with chronic obstructive pulmonary disease. Clin Sci Mol Med 54:295, 1978

15. Mann J, Bradley CA, Authonisen NR: Occlusion pressure in acute bronchospasm induced by methacholine. Respir Physiol 33:339, 1978

16. Lederer DH, Altose MD, Kelsen SG, Cherniack NS: Comparison of occlusion pressure and ventilatory responses. Thorax 32:212, 1977

17. Herrera M, Blasco J, Venegas J et al: Mouth occlusion pressure ($P_{0.1}$) in acute respiratory failure. Intensive Care Med 11:134, 1985

18. Sassoon CSH, Te TT, Mahutte CK et al: Airway occlusion pressure: an important indicator for successful weaning in patients with chronic obstructive pulmonary disease. Am Rev Respir Dis 135:107, 1987

19. Montgomery AB, Holle RHO, Neagley SR et al: Prediction of successful ventilator weaning using airway occlusion pressure and hypercapnic challenge. Chest 91:496, 1987

20. Bradburne RM, McCool FD: The respiratory muscles: structural and functional considerations. p. 257. In Tobin MJ (ed): The respiratory muscles. JB Lippincott, Philadelphia, 1990

21. Tobin MJ: Respiratory muscles in disease. Clin Chest Med 9:263, 1988

22. Smith PEM, Calverley PMA, Edwards RHT et al: Practical problems in the respiratory care of patients with muscular dystrophy. N Engl J Med 316:1197, 1987

23. Laroche CM, Green M: Respiratory muscle involvement in systemic disease. p. 409. In Tobin MJ (ed): The respiratory muscles. JB Lippincott, Philadelphia, 1990

24. Skatrud J, Iber C, McHugh W et al: Determinants of hypoventilation during wakefulness and sleep in diaphragmatic paralysis. Am Rev Respir Dis 121:587, 1980

25. Tobin MJ: State of the art: respiratory monitoring in the intensive care unit. Am Rev Respir Dis 138:1625, 1988

26. Moxham J: Tests of respiratory muscle function. p. 312. In Tobin MJ (ed): The respiratory muscles. JB Lippincott, 1990

27. Alexander C: Diaphragm movements and the diagnosis of diaphragmatic paralysis. Clin Radiol 17:79, 1966

28. Newson-Davis J, Goldman M, Loh L et al: Diaphragm function and alveolar hypoventilation. Q J Med 177:87, 1976

29. Estenne M, DeTroyer A: Respiratory muscle involvement in tetraplegia. p. 360. In Tobin MJ (ed): The respiratory muscles. JB Lippincott, Philadelphia, 1990

30. Allen SM, Hunt B, Green M: Fall in vital capacity with posture. Br J Dis Chest 79:267, 1985

31. Rochester DF: Tests of respiratory muscle function. Clinics Chest Med 9:249, 1988

32. Koulouris N, Mulvey DA, Laroche CM et al: Comparison of two different mouthpieces for the measurement of $P_I$max and $P_E$max in normal and weak subjects. Eur Respir J 1:863, 1988

33. Leech JA, Gheezo H, Stevens D et al: Respiratory pressures and function in young adults. Am Rev Respir Dis 128:17, 1983

34. Vincken W, Ghezzo H, Cosio MG: Maximal static respiratory pressures in adults: normal values and their relationship to determinants of respiratory function. Bull Eur Physiopathol Respir 23:435, 1987

35. Wilson SH, Cooke NT, Edwards RHT et al: Predicted normal values for maximal respiratory pressures in Caucasian adults and children. Thorax 39:535, 1984

36. Chen HI, Kuo CS: Relationships between respiratory muscles function and age, sex, and other factors. J Appl Physiol 66:943, 1989

37. Bendixin HH, Bunker JP: Measurements of inspiratory force in anesthetized dogs. Anesthesiology 23:315, 1962

38. Wescott DA, Bendixin HH: Neostigmine as a curare antagonist: a clinical study. Anesthesiology 23:324, 1962

39. Sahn SA, Lakshminarayan S: Bedside criteria for discontinuation of mechanical ventilation. Chest 63:1002, 1973

40. Tobin MJ: Weaning from mechanical ventilation. Current Pulmonology 11:47, 1990

41. Marini JJ, Smith TC, Lamb V: Estimation of inspiratory muscle strength in mechanically ventilated patients: the measurement of maximal inspiratory pressure. J Crit Care 1:32, 1986

42. Multz AS, Aldrich TK, Prezant DJ et al: Maximal inspiratory pressure is not a reliable test of inspiratory muscle strength in mechanically ventilated patients. Am Rev Respir Dis 142:529, 1990

43. Laporta D, Grassino A: Assessment of transdiaphragmatic pressure in humans. J Appl Physiol 58:1469, 1985

44. Miller J, Moxham J, Green M: The maximal sniff in the assessment of diaphragm function in man. Clin Sci 69:91, 1985

45. Faulkner JA, Maxwell LC, Ruff GL et al: The diaphragm as muscle: contractile properties. Am Rev Respir Dis 119(Suppl):89, 1979

46. Aldrich TK: Respiratory muscle fatigue: p. 329. In Tobin MJ (ed): The respiratory muscles. JB Lippincott, Philadelphia, 1990

47. Moxham J: Respiratory muscle fatigue: mechanisms, evaluation and therapy. Br J Anaesthesia 65:43, 1990

48. Bellemare F, Bigland-Ritchie B: Central components of diaphragm fatigue assessed by phrenic nerve stimulation. J Appl Physiol 62:1307, 1987

49. Aubier M, Farkas G, DeTroyer A, Roussos C: Detection of diaphragm fatigue in man by phrenic stimulation. J Appl Physiol 50:538, 1981

50. Meir A, Brophy C, Moxham J, Green M: Phrenic nerve stimulation in normal subjects and in patients with diaphragmatic weakness. Thorax 42:885, 1987

51. Petrofsky JS: Quantification through the surface EMG of muscle fatigue and recovery during successive isometric contraction. Aviat Space Environ Med 52:545, 1981

52. Bracewell RN: The Fourier transform. Sci Amer June:86, 1989

53. Schweitzer TW, Fitzgerald JW, Bowden JA, Lynne-Davies P: Spectral analysis of human inspiratory diaphragmatic electromyograms. J Appl Physiol 46:152, 1979

54. Gross D, Grassino A, Ross D, Macklem PT: Electromyogram pattern of diaphragmatic fatigue. J Appl Physiol 46:1, 1979

55. Gross D, Ladd HW, Riley EJ et al: The effect of training on strength and endurance of the diaphragm in quadriplegia. Am J Med 68:27, 1980

56. Jardim J, Farkas G, Prefaut C et al: The failing inspiratory muscles under normoxic and hypoxic conditions. Am Rev Respir Dis 124:274, 1981

57. Walsh JM, Romano S, Grassino A: The effect of diaphragm length on the EMG power spectrum. Clin Res 38:847A, 1990

58. Walsh JM, Ito T, Grassino A: A model to detect intermittent respiratory muscle fatigue. FASEB J 4:A291, 1990

59. Walsh JM, Ito T, Grassino A: Detecting intermittent muscle fatigue by the various of the median frequency. FASEB J 5:A1035, 1991

60. McGregor M, Becklake MR: The relationship of oxygen cost of breathing to respiratory mechanical work and respiratory force. J Clin Invest 40:971, 1961

61. Field S, Sanci S, Grassino A: Respiratory muscle oxygen consumption estimated by the diaphragm pressure-time index. J Appl Physiol 57:44, 1984

62. Collet PW, Perry C, Engel LA: Pressure-time product, flow, and oxygen cost of resistive breathing in humans. J Appl Physiol 58:1263, 1984

63. Bellemare F, Grassino A: Effect of pressure and timing of contraction on human diaphragm fatigue. J Appl Physiol 53:1190, 1982

64. Dodd DS, Kelly S, Collet PW, Engel LA: Pressure-time product, work rate, and endurance during resistive breathing in humans. J Appl Physiol 64:1397, 1988

65. Clanton TL, Dixon GF, Drake J, Gadek JE: Effects of breathing pattern on inspiratory muscle endurance in humans. J Appl Physiol 59:1834, 1985

66. McCool FD, McCann DR, Leith DE, Hoppin FG: Pressure-flow effects on endurance of inspiratory muscles. J Appl Physiol 60:299, 1986

67. Esau SA, Bellemare F, Grassino A et al: Changes in relaxation rate with diaphragmatic fatigue in humans. J Appl Physiol 54:1353, 1983

68. Esau SA, Bye TP, Pardy RL: Changes in rate of relaxtion of sniffs with diaphragmatic fatigue in humans. J Appl Physiol 55:731, 1983

69. Milic-Emili J: Recent advances in clinical assessment of control of breathing. Lung 160:1, 1982

70. Tobin MJ, Chadha TS, Jenouri G et al: Breathing patterns 1. Normal subjects. Chest 84:202, 1983

71. Tobin MJ, Chadha TS, Jenouri G et al: Breathing patterns 2. Diseased subjects. Chest 84:286, 1983

72. Tobin MJ: Noninvasive evaluation of respiratory movement. p. 29. In Nochomovitz ML, Cherniack NS (eds): Noninvasive respiratory monitoring. Churchill Livingstone, New York, 1986

73. Perez W, Tobin MJ: Separation of factors responsible for change in breathing pattern induced by instrumentation. J Appl Physiol 59:1515, 1985

74. Sackner MA, Krieger BP: Noninvasive respiratory monitoring. p. 663. In Scharf SM, Cassidy SS (eds): Heart-lung interactions in health and disease. Marcel Dekker, New York, 1989

75. Tobin MJ, Jenouri G, Lind B et al: Validation of respiratory inductive plethysmography in patients with pulmonary disease. Chest 83:615, 1983

76. Tobin MJ, Guenther SM, Perez W, Mador MJ: Accuracy of the respiratory inductive plethysmography during loaded breathing. J Appl Physiol 62:497, 1987

77. Sackner MA, Watson H, Belsito AS et al: Calibration of respiratory inductive plethysmography during natural breathing. J Appl Physiol 66:410, 1989

78. Yang K, Tobin MJ: A prospective study of predicting outcome of trials of weaning from mechanical ventilation. N Engl J Med 324:1445, 1991

79. Tobin MJ, Perez W, Guenther SM et al: The pattern of breathing during successful and unsuccessful trials of weaning from mechanical ventilation. Am Rev Respir Dis 134:1111, 1986

80. Gravelyn TR, Weg JR: Respiratory rate as an indicator of acute respiratory dysfunction. JAMA 244:1123, 1980

81. McFadden JP, Price RC, Eastwood HD et al: Raised respiratory rate in elderly patients: a valuable physical sign. Br Med J 284:626, 1982

82. Browning IB, D'Alonzo GE, Tobin MJ: Importance of respiratory rate as an indicator of respiratory dysfunction in patients with cystic fibrosis. Chest 97:1317, 1990

83. von Euler C: The functional organization of respiratory phase-switching mechanisms. Fed Proc 36:2375, 1977

84. Cohen MI, Feldman JL: Models of respiratory phase-switching. Fed Proc 36:2367, 1977

85. Clark FJ, von Euler C: On the regulation of depth and rate of breathing. J Physiol (Lond) 222:267, 1972

86. Milic-Emili J, Grunstein MM: Drive and timing components of ventilation. Chest 70:131, 1976

87. Grunstein MM, Younes M, Milic-Emili: Control of tidal volume and respiratory frequency in anesthetized cats. J Appl Physiol 35:463, 1973

88. Hirshman CA, McCullough RE, Weil JV: Normal values for hypoxic and hypercapnic drives in man. J Appl Physiol 38:1095, 1975

89. Sahn SA, Zwillich CW, Dick N et al: Variability of ventilatory responses to hypoxia and hypercapnia. J Appl Physiol 43:1019, 1977

90. Tobin MJ, Mador MJ, Guenther SM et al: Variability of resting respiratory drive and timing in healthy subjects. J Appl Physiol 65:309, 1988

91. Tobin MJ, Guenther SM, Perez W et al: Konno-Mead analysis of ribcage-abdominal motion during successful and unsuccessful trials of weaning from mechanical ventilation. Am Rev Respir 135:1320, 1987

92. Tobin MJ, Perez W, Guenther SM et al: Does ribcage abdominal paradox signify respiratory muscle fatigue? J Appl Physiol 63:851, 1987

93. Cohen C, Zagelbaum G, Gross D et al: Clinical manifestations of inspiratory muscle fatigue. Am J Med 73:308, 1982

94. Tobin MJ, Jenouri G, Birch S et al: Effect of positive end-expiratory pressure on breathing patterns of normal subjects and intubated patients with respiratory failure. Crit Care Med 11:859, 1983

95. Lennox S, Mengeot PM, Martin JG: The contributions of rib cage and abdominal displacements to the hyperinflation of acute bronchospasm. Am Rev Respir Dis 132:679, 1985

96. Hoffman RA, Ershowsky P, Krieger BP: Determination of auto-PEEP during spontaneous and controlled ventilation by monitoring changes in end-expiratory thoracic gas volume. Chest 96:613, 1989

MONITORING THE MECHANICS OF THE RESPIRATORY SYSTEM

JOHN J. MARINI, MD[†]

WHAT ARE MECHANICS AND HOW ARE THEY MEASURED?

The mechanical properties of the respiratory system are the characteristics that influence the energy cost of breathing. Because pressure gradients provide the forces driving gas flow and counterbalancing elastic recoil, the assessment of respiratory mechanics involves the measurement of flows, volumes (flow integrated over time), and pressure gradients. Indeed, the equation of motion of the respiratory system, an expression of these relationships, can be written as[1] (Fig. 1):

$$P = R\dot{V} + \frac{V}{C} + P_{ex}$$

In this equation, P is the pressure applied across the respiratory system, R is inspiratory resistance, C is inspiratory compliance, $\dot{V}$ and V are flow and volume inspired in excess of the end-expiratory value, and P_{ex} is end-expiratory alveolar pressure. Flow, the rate of volume change, can be directly measured with a variety of sensing instruments. Alternatively, flow can be determined indirectly by differentiating spirometric volume. The volumes of interest during routine assessment of respiratory system mechanics are those that exceed the (passive) equilibrium value. The equilibrium point of the respiratory system is the position at which the system is at rest, with end-expiratory alveolar pressure the same as the end-expiratory pressure at the airway opening. (Thus, when positive end-expiratory pressure (PEEP) is applied, the equilibrium position is displaced to that higher volume corresponding to PEEP.)

[†] Professor of Medicine, University of Minnesota, Director, Pulmonary and Critical Care Medicine, St. Paul-Ramsey Medical Center, Minneapolis/ St. Paul, Minnesota

Although regional mechanics are of unquestioned importance in determining ventilation and gas exchange, technology available at the bedside currently limits measurement to the global properties of the respiratory system.

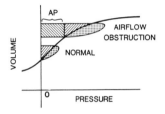

FIGURE 1 Relationship of transthoracic pressure to volume for a normal subject and for a patient with airflow obstruction. Cross-hatched areas are proportional to the elastic work of breathing. Stippled areas quantify the frictional (resistive) workload. Note that in the presence of dynamic hyperinflation, AP adds significantly to the elastic work of breathing. From Marini JJ: Ventilatory management of chronic obstructive pulmonary disease. p. 495. In Cherniack NS (ed): Chronic obstructive pulmonary disease. WB Saunders, Philadelphia, 1990. With permission.

Although regional mechanics are of unquestioned importance in determining ventilation and gas exchange, technology available at the bedside currently limits measurement to the global properties of the respiratory system.

Flow is most commonly measured by pneumotachography, and volume changes are tracked by integrating the resulting flow signal. Inductance plethysmography is another alternative.[2] Pressure changes relevant to the lungs must be assessed as the difference between the airway pressure (P_{aw}) and the pleural pressure (P_{pl}) that surrounds them. The esophagus provides a convenient site for measuring changes in intrapleural pressure. With the airway occluded, pressure measured at the airway opening serves also to estimate alveolar pressure. Because the lungs are inherently passive, their mechanical properties can be assessed during any form of spontaneous, pressure-assisted, or controlled ventilation. The mechanical properties of the chest wall, in contrast, can only be evaluated during controlled ventilation, when the actual pressure acting to distend that structure can be accurately measured.

In clinical practice, the monitoring of respiratory mechanics assumes greatest importance for the patient who is intubated and mechanically ventilated. Although readily available, airway pressure is of limited use unless assessed under passive conditions or supplemented by esophageal pressure (P_{es}). Most clinicians rarely consider esophageal pressure measurement, believing that it is neither needed nor well tolerated. In fact, some assessment of intrapleural pressure can be of great value in decision making, both for the respiratory and for the cardiovascular systems. Under conditions of controlled inflation, swings in central venous pressure (CVP) also provide a reliable, if somewhat imprecise, indicator of changes in intrathoracic pressure. (During vigorous spontaneous efforts, the reliability of the CVP may be somewhat less, but this question is relatively unstudied.) It must be emphasized that in the absence of P_{es} or some other estimate of P_{pl}, resistance, compliance, and the mechanics measures on which they are based cannot be reliably assessed from P_{aw} alone in patients making active efforts. Except as otherwise noted, the remaining discussion of this chapter will assume passive conditions and the availability of airway pressure, flow, and spirometric volumes.

MONITORING LUNG AND CHEST WALL MECHANICS

During spontaneous breathing and all conventional forms of mechanical ventilation, gas is driven to and from the alveoli by differences in pressure. Under passive conditions, all required power is provided by the mechanical ventilator. The difference between applied airway pressure and atmospheric pressure is the sum of two components: (1) the pressure needed to drive gas between the airway opening and the alveolus and (2) that required to hold the alveoli expanded against the combined elastic recoil of the lung and chest wall.[1] In a passively ventilated system, the elastic component is most easily assessed by measuring pressure at the airway opening under stop-flow (static) conditions.

STATIC PRESSURE–VOLUME RELATIONSHIPS

When flow stops at the end of tidal expiration, the pressures at the airway opening and alveolus are identical and the system is at equilibrium. The pressure (ΔP_L) required to expand the lung by a certain volume (ΔV) is the corresponding change in transpulmonary pressure (P_L = alveolar pressure [P_{alv}] − P_{pl}). Lung compliance ($C_L = \Delta V/\Delta P_L$), the inverse of elastance, indicates the pressure required per unit change in lung volume. Under passive conditions, the pressure needed to simultaneously expand the chest wall by the same ΔV is given by the average change in "intrathoracic" pressure (ΔP_{pl}), usually and most conveniently sampled in the esophagus. The distensibility of the relaxed chest wall is characterized by chest wall compliance ($C_W = \Delta V/\Delta P_{pl}$). Thus, the slope of the pressure–volume relationship for the total respiratory system (C_{RS}) is $\Delta V/\Delta P_{alv}$ (Fig. 2). In ventilator-derived calculations of compliance, ΔV must be measured at the inlet of the endotracheal tube, or total expired volume must be adjusted for the amount stored in compressible circuit elements during (pressurized) inspiration. Most conveniently, ΔV is taken as the tidal volume and ΔP_{alv} is the difference in alveolar pressure at the two extremes of the tidal cycle [the peak static plateau pressure (P_s) − the sum of PEEP and auto-PEEP].

Compliance measurements may have therapeutic and prognostic value in patients with acute failure to oxygenate the arterial blood (Fig. 3). When PEEP is applied incrementally, static compliance tends to reach its highest value coincident with maximal recruitment of lung units, reduction in shunt fraction, and improvement in oxygen delivery.[3,4] It is a good general principle not to use values of end-expiratory pressure or tidal volume that significantly depress thoracic compliance, unless safe transpulmonary pressures can be used and objective evidence of improved O_2 delivery is present.[5] Excessive pressures, as a rule >35

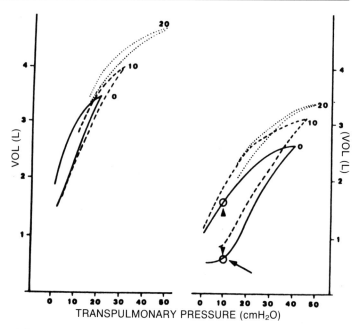

FIGURE 2 Static pressure–volume curves for two patients with ARDS at 0, 10, and 20 cmH_2O end-expiratory pressure. Without PEEP applied, the pressure–volume curve of the acutely edematous respiratory system often demonstrates hysteresis (arrowheads) and an inflection point (P_{flex}) on the inflation limb (arrow, right). At the highest level of PEEP (20 cm H_2O), P_{flex} is lost and the pressure–volume curve assumes a monotonic, flattened profile. No inflection point may be observed in severely affected patients or in those already recovered (left). Adapted from Benito S, Le Maire F: Pulmonary pressure-volume relationship in acute respiratory distress syndrome in adults: role of positive end-expiratory pressure. J Crit Care 5:27, 1990. With permission.

Excessive pressures, as a rule >35 cm H_2O between alveolus and pleural space (transalveolar pressure), risk barotrauma and hemodynamic compromise without tangible benefit to gas exchange or oxygen delivery.

cm H_2O between alveolus and pleural space (transalveolar pressure), risk barotrauma and hemodynamic compromise without tangible benefit to gas exchange or oxygen delivery.

Serial changes in the respiratory pressure–volume curve and computed static compliance also tend to reflect the worsening or resolution of acute lung injury.[6,7] Maximal depression of lung compliance in acute respiratory distress syndrome (ARDS) often requires 1–2 weeks to develop. Normal compliance of the respiratory system is $\approx$ 80–100 ml/cmH$_2$O. Severe disease is implicated when compliance falls to 30 ml/cmH$_2$O or less.

Both the number of aerated alveoli and their relative distention influence the compliance value. Therefore, caution must be exercised when attempting to use C_{RS} as an in-

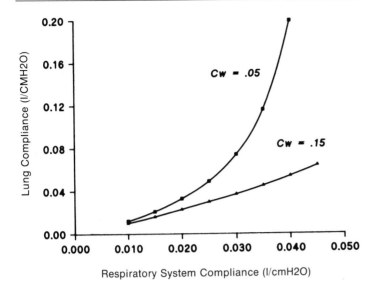

FIGURE 3 Relationship of lung compliance to respiratory system compliance for two different values of chest wall compliance. Note the extreme curvilinearity of this relationship under stiff chest wall conditions. From Marini JJ: Lung mechanics in the adult respiratory distress syndrome: recent conceptual advances and implications for management. Clin Chest Med 11(4):673, 1990. With permission.

dicator of underlying tissue elastance. Ideally, compliance would be referenced to a measure of absolute lung volume (V_{abs}) (such as FRC or TLC) to produce a "specific compliance," C_{RS}/V_{abs}.[8] (For example, identical pressures drive greatly different volumes into the normal lungs of elephants and mice. The C_L is influenced by this volume difference, whereas C_L/V_{abs} is not.) Even in the same individual, C_{RS} can change greatly near the extremes of the vital capacity range. Thus, most patients with hyperinflated lungs who are ventilated for acute exacerbations of asthma or chronic obstructive pulmonary disease (COPD) have a depressed C_{RS}, despite supernormal tissue distensibility when assessed in a lower volume range. This reduction in compliance is due, in part, to lung overdistention and, in part, to the inward recoil of the chest wall at high volumes. Furthermore, C_{RS} can be apparently depressed if the pressure component corresponding to dynamic hyperinflation is not considered.[9]

The C_{RS} may also be depressed at the lower extremes of lung volume if substantial atelectasis occurs, as during pulmonary edema.[10] As the chest expands, the number of recruited alveoli tends to increase, moving C_{RS} toward its

Ideally, compliance would be referenced to a measure of absolute lung volume (such as FRC or TLC) to produce a "specific compliance," C_{RS}/V_{abs}.

During acute respiratory failure, the presence of an inflection point of compliance change on the static pressure–volume curve appears to indicate recruitable lung and potential benefit from additional PEEP.

normal value. (The reverse phenomenon, derecruitment, occurs during tidal lung deflation, producing hysteresis of the static pressure–volume curve.) Thus, C_L and C_{RS} may appear to vary with increasing tidal volume, improving until alveolar units are fully recruited or tissue elastic limits are approached. During acute respiratory failure, the presence of an inflection point of compliance change (P_{flex}) on the static pressure–volume curve appears to indicate recruitable lung and potential benefit from additional PEEP.[7,11]

Although seldom calculated, thoracic elastance (E_{RS}), the reciprocal of C_{RS}, has certain advantages for clinical use.[12] Unlike the subcomponents of respiratory system compliance, elastances of the lung (E_L) and chest wall (E_W) add in series:

$$E_{RS} = E_L + E_W \qquad (1)$$

On the other hand, their respective compliances add in parallel:

$$\frac{1}{C_{RS}} = \frac{1}{C_L} + \frac{1}{C_W} \qquad (2)$$

Therefore, even though C_{RS} is often used to assess the elastic properties of the lung, the relationship of C_{RS} to C_L is not entirely straightforward (Fig. 3):

$$C_{RS} = \frac{C_L C_W}{(C_W + C_L)}$$

For this reason, changing chest wall compliance should be considered when attempting to evaluate the lung on the basis of total respiratory system behavior. The interpretation of elastance is considerably easier (Fig. 4).

Chest wall distensibility is often disturbed by abdominal distention, effusions, increased muscular tone, recent surgery, position changes, soft tissue injury, and many other factors common to the critical care setting. Such changes in chest wall compliance are important to consider in that they influence the interpretation of hemodynamic data (for example, the pulmonary artery occlusion or wedge pressure, P_W) as well as the calculations of chest mechanics data.

A given peak airway pressure has different hemodynamic and prognostic significance, depending on whether the lung or chest wall primarily accounts for that value.

The C_{RS} is the appropriate measure for calculating the effect of PEEP on lung volume. A given peak airway pres-

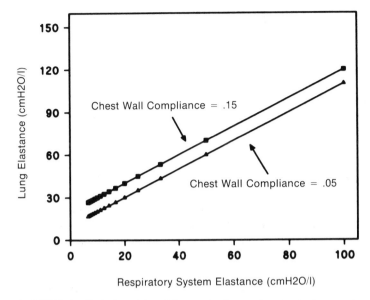

FIGURE 4   Relationship of lung elastance to respiratory system elastance for the same data depicted in Figure 3.

sure has different hemodynamic and prognostic significance, however, depending on whether the lung or chest wall primarily accounts for that value. The fraction of P_{ex} partitioned to the pleural space depends on the relative compliances of the lungs and chest wall[10,13]:

$$\Delta V_L = C_L[\Delta(P_{ex} - P_{pl})]$$
$$\Delta V_W = C_W(\Delta P_{pl})$$

and since $\Delta V_L = \Delta V_W$,

$$\Delta P_{pl} = \Delta P_{ex}\left(\frac{C_L}{(C_L + C_W)}\right) \qquad (3)$$

Equation 3 indicates that the *relative* stiffness of the lungs and chest wall determines the effect of PEEP on hemodynamics and measured P_W. Normally, $C_L \approx C_W$ over the tidal volume range, so that $\Delta P_{pl} \approx \frac{1}{2} \Delta P_{ex}$. Accordingly, about half of a given PEEP (or auto-PEEP) increment is normally reflected in the pleural pressure. With stiff lungs this "transmission" fraction falls to a lower value, and with a stiff chest wall (eg, obesity) it rises to a higher value.

USE OF THE AIRWAY PRESSURE TRACING TO CALCULATE EFFECTIVE COMPLIANCE AND RESISTANCE OF THE RESPIRATORY SYSTEM

Inspiratory Resistance and Thoracic Compliance

Digital technology has greatly expanded monitoring capability, especially during mechanical ventilation.

Digital technology has greatly expanded monitoring capability, especially during mechanical ventilation. During passive inflation, some systems now provide breath-to-breath estimates of R and C_{RS} as well as tracings of flow and airway pressure. All ventilators monitor pressure in the external airway. When a mechanical ventilator expands the chest of a passive subject using constant flow, calculations of total system compliance and resistance can be made from airway pressure alone. (During active efforts, P_{aw} must be supplemented by esophageal pressure to make the relevant calculations for the lung.)

As already noted, airway pressure must overcome the frictional and elastic forces opposing ventilation. The pressures required for these tasks are characterized by resistance (the pressure cost per flow unit) and compliance (the inverse of the pressure cost per unit volume).[14] These system characteristics can be gauged in several ways. When flow is transiently stopped at end inspiration, P_{aw} falls rapidly toward some value that represents an average of the peak alveolar pressure existing in regions with both higher and lower values. The difference between this end-inspiratory "stop flow," "plateau," or "peak static" (P_s) pressure and end-expiratory alveolar pressure (P_{ex}, the sum of PEEP and auto-PEEP) determines the component of end-inspiratory inflation pressure needed to overcome the elastic forces of tidal inflation (Fig. 5). When tidal volume (adjusted for gas compression) is divided by ($P_s - P_{ex}$), static effective compliance (C_{eff}) can be computed[15]:

$$C_{eff} = \frac{V_t - [(P_S - PEEP) \text{ (circuit compression factor)}]}{(P_S - P_{ex})}$$

During dynamic cycling, peak dynamic pressure (P_D) should be substituted for P_S to obtain the appropriate tidal volume correction for dynamic conditions. In clinical practice it is wise to determine the relationship of C_{eff} to tidal volume in order to avoid hyperinflation. At a minimum, the inspiratory dynamic airway pressure tracing should be carefully inspected for signs indicating overdistention. During constant flow, time is a direct analog of delivered

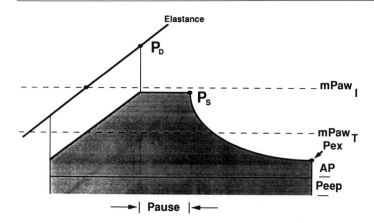

FIGURE 5   Airway and alveolar pressures during constant inspiratory flow (passive conditions). Assuming constant values for resistance and compliance, the slope of the airway pressure tracing is proportional to respiratory system elastance ($\Delta P/\Delta V$), the inverse of compliance. Expiratory volume and alveolar pressure decay exponentially. P_{ex} is the sum of applied PEEP and auto-PEEP. (mP_{awI}) reflects the work per liter of ventilation. mP_{awT} is mean airway pressure for the total cycle (which in this instance is somewhat less than mean alveolar pressure).

volume, so that the slope of the airway pressure tracing reflects dynamic elastance ($1/C_{RS}$) (Fig. 5). Unfortunately, even under constant flow conditions, it is not always possible to draw a single tangent to the P_{aw} inflation curve that characterizes the entire inspiratory period.

When a flow signal is not available, the mechanics of the system can still be readily assessed if either flow or inspiratory airway pressure are known to be constant. Other waveforms (decelerating flow, sinusoidal flow, etc) are less easy to work with. Constant flow, volume-cycled ventilation is perhaps the most widely employed mode in current practice, and a monitored flow signal is not often readily available. If the ventilator's performance characteristics are good and the flow values actually delivered nominal, estimates of R and C acceptable for clinical purposes can easily be made.

Under CF conditions, the pressure achieved just prior to the cessation of gas delivery, P_D, is the total pressure needed to drive gas to the alveolar level at the set flow rate and to expand the lungs and chest wall by the full tidal volume. The difference between P_D and P_S approximates the gradient of pressure driving end-inspiratory gas flow and varies with the resistance of the lungs, chest wall, and endotracheal tube. The term "resistance" usually refers to the ratio between the pressure necessary to drive flow (P_R)

and flow itself. However, P_R is usually a nonlinear function of flow, so that R does not remain constant across all flow rates: $P_R \approx kV^{\epsilon}$ ($1 \leq \epsilon \leq 2$). Thus, for unchanging geometry, computed resistance usually rises as flow increases, especially if flow is highly turbulent.

The ratio of delivered volume (compression-corrected) to the (P_D-PEEP) difference, the "dynamic characteristic,"[16] provides an index of the overall difficulty of chest expansion, provided that tidal volume and inspiratory flow rate stay unchanged and that inflation occurs passively. (Note that this is not a true dynamic compliance value, due to the kinetic nature of the measurement.) Because P_D is influenced by both the frictional and elastic properties of the thorax, it may be a simple yet valuable indicator of bronchodilator response.[17] Here, P_D reflects not only the decline in frictional work that occurs during effective bronchodilation but also any changes that may have occurred in V_E or dynamic hyperinflation.

Because P_D decays exponentially to P_S, the exact value assigned to P_S may depend on the duration of flow interruption. The point at which inspiratory flow first ceases [(zero flow (ZF)] invariably occurs before the plateau is fully achieved, so that the P_D-P_S difference usually exceeds the P_D-P_{ZF} difference by 10–20%. Values for end-inspiratory resistance computed using P_D-P_{ZF} are therefore smaller than those computed using the full P_D-P_S value, which includes pressure components related to volume redistribution and stress relaxation. The $V_t/(P_{ZF}$-$P_{ex})$ quotient yields an estimate of (inspiratory) dynamic compliance (C_{DYN}), a value invariably less than that commonly computed from the $V_t/(P_S$-$P_{ex})$ ratio (C_{STAT}). In normal subjects, R_{DYN}, a value influenced by tissue resistance as well as airway resistance, tends to remain stable or fall as flow rate increases, provided that airway opening pressure is measured beyond the tip of an endotracheal tube.[18] In patients with airflow obstruction, however, both R_{DYN} and R_{STAT} demonstrate the expected rise with flow increases.[19]

Expiratory Resistance

In obstructive disease, expiratory resistance exceeds inspiratory resistance, fluctuates to greater extent during the tidal cycle, and bears more direct relevance to air trapping.

In obstructive disease, expiratory resistance (R_{ex}) exceeds inspiratory resistance (R_{in}), fluctuates to greater extent during the tidal cycle, and bears more direct relevance to air trapping.[9,20] Although seldom computed, R_{ex} may be determined during passive exhalation from simultaneous recordings of exhaled airflow and tidal volume (V_t). A representative volume is selected (for example, $V = \frac{1}{2}V_t$) and the corresponding flow recorded. From the estimated upstream alveolar pressure at volume V: $[P_{alv(V)} \approx P_S - (V/$

C_{RS})], expiratory flow resistance, the quotient of alveolar minus airway opening pressure (P_{ao}) and flow, can be approximated at that point from the expression:

$$R_{ex} = \frac{P_{alv(V)} - P_{ao}}{\dot{V}} \text{ or } R_{ex} = \frac{P_S - [(V/C_{RS}) + P_{ao}]}{\dot{V}} \quad (4)$$

where V is the exhaled volume at the time of measurement. In theory, this method should provide a representative estimate of R_{ex}. However, no study is currently available to test its validity against an alternative (plethysmographic or flow interruptive) method.

Once the static (inflation hold) pressure is known and the corresponding C_{RS} value has been computed, expiratory resistance can also be estimated from the observed "time constant" of passive deflation. Ideally, the passive respiratory system deflates as a single compartment, allowing alveolar pressure to decay in purely exponential fashion from its starting value (P_S) (Fig. 6). If alveolar pressure, P(t), is known at any time t after deflation begins then:

$$P(t) \approx (P_S - PEEP)e^{-kt} + PEEP$$

where e is the base of natural logarithms (2.718) and k is the reciprocal of the expiratory time constant (τ). Solving this equation for $k = 1/R_x C$ estimates the time constant. When one time constant ($\tau = R_{ex}C$), expressed in seconds, has elapsed since the onset of deflation, $1/e = 1/2.718$, or

Once the static (inflation hold) pressure is known and the corresponding C_{RS} value has been computed, expiratory resistance can also be estimated from the observed "time constant" of passive deflation.

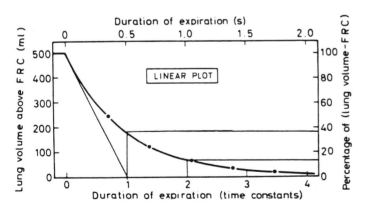

FIGURE 6 Expiratory exponential decay. Equal fractions of the volume remaining are exhaled in equal time intervals. Exhalation is nearly complete after four time constants (RC) have elapsed. A tangent to the volume time curve drawn at the onset of deflation intersects the time axis (zero volume) one time constant afterward. Adapted from Nunn JF: Applied respiratory physiology. Butterworths, Boston, 1977. With permission.

37%, of the starting volume (above PEEP) remains to be expelled. After three time constants, only 5% of the tidal volume remains. If both C_{RS} and the time constant (measured from a volume–time plot) are available, an average expiratory resistance can be computed from their quotient ($R_{ex} = \tau/C$).

In theory, this method for computing R_{ex} provides information unavailable from the inspiratory pressure data routinely used. However, the assumptions on which such estimates are based are often questionable, especially in patients with severe airflow obstruction. The lungs and chest wall rarely deflate as an ideal one-compartment system, and the expiratory pathway includes the external apparatus extending from the endotracheal tube past the exhalation valve to the expiratory port, as well as the patient's airway. For these and other reasons, expiratory resistance values calculated from the τ/C ratio must be considered crude estimates at best.

Flow Interruption Technique
The technique of interrupting expiratory airflow repeatedly has recently been adapted to determine the mechanics of the respiratory system in acutely ill patients receiving mechanical ventilation.[19] Following end-inspiratory airway occlusion, a series of brief ($\approx$0.2 s) interruptions of expiratory flow is performed during passive deflation (Fig. 7). Multiple post-interruption plateaus of airway pressure are thereby generated, yielding estimates of alveolar pressure that can be used in conjunction with flow and volume to compute R_{ex} and C_{RS}. The interrupter method can be applied to paralyzed or anesthetized patients, either manually or by using a highly responsive solenoid valve system. Flow interruption is not practical to apply to patients with high minute ventilation requirements or to those who respond by muscular contraction.

Although a post-interruption plateau is achieved almost immediately in most normal subjects and in patients with restrictive disease, patients with severe airflow obstruction exhibit a substantial delay before complete equilibration is achieved. Interestingly, those with dynamic expiratory flow limitation demonstrate high flow transients immediately after occlusion release. Other signs of dynamic airway compression include a linear and/or biphasic flow profile, as well as failure of added resistance to influence flow rate. Such observations may have clinical relevance in that expiratory airflow limitation during passive deflation indicates dynamic hyperinflation and may portend both a beneficial response to added PEEP and continued ventilator

Expiratory airflow limitation during passive deflation indicates dynamic hyperinflation and may portend both a beneficial response to added PEEP and continued ventilator dependence.

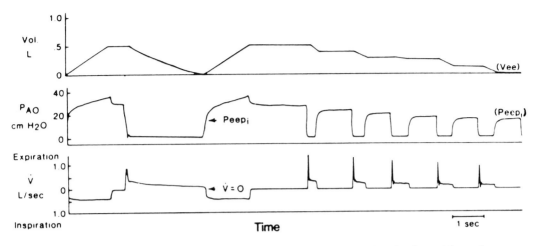

FIGURE 7   Multiple airway occlusions performed during exhalation in the setting of severe airflow obstruction. The post-occlusion spikes of flow, in conjunction with the linear expiratory flow profile, indicate flow limitation due to dynamic airway compression. From Hubmayr RD, Gay PC, Tayyab M: Respiratory system mechanics in ventilated patients: techniques and indications. Mayo Clin Proc 62:358, 1987. With permission.

dependence.[17,21] Flow-limiting dynamic airway compression during tidal breathing may also contribute to dyspnea.[22]

Endotracheal Tube and Expiratory Valve Resistance

The endotracheal tube is often a major determinant of the total resistance to airflow.[19,23] Depending on tube type, length, diameter, patency, and angulation, computed values for inspiratory resistance may be dominated by the resistive properties of the artificial airway. Tube resistance *in vivo* may be much higher than that of the same tube prior to insertion,[24] a fact of particular importance for patients with copious airway secretions. Marked flow dependence of resistance may also be demonstrated in certain patients, a phenomenon usually ascribed to turbulence developing in a narrow or partially occluded tube.[19] If endogenous (bronchial) resistance must be determined precisely, airway pressure should be sensed beyond the carinal tip of the endotracheal tube. This can be done with an intra- or extraluminal catheter or with a tube specially designed for measuring pressure at this site during jet ventilation. Overall, expiratory resistance is influenced not only by the endotracheal tube and the endogenous properties of the airway (already noted to be higher than during inspiration), but also by the flow impedance of the exhalation valve.

Depending on tube type, length, diameter, patency, and angulation, computed values for inspiratory resistance may be dominated by the resistive properties of the artificial airway.

AUTO-PEEP (INTRINSIC PEEP) EFFECT

Dynamic hyperinflation and the auto-PEEP phenomenon occur when time intervals between successive tidal inflations are not sufficient to reestablish the equilibrium position of the respiratory system.[9,25] When a mechanical ventilator powers inflation, alveolar pressure remains continuously positive through both phases of the ventilatory cycle. Airflow does not cease at end exhalation but continues very slowly as alveolar pressure gradually decompresses through critically narrowed airways. During

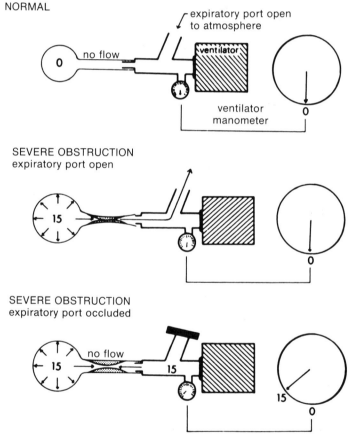

FIGURE 8   The auto-PEEP effect and its measurement by end-expiratory port occlusion. Auto-PEEP is defined as the positive-flow driving difference between alveolar pressure and applied pressure at end exhalation. AP can be quantified by central airway pressure within 0.5–1.5 seconds of expiratory port occlusion at end exhalation. From Pepe PE, Marini JJ: Occult positive end-expiratory pressure in mechanically ventilated patients with airflow obstruction. Am Rev Respir Dis 126:166, 1982. With permission.

Auto-PEEP is defined as the positive-flow driving difference between alveolar pressure and applied pressure at end exhalation.

apnea, as long as 40 seconds can elapse before flow completely stops. Auto-PEEP can be defined as the positive, flow-driving difference between alveolar and airway opening pressures at end expiration (Fig. 8). An auto-PEEP effect may be seen in virtually any circumstance causing a high demand for ventilation, even in patients without severe airflow obstruction. In patients without severe intrinsic airflow obstruction, auto-PEEP is largely the result of the high ventilation requirement and the resistance posed by the endotracheal tube and exhalation valve. Calculated airflow resistance may also be high when a substantial loss of patent air channels has occurred, as in the adult respiratory distress syndrome. Active muscular effort often contributes to the expiratory driving force and may cause alveolar pressure to remain positive at end exhalation, even without notable hyperinflation (Fig. 9). An auto-PEEP phenomenon has also been well described during high-frequency ventilation.[26]

The auto-PEEP effect has numerous hemodynamic and mechanical consequences. Barotrauma is an obvious risk. Furthermore, the hemodynamic problems associated with the auto-PEEP effect may be more severe than those incurred with PEEP of a similar level because obstructive lung disease enhances (while restrictive disease impairs) transmission of alveolar pressure to the pleural space. Auto-PEEP also adds to the work of breathing, presenting an increased threshold load to spontaneous inspiration and depressing the effective triggering sensitivity of the ventilator.[27-29] The addition of counterbalancing positive end-expiratory pressure (PEEP or CPAP) to patients with quantifiable auto-PEEP and expiratory flow limitation may im-

Auto-PEEP adds to the work of breathing, presenting an increased threshold load to spontaneous inspiration and depressing the effective triggering sensitivity of the ventilator. The addition of counterbalancing positive end-expiratory pressure (PEEP or CPAP) to patients with quantifiable auto-PEEP and expiratory flow limitation may improve subject comfort by relieving dyspnea and the work of breathing without markedly increasing lung volume or peak cycling pressure.

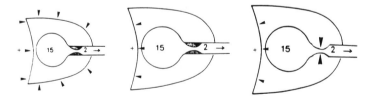

FIGURE 9   Three forms of auto-PEEP. Auto-PEEP can exist without dynamic hyperinflation (left panel) when vigorous expiratory muscle contraction persists to end expiration. Under conditions of passive inflation, auto-PEEP implies dynamic hyperinflation either without (middle) or with (right) expiratory flow limitation. In the presence of dynamic airway collapse, the addition of a modest amount of PEEP may improve effective triggering sensitivity and work of breathing. From Marini JJ: Lung mechanics in the adult respiratory distress syndrome: recent conceptual advances and implications for an arrangement. Clin Chest Med 11(4):673, 1990. With permission.

prove subject comfort by relieving dyspnea and the work of breathing without markedly increasing lung volume or peak cycling pressure.[29] If flow limitation is not present, however, adding PEEP simply presents a backpressure to expiratory gas flow and risks further hyperinflation without apparent benefit. As a general rule, PEEP more than sufficient to counterbalance auto-PEEP should not be added to patients with airflow obstruction. Furthermore, adding PEEP to already hyperinflated patients with airflow obstruction who are *passively* ventilated would appear to have little therapeutic rationale at the present time. If peak static pressure rises significantly in response to PEEP, additional hyperinflation is occuring and adding PEEP, therefore, is ill advised.

At the bedside, auto-PEEP can be estimated several ways (Table 1). Dynamic hyperinflation and auto-PEEP are suspected when significant flow persists to the very end of exhalation. Auto-PEEP (AP) is theoretically equivalent to the following expression:

$$AP = \frac{V_t}{[C(e^{t_e/RC} - 1)]}$$

where t_e is expiratory time and RC is the average exhalation time constant. If both end-expiratory resistance and flow were known, AP could be approximated as their quotient. Unfortunately, this is seldom the case. However, during passive ventilation, AP can be quantified by occluding the expiratory port of the ventilator at the end of the period allowed for exhalation between mechanical breaths [the end-expiratory port occlusion method (Fig. 8)].[25] This value averages all end-expiratory alveolar pressures, underestimating the highest and overestimating the lowest that actually exist. For accuracy, occlusion must occur at the appropriate time and persist for 0.5 seconds or longer—timing that is easiest to achieve during controlled ventilation. Delay of ventilator cycling can be achieved by markedly reducing frequency at the time of measurement. Several ventilators currently available facilitate prolongation of the exhalation phase by maintaining closure of the exhalation valve at the end of the set expiratory time, delaying the next breath and simplifying the measurement.

In my practice, I have made use of the fact that auto-PEEP must approximate the difference between end-inspiratory static pressure (plateau pressure) and the sum of (V_t/C and PEEP):

$$AP = P_S - \left(\frac{V_t}{C} + PEEP\right)$$

TABLE 1   Techniques for Estimating Auto-PEEP

1. End-expiratory port occlusion
2. Applied PEEP "counterbalancing"
3. Post maneuver change in P_s
4. $P_s - [(V_T/C) + PEEP]$
5. Proto-inspiratory "counterbalancing"
   Controlled (P_{aw})
   Spontaneous (P_{es})

During passive constant-flow conditions, C_{RS} can be estimated from the average slope of the inspiratory airway pressure curve. (As already noted, accurate measurement of C_{RS} requires prior knowledge of AP.) P_{ZF} may be a more appropriate end-inspiratory value to use than P_S under dynamic tidal conditions (without a pause applied). The validity of this assumption, however, has not been formally tested.

Recording the change in peak static pressure that occurs during passive ventilation as the delivered minute ventilation is dramatically reduced can be used to estimate AP. Alternatively, because the pressure associated with dynamic hyperinflation is the quotient of trapped volume and compliance, recording the volume change provides invaluable information.

Alternative methods to quantify AP directly require specialized sensing equipment and displays. During controlled inflation, AP can theoretically be measured by noting the airway pressure at which inspiratory flow begins.[9] During spontaneous efforts, the deflection of esophageal pressure needed to initiate inspiratory flow can be used to quantify the pressure needed to counterbalance the expiratory action of elastic recoil. This counterbalancing pressure, however, tends to be lower than the AP measured under passive conditions, for two reasons. First, the pressure required to initiate inspiratory flow is the pressure counterbalancing those units with the least AP. Furthermore, it does not account for the contribution to AP made by chest wall recoil at hyperexpanded volumes; only lung recoil is counterbalanced by changes in P_{es}.

Finally, it has been suggested that AP can be estimated as the lowest PEEP level that causes a detectable increase in lung volume, measured by impedance plethysmography.[30] For patients with dynamic airway compression, this may be approximately correct; for those without dynamic airway compression, it is unlikely to be correct.[31]

MEASURING ESOPHAGEAL PRESSURE

With rare exception, fluctuations of global pleural pressure are sensed in the esophagus using a well-positioned balloon catheter. Esophageal pressure recording enables estimation of the force generated during spontaneous breathing and facilitates partitioning of transthoracic pressure into its lung and chest wall components during passive inflation.

Esophageal pressure recording enables estimation of the force generated during spontaneous breathing and facilitates partitioning of transthoracic pressure into its lung and chest wall components during passive inflation.

Technique

Esophageal pressure is measured with a latex balloon (≈ 10 cm long) positioned in the lower or middle third of the esophagus[32] and affixed to a multiperforated catheter stent. A spiral arrangement of the catheter holes is desirable. The 10 cm length samples an adequate portion of the esophagus while minimizing artifact. (A shorter balloon can be influenced by regional pressure distortions arising near the heart and posterior mediastinum. A longer balloon may extend into the upper esophagus, a region that poorly reflects changes in global intrapleural pressure.[32,33]) A balloon volume of 0.2–0.5 ml transmits changes in intrathoracic pressure accurately during spontaneous cycles, while larger balloon volumes may stimulate esophageal contractions. However, to maintain sensitivity during positive pressure breathing cycles, a relatively large balloon volume (0.5–1.0 ml) is usually required. Larger volumes in this range prevent the balloon from collapsing against the catheter stent and damping the pressure signal. In the upright position P_{es} reflects the absolute value of global intrathoracic pressure with acceptable accuracy, but in the supine posture P_{es} overestimates the average resting intrathoracic pressure. Because the esophagus is a posterior structure, the weight of the mediastinal contents on the sensing balloon produces this artifact, which may be reduced or eliminated by assuming the lateral decubitus position.[34] Although P_{es} overestimates average pleural pressure in recumbency, changes in intrathoracic pressure are tracked well by a balloon in appropriate position.[35] The impact of a coexisting nasogastric or feeding tube on the accuracy of P_{es} has not been well studied; however, experiments in our laboratory suggest that a multiperforated esophageal balloon catheter continues to reflect changes in intrathoracic pressure with accuracy acceptable for clinical purposes.

To position the esophageal balloon during spontaneous breathing, one must first pass it into the stomach, a site identified by positive deflections of pressure during forceful inspiratory efforts (sniff test). The balloon is then withdrawn gradually until negative pressure deflections first appear, signaling the entry of the uppermost hole of the balloon-enveloped portion of the catheter into the intrathorcic compartment. (Multiperforated catheters tend to transmit the most negative pressure to which the balloon is exposed.) The catheter is then withdrawn a distance equivalent to the balloon length (≈ 10 cm) to ensure that the entire sensing area rests in the lower and mid-esophagus.[32] Appropriate position can be confirmed by mea-

Although P_{es} overestimates average pleural pressure in recumbency, changes in intrathoracic pressure are tracked well by a balloon in appropriate position.

suring airway and esophageal pressure deflections simultaneously during spontaneous efforts against an occluded airway.[36] When airway occlusion prevents gas from flowing into the lungs, no pressure can dissipate against resistance during breathing efforts and lung volume remains unchanged. It follows that, on average, no pressure gradient should develop between the occluded airway opening and the pleural space. Deflections of airway and esophageal pressure should therefore agree, within approximately 10% (Fig. 10).[35] Precise balloon placement is difficult if spontaneous efforts are not present. Using approximate anatomical guidelines, the balloon tip is usually advanced about 40 cm from the nostril.

Combined nasogastric tube and esophageal balloon catheters that serve a dual clinical purpose have been commercially available for a number of years. These catheters appear to track changes in intrathoracic pressure quite well, while simultaneously providing a channel for aspirating stomach contents or administering liquid feedings.[37]

Uses of Esophageal Pressure

Changes in esophageal pressure offer useful information when interpreting the end-expiratory wedge pressure under conditions of vigorous hyperpnea or elevated alveolar pressure (PEEP, AP).[38] As already noted, the P_{es} tracing allows calculation of lung compliance, airway resistance, and AP during spontaneous breathing and therefore helps partition the total impedance of the respiratory system into its lung and chest wall components. ΔP_{es} reflects the magnitude of patient effort during spontaneous or machine-aided breathing cycles. Although seldom employed clinically for this purpose, ΔP_{es} can be used to compute the work of breathing across the lung and external circuit or to calculate the product of developed pressure and the duration of inspiratory effort (the pressure–time product). Fluctuations in central venous pressure can be used for a similar purpose,[39] but the vascular pressure tracing is variably damped and therefore yields a low-range estimate of effort.

Transdiaphragmatic Pressure

Transdiaphragmatic pressure (P_{di}), the difference between P_{es} and gastric pressure (P_{ga}), is generated by a single inspiratory muscle (the diaphragm) and is used primarily in the research setting to quantify its effective contractile force.[40] although P_{di} is seldom used clinically, it is occa-

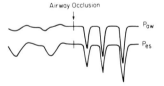

FIGURE 10 During total occlusion of the external airway, a well-positioned esophageal balloon should transmit a pressure deflection nearly equivalent to that within the central airway. (This is true regardless of the accuracy of P_{es} as an estimate of absolute pleural pressure.)

sionally employed in conjunction with phrenic nerve stimulation or voluntary effort (eg, inspiration to total lung capacity, Müeller maneuver, forceful sniffing) to investigate the possibility of diaphragmatic paralysis.

INFLATION IMPEDANCE: VALUE OF CONTINUOUSLY MONITORING P_{aw}

A continuous tracing of airway pressure provides useful information commonly neglected at the bedside.

A continuous tracing of airway pressure provides useful information commonly neglected at the bedside. For convenience, airway pressure can be monitored using the transducer and display equipment normally used for measuring pressures in the pulmonary vasculature. An air-filled transducer dedicated to gas pressure measurement must be exclusively assigned to this purpose, however, in order to eliminate the risk of air embolism. Apart from enabling the estimation of R and C_{RS}, the waveform of inspiratory airway pressure traced during a controlled machine cycle provides a graphic representation of the inflation work performed by the ventilator at the particular combination of tidal volume and flow settings used (Fig. 11). As already noted, time and volume are linear analogs when inflation occurs passively under constant flow conditions. The slope of the airway pressure curve therefore reflects dynamic compliance, and the area under the pressure–time curve is proportional to the pressure–volume work performed per breath by the machine.[14] The mean inflation pressure ($\bar{P}_i$) is the work per liter of ventilation for the

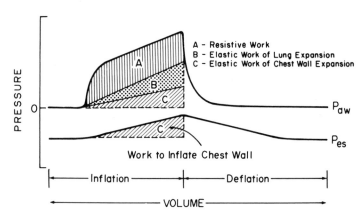

FIGURE 11   Work to inflate the lung and chest wall during a passive machine cycle delivered with constant flow. The pressure–volume area is composed of subcomponents related to various forms of frictional and elastic work. From Marini JJ: Strategies to minimize breathing effort during mechanical ventilation. Crit Care Clin 6(3):635, 1990. With permission.

particular combination of tidal volume and flow settings in use. Provided that flow and tidal volume do not change, $\overline{P}_i$ indexes the average impedance to chest inflation. (Under passive, constant flow conditions, $\overline{P}_i$ can also be estimated from P_D and P_S without recording the pressure tracing by using the approximation:

$$\overline{P}_i = P_D - \frac{[P_S - (PEEP + AP)]}{2}$$

Mean airway pressure for the entire breathing cycle, a value correlated with gas exchange efficiency, hemodynamic compromise, fluid retention, and the incidence of barotrauma, can be estimated as the product of $\overline{P}_i$ and the inspiratory time fraction, adjusted for the effect of applied PEEP:

$$\overline{P_{aw}} = \overline{P}_i \left(\frac{t_i}{t_{tot}}\right) + PEEP \left(1 - \frac{t_i}{t_{tot}}\right)$$

Mean alveolar pressure ($\overline{P_{alv}}$) deviates from mean airway pressure only when expiratory (R_x and inspiratory (R_i) resistance differ significantly (Fig. 12)[41]:

$$\overline{P_{alv}} = \overline{P_{aw}} + (R_x - R_i)\left(\frac{\dot{V}_E}{60}\right)$$

As this equation implies, mean alveolar pressure may greatly exceed mean airway pressure under conditions of high minute ventilation requirement and relatively high expiratory resistance.

Mean alveolar pressure may greatly exceed mean airway pressure under conditions of high minute ventilation requirement and relatively high expiratory resistance.

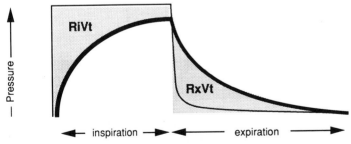

FIGURE 12   Airway (fine line) and alveolar (heavy line) pressures during pressure preset ventilation. Alveolar pressure builds and decays exponentially during inspiration and expiration, respectively. Flow is driven by the difference between airway and alveolar pressures on inspiration (shaded) as by alveolar pressure alone on expiration (shaded) mP$_{aw}$ and mP$_{alv}$ pressures are equivalent if R_iV_t equals the R_xV_t. Therefore, mP$_{aw}$ = mP$_{alv}$ if $R_i = R_x$.

MONITORING BREATHING EFFORT

MEASURES OF RESPIRATORY MUSCLE ACTIVITY

Oxygen Consumption of the Respiratory System

Two patients with different chest configurations, patterns of muscle activation, or degrees of coordination among the muscles of inspiration and expiration may perform identical external work but consume vastly different amounts of oxygen in the process.

Although the resting oxygen consumption rate of the ventilatory muscles during spontaneous breathing is usually less than 5% of the total body requirement, the energetic cost of breathing during acute respiratory failure may raise that percentage ten-fold.[42] Were it possible, selectively measuring the oxygen consumption rate of the ventilatory pump ($\dot{V}O_2R$) would estimate breathing effort at the basic level of cellular metabolism. Although difficult to measure, $\dot{V}O_2R$ theoretically accounts for all factors that tax the respiratory muscles, integrating the stresses imposed by external workload (W_B) and those related to any lack of efficiency (E) of the conversion mechanism: $\dot{V}O_2R = W_B/E$.[43] Two patients with different chest configurations, patterns of muscle activation, or degrees of coordination among the muscles of inspiration and expiration may perform identical external work but consume vastly different amounts of oxygen in the process.

Because $\dot{V}O_2R$ cannot be measured directly, total body oxygen consumption ($\dot{V}O_2$) is tracked as ventilatory stresses (for example, resistance or CO_2 inhalation) are imposed or relieved, thereby perturbing the respiratory system. Without question, there is considerable "background-to-signal" and "noise-to-signal" interference in such computations, and consequently $\dot{V}O_2$ does not lend itself to assessing breathing effort in the quasi-stable, critically ill patient. Furthermore, high levels of inspired oxygen present a major technical challenge. Unless extreme care is taken, these problems cannot be reliably overcome with present technology.

Electromyography

In current intensive care unit practice, the combination of transcutaneous nerve stimulation and electromyography (EMG) recording is often used to monitor the depth of pharmacologic paralysis during mechanical ventilation. Electromyography can also be used to assess respiratory muscle activity. The amplitude of an integrated, rectified electromyographic signal varies directly with the tension developed by the muscle it monitors.[44] In the laboratory setting, diaphragmatic EMG is best sensed by an electrode anchored at the gastroesophageal junction.[45] Unfortunately, such electrodes are difficult to position and cannot be left in place for long periods. Furthermore, unless filtered out, the amplitude of the electrocardiographic (ECG) signal can complicate quantitative interpretation of the integrated value. Surface EMG is more convenient, but specificity of the probe for the small area of underlying muscle limits its utility as a global measure of ventilatory effort. Furthermore, the integrated surface EMG fails to discriminate between the activation of inspiratory and expiratory muscles, between tonic and phasic activity, or between respiratory and nonrespiratory muscle activity. Finally, because the amplitude of the EMG varies widely with site preparation, electrode location, and patient anatomy, no absolute standards exist for comparing breathing effort across patients.[45] Like $\dot{V}O_2R$, the EMG is limited to tracking *relative* changes in the activity of the ventilatory system. Despite these drawbacks, EMG of the sternocleidomastoid muscle, an accessory muscle of respiration activated only when the system is under significant stress, holds great potential as a practical means of monitoring ventilatory effort.[46]

Direct Measures of External Mechanical Output

Work of Breathing
The mechanical work of breathing (a term defined by the laws of physics) and breathing effort are not synonymous terms. As already noted, if the breathing pattern is inefficient, great effort can be expended without developing forceful pressures or accomplishing measurable external mechanical work. Nonetheless, certain pressures and volumes are precisely measurable, and for the same patient tend to fluctuate in the same direction as breathing effort.

The mechanical work of breathing and breathing effort are not synonymous terms.

Quantifying Total Work of Chest Inflation
The mechanical work of inspiration is performed when volume is moved by a pressure gradient applied across the lung. At any volume above the equilibrium position, the total pressure difference applied is distributed in accordance with the simplified "equation of motion" of the respiratory system[1]:

$$P_i = R(\dot{V}) + \frac{V}{C}$$

The average pressure ($\overline{P}_i$) developed during tidal inflation can be approximated:

$$\overline{P}_i \approx R_i \left(\frac{V_t}{t_i}\right) + \frac{V_t}{2C} + P_{ex} \qquad (5)$$

In this expression, P_{ex} is the end-expiratory alveolar pressure, and t_i and V_t are inspiratory time and tidal volume. $\overline{P}_i$ (the average transstructural pressure) is numerically equivalent to the work per liter of ventilation.[47] Thus, if R_i, C, t_i, and V_t are known for the spontaneously breathing subject, the *external* work rate can be easily estimated. Work per tidal breath can be quantified from the area enclosed within a plot of transmural inflation pressure against inspired volume or from the integrated product of P_i and $\dot{V}$:

$$W_B = \int_0^{t_i} P_i \dot{V} dt$$

Total inspiratory mechanical work per minute (power) is the product of P_i and $\dot{V}_E$, or of W_B and f, the breathing frequency. If inflation is achieved with constant flow, P_i is approximated by the inflation pressure at midcycle (Fig. 11). With pressures and volumes expressed in their customary units, a convenient work unit is the joule or watt-second (1 joule $\approx$ 10 cmH$_2$O l). One kilogram meter (kgm), another work unit, equals about 10 joules.

To accurately estimate the work rate of spontaneous breathing, flow delivery during passive inflation must approximate the mean inspiratory flow rate of spontaneous breathing and its flow waveform, and the delivered tidal volume must also be the same. Unfortunately, such preconditions are seldom accomplished without deep sedation or paralysis. A number of approximations appear to compensate satisfactorily for differences between machine delivered and spontaneous cycles.[48]

Patient Work During Spontaneous and Machine-Aided Cycles
Triggered Volume-limited Machine Cycles. During flow-controlled, volume-cycled ventilation, patient effort has generally been assumed negligible whenever the machine aids the breathing cycle. This assumption is undoubtedly correct during controlled ventilation, but recent data indicate that it is often invalid during patient-triggered, machine assisted (Assist-Control) inflation.[49,50] Relaxation does not occur abruptly once the machine cycle begins. Rather, effort continues in proportion to respira-

If R_i, C, t_i, and V_t are known for the spontaneously breathing subject, the external work rate can be easily estimated.

Relaxation does not occur abruptly once the machine cycle begins.

tory drive and muscle strength.[50] Stated differently, the patient and machine work together to move the tidal volume at the specified rate. Assuming that similar external work is required to inflate the chest under passive and active conditions, the external work performed by the patient can be quantified from the difference in machine's work component in these two circumstances (Fig. 13). Similarity of the total mechanical workload can be assumed when impedance does not change and flow and tidal volume remain constant. When the ventilation requirement or sense of dyspnea is high, or when the ventilator is poorly adjusted, exertion levels during machine assistance may approach those of unsupported breathing. Interestingly, the impedance characteristics of the chest (R and C) do not influence the patient's effort significantly during assist-control cycles, provided that the ventilator satisfies the patient's demand for inspiratory flow.

Any factor that amplifies respiratory drive adds to the patient's work of breathing during these triggered machine cycles. Trigger sensitivity, peak flow setting, tidal volume, and end-expiratory pressure are the key physician-con-

When the ventilation requirement or sense of dyspnea is high, or when the ventilator is poorly adjusted, exertion levels during machine assistance may approach those of unsupported breathing.

Trigger sensitivity, peak flow setting, tidal volume, and end-expiratory pressure are the key physician-controlled variables.

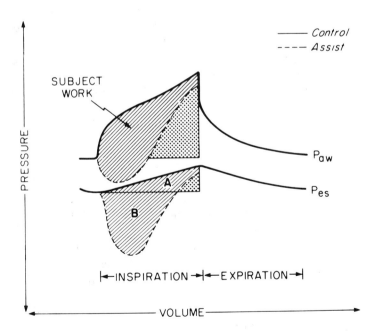

FIGURE 13   Two methods of computing subject work during machine-assisted cycles from active and passive P_{aw} and P_{es}. Area A represents subject work done across the chest wall, whereas area B represents subject work expended across the lung and external circuit. Modified from Marini JJ: Monitoring during mechanical ventilation. Clin Chest Med 9(1):73, 1988. With permission.

trolled variables. Clues to patient exertion during triggered machine cycles are available from inspection of the deformed and variable airway pressure tracing. When an airway pressure tracing is not used, the only hint of vigorous inspiratory effort may be the stuttering rise of the ventilator's manometer needle toward its peak value, usually varying over time. P_D itself may not be far different from the expected value, as patient effort weakens as lung volume increases toward the end of the inflation cycle.

Although the work of breathing can be estimated using the equation of motion, an esophageal balloon is required to directly measure mechanical work across the lung during spontaneous or pressure-supported breathing cycles.

Spontaneous Breathing Cycles. Although the work of breathing can be estimated using the equation of motion (see Equation 5), an esophageal balloon is required to directly measure mechanical work across the lung during spontaneous or pressure-supported breathing cycles. The fluctuation in the segment of pleural pressure tracing that spans inspiration tracks patient effort against the impedance of the lung and external circuit. Care must be taken to include any component attributable to AP. (When PEEP or continuous positive airway pressure [CPAP] is used, fluctuations of pressure should be referenced to the elevated baseline value of P_{es}.) Inspiratory work can be quantified by electronically integrating the product of P_{es} and flow or by measuring the area within a plot of P_{es} against inspired volume. The work done in expanding the chest wall cannot be directly measured during active breathing and must be estimated from published values of chest wall compliance, or preferably from the inflation characteristic of the passive chest wall ($P_{es} \cdot V$) traced during controlled (relaxed) inflation. The pressure required to inflate the passive chest wall is largely independent of the flow profile.

Pressure-supported Cycles. During ventilation with pressure support (PSV), the pressure contour remains essentially unchanged cycle-to-cycle, but the flow profile varies with changes in impedance and patient effort. Consequently, total work varies. Under these circumstances, airway pressure tracks only machine work and cannot be used directly in assessing patient effort. The patient's component of the total inspiratory work of breathing can be gauged, nonetheless, using plots of esophageal pressure and inspired volume during passive and pressure-supported inflations of similar depth and duration. The patient's work during the pressure-supported breath can be roughly estimated as the difference between the total work required from the machine–patient system (gauged from the equation of motion) and the amount of work provided by the machine alone $\approx P_S \cdot V_t$.

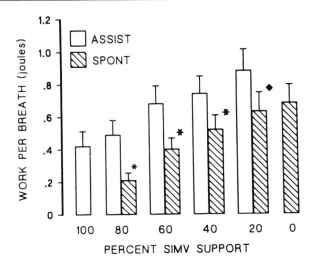

FIGURE 14   Work per breath during SIMV. Note that work out-put per breath was significantly greater (* $P < 0.05$) for ma-chine-assisted cycles at each level. From Marini JJ, Smith TC, Lamb VJ: External work output and force generation during synchronized intermittent mechanical ventilation: effect of ma-chine assistance on breathing effort. Am Rev Respir Dis 138:1169, 1988. With permission.

Pressure–Time Product and Pressure–Time Index

Isometric components of muscle tension (which consume oxygen without contributing to volume change) fail to reg-ister as externally measured work, accounting in large part for the lack of agreement between $\dot{V}O_2R$ and W_B.[51] A pres-sure–time product (PTP = $\overline{P}_i \cdot t_i$) parallels effort and $\dot{V}O_2R$ more closely than W_B because it includes the "isometric" component of muscle pressure and is less influenced by the impedance to contraction.[52] Comparison of work and pressure–time products during the intermittent unloading of synchronized intermittent mandatory ventilation (SIMV) brings these considerations into sharp relief.[53] Here, calculation of workload would erroneously suggest effort to be greater during machine-aided cycles (Fig. 14). In fact, for the dyspneic subject, the pressure time products are similar.

When P_i is referenced to the maximal isometric pressure that can be generated at FRC (Pmax) and inspiratory time is expressed as a fraction of total cycle length (t_{tot}), a po-tentially useful effort index (pressure–time index [PTI]) is derived[36]:

$$PTI = \overline{P}_i/P_Imax \times t_i/t_{tot}$$

During full cooperation, values of PTI that exceed ≈ 0.15 identify highly stressful breathing workloads that may induce fatigue.

During full cooperation, values of PTI that exceed ≈ 0.15 identify highly stressful breathing workloads that may induce fatigue. The PTI can therefore be regarded as an (inverse) indicator of endurance. Unfortunately, whereas $\bar{P}_i$ is relatively simple to estimate, P_Imax is very difficult to measure in critically ill subjects. Techniques that enforce breathing effort, such as the use of a one-way valve in conjunction with drive stimulation by CO_2 inhalation[54] may eventually prove useful in this assessment.

Influence of AP on W_B Because pressure sufficient to counterbalance AP must be applied before flow can be initiated, AP imposes an inspiratory threshold load. Furthermore, a "block" of external work (Fig. 1) dimensioned by AP forms an important part of the total pressure–volume work described by the equation of motion (equation 5):

$$W_B = \bar{P}_i \cdot V_t$$

$$W_B \approx R \left(\frac{V_t^2}{t_i} \right) + \left(\frac{V_t^2}{2C} \right) + (AP)\, V_t$$

(During work calculations of triggered machine cycles, the additional work imposed by AP is accounted for in the proportional elevation of the baseline control curve.) The threshold load imposed by AP effectively reduces the trigger sensitivity of the machine to a value equal to the sum of AP and the set value. Recent experimental work indicates that judicious use of low levels of CPAP or PEEP can help restore trigger sensitivity and reduce the work of breathing.[28,29,55]

SPIROMETRIC MEASUREMENTS

VITAL CAPACITY

In acute disorders of neuromuscular function, VC tends to be preserved relative to P_Imax for two primary reasons. First, the pressure–volume relationship of the thorax is convex to the volume axis. Second, whereas many seriously ill patients can generate brief spikes of inspiratory pressure, few can or will sustain inspiratory effort long enough to achieve the plateau of their volume curve. Depending on the information desired from the VC, a "stacked" VC may be useful in this setting (Fig. 15).[56] The stacking technique measures volume on the inspiratory limb and uses a one-way valve to enable the patient to rest

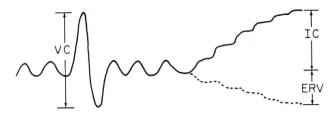

FIGURE 15   Vital capacity (VC) measured by conventional and "stacked" spirometry. Inspiratory capacity (IC) and expiratory reserve volume (ERV) can be measured using an appropriately directed one-way valve during spontaneous breathing.

at an elevated volume between inspiratory efforts. The patient need not cooperate fully with testing—the naturally escalating inspiratory drive to breathe evokes forceful effort, especially when stimulated by inspired CO_2 or dead space rebreathing. For the same achieved volume, the peak esophageal pressures developed during breath stacking and during the standard inspiratory capacity (IC) maneuver are similar. Use of the breath-stacking technique may also allow more effective incentive spirometry, particularly with respect to the duration of hyperinflation.[57] A large discrepancy between the depth and duration of the conventional and breath-stacked VC may be seen in patients to weak, too uncooperative, or too air hungry to sustain a single inspiratory effort. Although a stacked VC may reflect the elastic properties of the lungs and chest wall more accurately than a conventional VC maneuver, its ability to accurately reflect muscle strength has yet to be determined.

As the supine position is assumed, vital capacity falls by less than 20% in normal individuals and by only slightly more in patients with unilateral diaphragmatic paralysis. A positional change in VC > 30% suggests bilateral diaphragmatic dysfunction or paralysis, particularly if paradoxical abdominal motion and orthopnea are observed. Although fluoroscopy can be helpful in detecting *unilateral* diaphragmatic paralysis, there are many false negative tests. Fluoroscopy is even more unreliable when both leaves of the diaphragm are dysfunctional. When suspected, diaphragmatic dysfunction can be confirmed best using esophageal and gastric pressure measurements to compute transdiaphragmatic pressure during deep breaths or forceful efforts (Table 2).

OTHER SPIROMETRIC DATA

Few critically ill patients can perform forced spirometry adequately. Nonetheless, measurements of peak flow and FEV_1, useful in guiding management decisions, can gen-

Use of the breath-stacking technique may allow more effective incentive spirometry, particularly with respect to the duration of hyperinflation.

TABLE 2	Diaphragm Weakness

Orthopnea
Paradoxical abdominal
  motion
ΔVC, sitting to supine
  >30%
Transdiaphragmatic
  pressure
    <25 cmH_2O at TLC
    <60 cmH_2O maximal

erally be obtained in asthmatic subjects and those with ex-acerbated COPD. Furthermore, a great deal of useful data is often available on the spirogram or flow tracing of tidal breathing. Persistent flow at end expiration indicates the presence of AP, and a linear or kinked flow profile suggests flow limitation during tidal exhalation.[58] During sponta-neous ventilation, a ratio of frequency to tidal volume that exceeds 100 breaths/min/l documents a pattern of rapid shallow breathing that is unlikely to be sustained. The abil-ity of a patient to double resting minute ventilation indi-cates a considerable reserve of muscular power. Delay of a ventilator-delivered breath during passive ventilation al-lows measurement of the volume of trapped gas.[59]

MONITORING STRENGTH AND MUSCLE RESERVE

The ability of the patient to sustain independent breathing must not be judged on the basis of any absolute value for workload, but rather on workload interpreted against the background of muscular strength and endurance.

The output demanded of the ventilatory muscles is dictated by the product of $\dot{V}_E$ and the work or oxygen cost per liter of ventilation (discussed previously). However, the ability of the patient to sustain independent breathing must not be judged on the basis of any absolute value for workload, but rather on workload interpreted against the background of muscular strength and endurance. Without full patient cooperation it is questionable that any measure of strength can reflect the full capability for pressure development. The two measures of respiratory muscle strength most com-monly employed in the clinical setting are the vital capacity (just discussed) and the maximum inspiratory pressure (MIP) generated against an occluded airway.[23]

MAXIMAL INSPIRATORY PRESSURE

Assuming full cooperation, a symmetrical reduction in in-spiratory and expiratory maximal respiratory pressures strongly suggests generalized muscle weakness. (Al-though maximal expiratory pressures are seldom measured in critically ill patients, a good qualitative indication of ex-piratory muscle strength can sometimes be observed in the vigor of the coughing effort.) When recording the MIP, lung volume should be trapped in the range between re-sidual volume and FRC to optimize the mechanical advan-tage of the inspiratory muscles.[60-62] In poorly cooperative subjects, it is equally important to wait sufficient time to elicit a near maximal increase in respiratory drive.

Approximately 20 seconds or 10 breathing efforts are re-quired to elicit the maximal pressure response from a poorly cooperative patient.[63] The patient must neither be overventilated nor overstressed before data recording, and occlusion of the airway must occur at FRC or lesser volume. Introducing a one-way valve that selectively permits expiration ensures that inspiratory efforts initiated late in the series occur at a volume between FRC and residual volume. With each breathing effort, additional air is pumped from the thorax, improving the mechanical advantage of the inspiratory muscles and amplifying respiratory drive.[60,64] Measured in this way, the MIP of most patients on mechanical ventilation exceeds -40 mmHg (-52 cmH$_2$O), even as they remain ventilator dependent.[63]

References

1. Otis AB, Fenn WO, Rahn H: Mechanics of breathing in man. J Appl Physiol 2:592, 1950

2. Chadha TS, Watson H, Birch S et al: Validation of respiratory inductive plethysmography using different calibration procedures. Am Rev Respir Dis 125:644, 1982

3. Blanch L, Fernandez R, Benito S et al: Effect of PEEP on the arterial end-tidal carbon dioxide gradient. Chest 92:451, 1987

4. Suter PM, Fairley HB, Isenberg MD: Optimum end-expiratory pressure in patients with acute pulmonary failure. N Engl J Med 292:284, 1975

5. Suter PM: Appropriate lung distention for gas exchange in ARDS. Chest 85:4, 1984

6. Lamy M, Fallat RJ, Koeniger E et al: Pathologic features and mechanics of hypoxemia in adult respiratory distress syndrome. Am Rev Respir Dis 114:267, 1976

7. Matamis D, LeMaire F, Harf A et al: Total respiratory pressure volume curves in the adult respiratory distress syndrome. Chest 86:58, 1984

8. Comroe JH: Physiology of respiration. Yearbook Medical Publishers, Chicago, 1974

9. Rossi A, Gottfried SB, Zocchi L et al: Measurement of static compliance of the total respiratory system in patients with acute respiratory failure during mechanical ventilation: the effect of intrinsic positive end-expiratory pressure. Am Rev Respir Dis 131:672, 1985

10. O'Quin R, Marini JJ, Culver BH, Butler J: Transmission of airway pressure to the pleural space during lung edema and chest wall restriction. J Appl Physiol 59(4):1171, 1985

11. Benito S, LeMaire F: Pulmonary pressure-volume relationship in acute respiratory distress syndrome in adults: role of positive end-expiratory pressure. J Crit Care 5:27, 1990

12. Kaz JA, Zinn SE, Ozanne GM et al: Pulmonary, chest wall, and lung-thorax elastances in acute respiratory failure. Chest 80:304, 1981

13. Chapin JC, Downs JB, Douglas ME et al: Lung expansion, airway pressure transmission and positive end-expiratory pressure. Arch Surg 114:1193, 1979

14. Marini JJ, Rodriguez RM, Lamb VJ: Bedside estimation of the inspiratory work of breathing during mechanical ventilation. Chest 89(1):56, 1986

15. Capps JS, Hicks GH: Monitoring non-gas respiratory variables during mechanical ventilation. Respir Care 32:558, 1987

16. Bone RC: Monitoring ventilatory mechanics in acute respiratory failure. Respir Care 28:597, 1983

17. Gay PC, Rodarte JR, Tayyab M et al: Evaluation of bronchodilator responsiveness in mechanically ventilated patients. Am Rev Respir Dis 136:880, 1987

18. Bates JTM, Rossi A, Milic-Emili J: Analysis of the behavior of the respiratory system with constant inspiratory flow. J Appl Physiol 58:1840, 1985

19. Gottfried SB, Rossi A, Higgs BD et al: Noninvasive determination of respiratory system mechanics during mechanical ventilation for acute respiratory failure. Am Rev Respir Dis 131:672, 1985

20. Rossi A, Gottfried SB, Higgs BD et al: Respiratory mechanics in mechanically ventilated patients with respiratory failure. J Appl Physiol 58:1849, 1985

21. Kimball WR, Leith DE, Robins AG: Dynamic hyperinflation and ventilator dependence in chronic obstructive pulmonary disease. Am Rev Respir Dis 126:991, 1982

22. O'Donnell DE, Sanii R, Anthonisen NR, Younes M: Effect of dynamic airway compression on breathing pattern and respiratory sensation in severe chronic obstructive pulmonary disease. Am Rev Respir Dis 135:912, 1987

23. Sahn SA, Lakshminarayan S, Petty TL: Weaning from mechanical ventilation. JAMA 235:2208,1976

24. Wright PW, Marini JJ, Bernard GR: In vitro versus in vivo comparison of endotracheal tube airflow resistance. Am Rev Respir Dis 140(1):10, 1989

25. Pepe PE, Marini JJ: Occult positive end-expiratory pressure in mechanically ventilated patients with airflow obstruction. Am Rev Respir Dis 126:166, 1982

26. Simon BA, Weinmann C, Mitzner W: Mean airway pressure and alveolar pressure during high frequency ventilation. J Appl Physiol 57:1069, 1984

27. Fleury BD, Murciano D, Talamo C et al: Work of breathing in patients with chronic obstructive pulmonary disease in acute respiratory failure. Am Rev Respir Dis 131:822, 1985

28. Smith TC, Marini JJ, Lamb VJ: The effect of PEEP on auto-PEEP (Abstr). Chest 89:443S, 1986

29. Smith TC, Marini JJ, Lamb VJ: The inspiratory threshold load resulting from airtrapping during mechanical ventilation (Abstr). Am Rev Respir Dis 135:A52, 1987

30. Hoffman RA, Ershowsky P, Krieger BP: Determination of auto-PEEP during spontaneous and controlled ventilation by monitoring dogs in end expiratory thoracic gas volume. Chest 96(3):613, 1989

31. Marini JJ: Should PEEP be used in airflow obstruction? (editorial) Am Rev Respir Dis 140(1):1, 1989

32. Macklem PT: Procedures for standardized measurements of lung mechanics. National Health Institute, Division of Lung Disease, Bethesda, 1974

33. Knowles JH, Henry SK, Rahn H: Possible errors using esophageal balloon in determination of pressure-volume characteristics of the lung and thoracic cage. J Appl Physiol 14:525, 1959

34. Craven KD, Wood LDH: Extrapericardial and esophageal pressures with positive end-expiratory pressure in dogs. J Appl Physiol 51:798, 1981

35. Baydur A, Behrakis K, Zin A et al: A simple method for assessing the validity of esophageal balloon technique. Am Rev Respir Dis 126:788, 1982

36. Bellemare F, Grassino A: Effect of pressure and timing of contraction on human diaphragm failure. J Appl Physiol 53:1190, 1982

37. Gillespie DJ: Comparison of intraesophageal balloon pressure measurements with a nasogastric-esophageal balloon system in volunteers. Am Rev Respir Dis 126:583, 1982

38. Marini JJ: Hemodynamic monitoring using the pulmonary artery catheter. Crit Care Clin 2(3):551, 1986

39. Smiseth OA, Refsum H, Tyberg JV: Pericardial pressure assessed by right atrial pressure: a basis for calculation of left ventricular transmural pressure. Am Heart J 108:603, 1984

40. Nunn JF: Applied respiratory physiology. Butterworths, Boston, 1977

41. Marini JJ: Lung mechanics in the adult respiratory distress syndrome: recent conceptual advances and implications for management. Clin Chest Med 11(4):673, 1990

42. Field S, Kelly SM, Macklem PT: The oxygen cost of breathing in patients with cardiorespiratory disease. Am Rev Respir Dis 126:9, 1982

43. Roussos C, Campbell EJM: Respiratory muscle energetics. p. 481. In Fishman AP, Macklem PT, Mead J (eds): Handbook of physiology. American Physiological Society, Bethesda, 1986

44. Bigland B, Lippold OCJ: The relation between force, velocity and integrated electrical activity in human muscles. J Physiol (Lond) 123:214, 1954

45. Loring SH, Bruce EW: Methods for study of the chest wall. p. 415. In Fishman AP, Macklem PT, Mead J (eds): Handbook of physiology. American Physiological Society, Bethesda, 1986

46. Moxham J, Wiles CM, Newham D et al: Sternomastoid muscle function and fatigue in man. Clin Sci Mol Med 59:463, 1980

47. Marini JJ: The role of the inspiratory circuit in the work of breathing during mechanical ventilation. Respir Care 32(6):419, 1987

48. Truwit JD, Marini JJ, Lamb VJ: The work of spontaneous breathing can be predicted noninvasively during mechanical ventilation (Abstr). Am Rev Respir Dis 137:64, 1988

49. Marini JJ, Capps JS, Culver BH: The inspiratory work of breathing during assisted mechanical ventilation. Chest 87(5):612, 1985

50. Marini JJ, Rodriguez RM, Lamb VJ: The inspiratory workload of patient-initiated mechanical ventilation. Am Rev Respir Dis 134:902, 1986

51. McGregor M, Becklake M: The relationship of oxygen cost of breathing to respiratory mechanical work and respiratory force. J Clin Invest 40:971, 1961

52. Roussos C: Energetics. p. 437. Roussos C, Macklem PT (eds): The thorax. Marcel Dekker, New York, 1985

53. Marini JJ, Smith TC, Lamb VJ: External work output and force generation during synchronized intermittent mechanical ventilation: effect of machine assistance on breathing effort. Am Rev Respir Dis 1988

54. Truwit JD, Lamb VJ, Marini JJ: Validation of a technique to assess maximal inspiratory pressure in poorly cooperative patients (Abstr). Am Rev Respir Dis 139(4):A98, 1989

55. Simkovitz P, Brown K, Goldberg P et al: Interaction between intrinsic and externally applied PEEP during mechanical ventilation (Abstr). Am Rev Respir Dis 135:A202, 1987

56. Marini JJ, Rodriguez RM, Lamb VJ: Involuntary breath stacking: an alternative method for vital capacity estimation in poorly cooperative subjects. Am Rev Respir Dis 134:694, 1986

57. Baker WL, Lamb VJ, Marini JJ: Breath-stacking increases the depth and duration of chest expansion by incentive spirometry. Am Rev Respir Dis 141:343, 1990

58. Truwit JD, Marini JJ: Evaluation of thoracic mechanics in the ventilated patient. Part 1: Primary measurements. J Crit Care 3(2):133, 1988

59. Tuxen DV, Lane S: The effects of ventilatory pattern on hyperinflation, airway pressures, and circulation in mechanical ventilation of patients with severe airflow obstruction. Am Rev Respir Dis 136:872, 1987

60. Black LF, Hyatt RE: Maximal respiratory pressures: normal values and relationship to age and sex. Am Rev Respir Dis 99:696, 1969

61. Black LF, Hyatt RE: Maximal static respiratory pressure in generalized neuromuscular disease. Am Rev Respir Dis 103:641, 1971

62. Byrd RB, Hyatt RE: Maximal static respiratory pressures in chronic obstructive lung disease. Am Rev Respir Dis 98:848, 1968

63. Marini JJ, Smith TC, Lamb VJ: Estimation of inspiratory muscle strength in mechanically ventilated patients: the measurement of maximal inspiratory pressure. J Crit Care 1(1):32, 1986

64. Godfrey S, Campbell EJM: The control of breath holding. Respir Physiol 4:385, 1968

COMPUTERIZATION AND QUALITY CONTROL OF MONITORING TECHNIQUES

REED M. GARDNER, PhD[†]

Webster defines quality as: "The degree of excellence which a thing possesses."[1] Demming, a pioneer in producing high quality products who helped the Japanese become world leaders in producing quality products, points out that "Reliable service reduces costs. Delays and mistakes raise costs."[2] Berwick tells us that "Real improvement in quality depends, according to the Theory of Continuous Quality Improvement, on understanding and revising the production process on the basis of data about the processes themselves. Every process produces information on the basis of which the process can be improved."[3] In a monograph written for the American Hospital Association, James tells us that quality is roughly equivalent to medical outcomes.[4] He further states that quality is "one of those things that is very difficult to define, but that anyone can recognize—I know it when I see it." These and others have shown that medicine, like any other "process," can be improved and that among other things the transfer of information is a key to improving the health care system. In about 1770 the great English writer Samuel Johnson said "Men more frequently need to be reminded than informed."

Recently in the *New York Times* (January 13, 1991), Glenn Rifkin pointed out what quality means in terms of some everyday examples (Fig. 1).[5] It is interesting to compare the performance of different elements of our society. Not of much surprise, and in fact almost to our delight, we see that tax advice by telephone from the Internal Revenue Service is very error prone—about 15% of the time! The average company has approximately a 1% error rate, while

Reliable service reduces costs. Delays and mistakes raise costs.

† Professor of Medical Informatics, University of Utah, Co-Director of Medical Computing, LDS Hospital, Salt Lake City, Utah

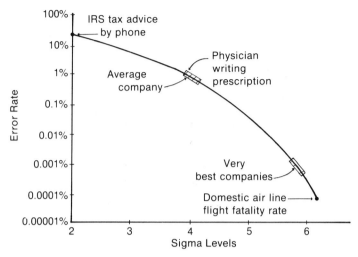

FIGURE 1   Error rates for some everyday tasks. Sigma levels = standard deviations from mean. Adapted from Rifkin G: Pursuing zero defects under the six sigma banner. The New York Times, January 13, 1991, p. 9. With permission.

the least error-prone have an error rate of less than 0.001%. Note that physicians writing prescriptions have close to a 1% error rate, the same as the average company. Domestic airlines have the lowest error rate.

Brennan and Leape and their colleagues have recently outlined the incidence of adverse events in hospitals.[6,7] They found what others have also found, namely, that errors in medical practice are common.[7] The researchers found that many factors increase the risk that a patient will have an adverse event during hospitalization and that a major determinant is the complexity of the disease or treatment. Complex patients are more likely to have adverse events. Clearly, patients in the Intensive Care Unit (ICU) are the most ill and have the most procedures performed on them of any patients in the hospital. Therefore, it is not surprising that the need for high quality care with the fewest errors should be the goal of everyone caring for patients in the ICU. How can this be achieved? Leape et al. state that "As knowledge increases, in theory more adverse events will become preventable" and that "Automatic 'fail-safe' systems—such as a computerized system that makes it impossible to order or dispense a drug to a patient with a known sensitivity—are likely to have an increasing role."[7] McDonald has stated that most adverse events are preventable, particularly those due to errors or negligence.[8] As noted in Figure 1, the airline industry has made dramatic progress in minimizing the number of errors and, consequently, deaths. The "flight recorder" has been one of the contributors to this achievement and shows that at-

McDonald has stated that most adverse events are preventable, particularly those due to errors or negligence.

tention to systematic causes and consequences of errors has been worthwhile. The United States Army has developed a procedure to study and reduce human errors known to be the largest cause of aircraft accidents[9]; they call it the 3W approach. 3W stands for *What* happened?, *What* was the cause?, and *What* you do about it? Medicine should look at this procedure to determine how helpful it would be in preventing unwanted incidents and deaths.[6,7,9] Computers might be able to help in this process. The remainder of this chapter will deal with experience in using computers to improve the process of care.

HOW CAN COMPUTERS HELP?

Several areas where computers are being used to improve the quality of patient care are discussed below.

DATA ACQUISITION

The use of microcomputers in bedside monitors has revolutionized the acquisition, display, and processing of physiological data. Few bedside monitors or ventilators are marketed today that do not use at least one microcomputer. Sensors convert biological signals (such as pressure, flow, or mechanical movement) into electrical signals, while some biological signals, such as the electrocardiogram (ECG) are already in electrical form. These signals are "digitized" and processed to extract features from the waveforms; for example, determining heart rate from an ECG or arterial pressure pulse or deriving systolic, diastolic, and mean pressure from an arterial pressure waveform. These same computers can monitor the signal qualify of the waveforms and alert nurses or physicians when there is poor skin contact with an ECG lead or poor signal quality from a finger or ear probe of a pulse oximeter (see Fig. 3). As a consequence, alarms in bedside monitors are now much "smarter" and raise fewer false alarms. Automated data acquisition now allows nurses and physicians to have data almost continuously.

The use of microcomputers in bedside monitors has revolutionized the acquisition, display, and processing of physiological data.

DATA ANALYSIS

Increased sophistication of pulmonary, hemodynamic, and renal monitoring has resulted in the need to calculate derived parameters. In many ICUs today, this task is performed by nurses using a pocket calculator or perhaps even a programmable calculator. Unfortunately, entry of data from multiple sources and reentry of data by hand into the calculators results in delays and errors. Clearly, a computer system could enhance this process by making the calculations automatically and without error.

DATA COMMUNICATIONS

Communication is one of the most important tasks of health care professionals.

Communication is one of the most important tasks of health care professionals. Data underlie every medical decision, and except for the personal observations made by and acted upon by physicians at the bedside, data must be communicated. Often, the data are communicated through several people and via several media before getting to the medical decision maker. Each step in the process, especially if it involves people and handwritten records, can result in delays and errors. Clearly, computers are fast and accurate at recording and communicating data. Using the computer's capabilities, multiple users can have access to the patient data from multiple locations presented in a format that is optimized for their use.

DATA INTEGRATION

In the modern ICU it is not unusual for a patient to be connected to several computerized monitoring devices (Fig. 2).[10] For some of these data sources, such as intake and output, data are manually entered into the computer; for others they are electronically transmitted from locations such as the clinical laboratory. Results from a study that evaluated data used by physicians in ICU teaching rounds illustrates that data from multiple sources are used in decision making.[11] Laboratory data made up 42% of the data used to make treatment decisions; infusions, medications, and intake-output data account for 22%, nurse observations 21%, data from the bedside monitor 13%, and data from other sources 2%. To be effective and complete, physicians must integrate data from many sources. Most past attempts at computerization of ICUs have attempted to only deal with data from the bedside monitors.

The computer is an extraordinary tool for collection and integration of clinical patient data.

The computer is an extraordinary tool for collection and integration of clinical patient data. With the use of computer communications networks, as soon as data are available from a blood gas or clinical laboratory, data from these

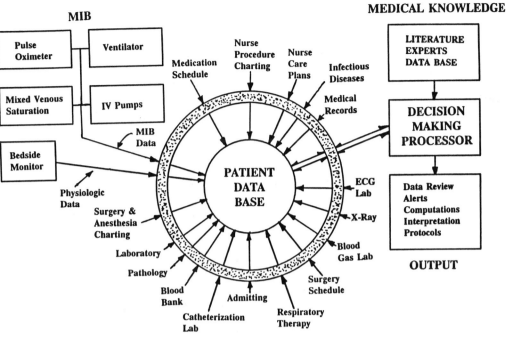

FIGURE 2   Diagram of a computerized intensive care unit data collection system. MIB = Medical Information Bus. Adapted from Gardner RM, Bradshaw KE, Hollingsworth KW: Computerizing the intensive care unit: current status and future directions. J Cardiovasc Nurs 4:68, 1989. With permission.

sources are available in the ICU. Delays are avoided, transcription errors are eliminated, and time can be saved.

DECISION MAKING ASSISTANCE

Medical decision making has traditionally been considered a scientific, as well as intuitive, process. In recent years, however, formal methods for decision making have been applied to medical problem solving and computer-assisted medical decision making has gained wider acceptance. Indeed, discussion of artificial intelligence (AI) is commonplace in medicine today (see the following chapter entitled *Use of Monitoring Information in Decision Making*). Computers can be used to interpret data, for example, interpretation of ventilatory status based on blood gas reports. Computers can also be used to alert physicians, nurses, or therapists when a medication may be contraindicated or a laboratory result is a threat to life.[13,14] As noted by Morris, computers can also be used guide patient treatment using protocols.[12,15–17]

Computer-assisted medical decision making has gained wider acceptance.

Computers can be used to alert physicians, nurses, or therapists when a medication may be contraindicated or a laboratory result is a threat to life.

COMPUTER-BASED CHARTING

The patient record remains the principal instrument for ensuring the continuity of care.

The patient record remains the principal instrument for ensuring the continuity of care.[10] The medical record for every patient is a document that begs to be computerized.[18,19] For patients in ICU, and those undergoing anesthesia and surgery, this need is especially urgent. Information in the medical record should be easily retrievable and reviewable in a temporal relationship to associated data. Records having these characteristics would facilitate the routine processing of data required for medical decisions. Traditional manually recorded medical records lack these attributes.[19] Therefore, many investigators have attempted to computerize the medical record and make it "paperless." However, the hospital medical record has been difficult to computerize—far more difficult than either bank records or airline reservations.

With the "on-line" bedside monitoring situation, historically each supplier of monitoring equipment has wanted to "do it all." Each vendor wanted to provide *every* monitoring device for *every* bedside. Unfortunately, none of the vendors are large enough, flexible enough, or innovative enough to invent *all* the new monitoring devices. As a result, there is a veritable "Tower of Babel" situation with data flowing from bedside devices.

Bedside monitoring devices today are being designed with microprocessors as the principal tool to solve the complex measurement tasks. Even small, portable infrared sensor-based devices "shined" into the eardrum to quickly, noninvasively, and accurately measure patient temperature are microprocessor based. Thus, the challenge is to acquire, store, report and use this data for diagnostic and therapeutic decision making. To facilitate automatic data acquisition from the multitude of devices located at the bedside, the medical, nursing, respiratory therapy, and medical informatics staffs at LDS Hospital in Salt Lake City have integrated data flowing from bedside physiological monitors using the Medical Information Bus (MIB) (See Fig. 2). Devices such as infusion pumps, pulse oximeters, mixed venous saturation monitors, and ventilators have been interfaced to the MIB. The MIB is being standardized by the Institute of Electrical and Electronic Engineers (IEEE) with their MIB standards committee IEEE P1073 established in 1984.[20]

Recently at LDS Hospital, computers have replaced manual charting for respiratory therapy.[21] To be effective, such systems must provide easy methods for data entry and review, give accurate and descriptive documentation, automate several functions with a single input (billing, reporting, valid data checks, alerting). The system is now used routinely in ICU, and throughout the hospital.[22-25] Each day more than 18,000 data items are entered into the computer system. Very few (< 1%) of the data items entered give cause for alarm or immediate action.

QUALITY IMPROVEMENT

Quality assurance, measurement of outcomes, and documentation of performance are growing requirements for modern hospitals. Because of the low incidence yet potentially fatal consequences of missing or not acting on potentially life-threatening events, computers are becoming indispensable in care of the acutely ill.[3,4,25,26] Currently, our respiratory care quality assurance program uses the enhanced capabilities of our integrated computerized database.[26] Data from the blood gas laboratory, microbiology laboratory, clinical chemistry laboratory, the Admit Discharge, Transfer module, and the respiratory therapy charting are used.[25,26] Manual chart review is by necessity retrospective and usually performed on "samples" of patient charts. As a consequence, it may take weeks to discover errors in treatment with the result that little can be done to correct errors.

To fill this need, a Medical Director's ALERT report is generated each day just before morning rounds. Nine different events for each patient receiving respiratory care are reviewed each day.[26] Table 1 shows some recent results from the ALERT report.

A similar analysis was made for the blood gas laboratory data. Each month approximately 4,000 blood gas tests are run. Table 2 shows that nearly 99% of the results are not life-threatening. Thus, only about 48 analyses (1.2%) each month require immediate action and follow up.

Not only can computer systems save respiratory therapists and technicians time, they also strengthen the ability of medical directors to improve the quality of patient care.

Because of the low incidence yet potentially fatal consequences of missing or not acting on potentially life-threatening events, computers are becoming indispensable in care of the acutely ill.

Not only can computer systems save respiratory therapists and technicians time, they also strengthen the ability of medical directors to improve the quality of patient care.

TABLE 1   Medical Director's ALERTs

	Percentage
$F_IO_2 \geq 60\%$ (ICU)	50%
PEEP >10 cm H_2O	20%
Cuff pressure >27 cm H_2O	14%
Peak pressure >60 cm H_2O	6%
Temperature >39°C	6%
$F_IO_2 \geq 60\%$ (Non-ICU)	4%

TABLE 2   Blood Gas ALERTs (Approximately 4,000 Blood Gas Analyses Per Month)

		n	%
Blood gases OK		3,952	98.8%
Blood gases results life-threatening		48	1.2%
pH	<7.30	20	0.50%
PO_2	<55 mmHg	17	0.43%
pH	>7.54	9	0.23%
CoHb	>5%	2	0.05%

As a consequence, policy and procedure reviews have been strengthened to provide an overview of the performance of each staff member.[26] Thus, the goal of Continuous Quality Improvement is being accomplished.[3,4,26] In addition, some of the goals set forward by the Joint Commission on Accreditation of Healthcare Organizations (JCAHO) and others recommending improvements in quality of care are being carried out with the aid of computers.[27–30]

COMPUTERIZED RESPIRATORY MONITORING

FUTURE CHALLENGES AND OPPORTUNITIES

Computerized bedside monitors, ventilators, pulse oximeters, and mixed venous oximeters have provided us with a flood of data. However, much like floods of water can overwhelm us, so can floods of data overwhelm computer storage capabilities and overload the computers and humans that must use the data for decision making. Artifacts and noise in the data stream continue to be a problem for automated and human data collection. The issue of data "ownership" and sharing also becomes a problem. For example, with pulse oximeters we find that saturations are independently stored in computer records by respiratory therapists, nurses, and blood gas technicians. All of these "non-computer" problems must be resolved before optimal data collection and decision making can be applied.

To illustrate these issues, we recently collected data for 12 hours from a patient on a ventilator. Figure 3 is a plot of the pulse oximeter oxygen saturation for this 12-hour period. Figure 3A shows the raw data available from the pulse oximeter at 30-second intervals, and Figure 3B illus-

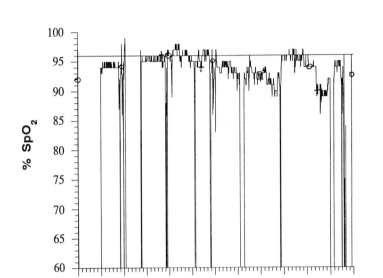

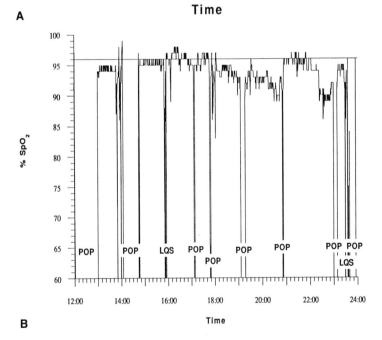

FIGURE 3 Plot of oxygen saturation data coming from a pulse oximeter every 30 seconds for a 12-hour period obtained through the MIB. (A) Raw saturation data with data manually charted by nurses (○) and respiratory therapists (+). (B) Same data as (A) but with markings of POP and LQS. (*Figure continues.*)

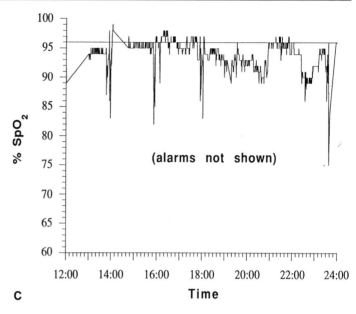

FIGURE 3 (*continued*)   (C) Same data as in (A) but with time intervals with POP or LQS eliminated.

trates the times when the probe (on the ear) was either off the patient (POP = probe off patient) or had a low quality signal (LQS). Figure 3C illustrates how having knowledge about signal quality can minimize the noise or artifact in the information presented. Figure 4A is a plot of the raw pulse rate data obtained from the same pulse oximeter and Figure 4B is the data after taking into consideration the knowledge about signal quality. These data illustrate the problem of data overload, artifact, and ownership.

OVERLOAD: For the 12 hours of saturation and heart rate data flowing from the pulse oximeter registered every 30 seconds, there are about 60,000 bytes of data stored in the computer—approximately twice the number of characters presented in this chapter.

ARTIFACT: From Figure 3A and 4A it is clear that artifacts are the major problem that must be resolved.

OWNERSHIP: Figure 3A also shows by the + and O marks where therapists and nurses, respectively, have charted oxygen saturation data. The nurses charted at about a 2-hour interval and the therapist charted at more irregular time periods. Their measurements have a reasonable correspondence with the "true" value for the times noted.

Figure 5 is a plot of the spontaneous respiratory rate for the same patient for the same time interval as in Figures

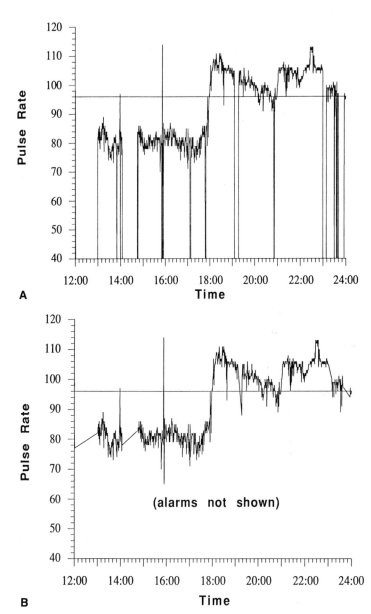

FIGURE 4   Plot of heart rate data coming from a pulse oximeter every 30 seconds for a 12-hour period obtained through
the MIB. (A) Raw heart rate data. (B) Same data as in (A) but
with time intervals with POP or LQS eliminated.

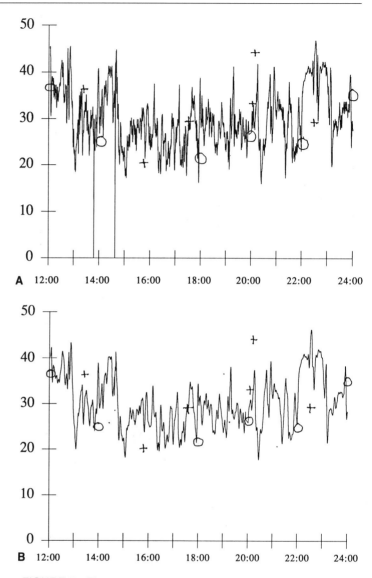

FIGURE 5   The spontaneous respiratory rate for the same patient as in Figs. 3 and 4 and obtained from the ventilator via MIB. These data were obtained every 10 seconds. (A) Plot of the raw data and those charted by respiratory therapists (+) and nurses (○). (B) Plot of a 3-minute average of the spontaneous respiratory rate. (*Figure continues.*)

3 and 4. The problems discussed above are further exacerbated with ventilator data.

OVERLOAD: The data space required to store the data from the ventilator with all its parameters is over 375,000 bytes of data for this 12-hour period.

ARTIFACT: The respiratory rate signal from the ventilator

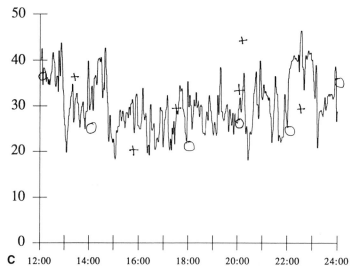

FIGURE 5 (*continued*)   (C) Plot of a 3-minute median of the spontaneous respiratory rate.

clearly has considerable noise (Fig. 5A). Taking either a 3-minute mean (Fig. 5B) or a 3-minute median (Fig. 5C) of the respiratory rate smooths the data. However, note that the values selected and manually charted by the respiratory therapists and nurses appear to be taken as "instantaneous" observations and not based on watching for a minute or so and "averaging" the results. Based on this and other observations, concern arises about the quality of data recorded by human observers.

OWNERSHIP: With ventilator data, as with pulse oximeter data, nurses and therapists chart the information. Their observations, even when taken within similar time windows, seem to have large variability.

We have proven the basic premise of the MIB in clinical applications. However, sociological, physiological, data selection, artifact reduction, and medic-legal issues must still be addressed. For example, consider the emotional issue of taking something away when a process becomes automated. If an individual is charting data and must write it down, this process usually causes the individual to "think" about or process the data. By having the computer take over this task, is something lost? What data should be used? How should it be integrated and communicated?

With newer monitors, three or four devices may be giving the same information, such as heart rate. Which are correct and which should be logged? Despite the fact that people think that they are the most accurate "data loggers," evidence clearly indicates that humans do make data

Concern arises about the quality of data recorded by human observers.

measurement and logging errors. Finally, the people factors and data selection strategies are more difficult than the engineering interface and computer science data acquisition requirements. These issues provide challenges and opportunities for making future progress in patient charting and patient care.

ACKNOWLEDGMENTS

The author wishes to acknowledge the efforts and cooperation of several colleagues and graduate students who have contributed to this work: graduate students Thomas A. Oniki and Hsueh-Fen W. Young, Director of Clinical Engineering William L. Hawley, and Thomas D. East, PhD, for their help with Medical Information Bus data collection. Thanks are also extended to physicians C. Gregory Elliott, Medical Director of Respiratory Care, Terry P. Clemmer, Director of the Shock Trauma Unit, and Alan H. Morris, Director of Medical Research for the Pulmonary Division for their vision and involvement in computerizing much of the patient care process at LDS Hospital.

References

1. Webster's new world dictionary. 2nd ed. Simon and Schuster, New York, 1980

2. Demming WE: Quality, productivity, and competitive position. Massachusetts Institute of Technology Center for Advanced Engineering Study, Cambridge, Mass, 1982

3. Berwick DM: Continuous improvement as an ideal in health care. N Engl J Med 320:53, 1989

4. James BC: Quality management for health care delivery. The Hospital Research and Education Trust of the American Hospital Association, Chicago, 1989

5. Rifkin G: Pursuing zero defects under the six sigma banner. The New York Times, January 13 1991, 9

6. Brennan TA, Leape LL, Laird NM et al: Incidence of adverse events and negligence in hospitalized patients: results of the Harvard Medical Practice Study I. N Engl J Med 324:370, 1991

7. Leape LL, Brennan TA, Laird NM et al: The nature of adverse events in hospitalized patients: results of the Harvard Medical Practice Study II. N Engl J Med 324:377, 1991

8. McDonald CJ: Protocol-based computer reminders, the quality of care and the non-perfectability of man. N Engl J Med 295:1351, 1976

9. Ricketson DS, Brown WR, Graham KN: 3W approach to the investigation, analysis, and prevention of human-error aircraft accidents. Aviat Space Environ Med 51:1036, 1980

10. Gardner RM, Bradshaw KE, Hollingsworth KW: Computerizing the intensive care unit: current status and future directions. J Cardiovasc Nurs 4:68, 1989

11. Bradshaw KE, Gardner RM, Clemmer TP et al: Physician decision-making: evaluation of data used in a computerized ICU. Int J Clin Monit Comput 1:81, 1984

12. Morris AH: Use of monitoring information in decision-making. Contemp Management Crit Care 1(4):213

13. Bradshaw KE, Gardner RM, Pryor TA: Development of a computerized laboratory alerting system. Comp Biomed Res 22:575, 1989

14. Tate KE, Gardner RM, Weaver LK: A computerized laboratory alerting system. MD Comput 7:296, 1990

15. Sittig DF, Pace NL, Gardner RM: Implementation of a computerized patient advice system using the HELP clinical information system. Comp Biomed Res 22:474, 1989

16. Sittig DF, Gardner RM, Morris AH, Wallace CJ: Clinical evaluation of computer-based respiratory care algorithms. Int J Clin Monit Comput 7:177, 1990

17. Henderson S, Crapo RO, East TD et al: Computerized clinical protocols in an intensive care unit: how well are they followed? p. 284. Symposium on Computer Applications in Medical Care. IEEE Press, Los Alamitos, California, 1990

18. Automated medical records hold promise to improve patient care. GAO/IMTEC-91-5 General Accounting Office US Government, January 1991

19. McDonald CJ, Tierney WM: Computer-stored medical records: their future role in medical practice. JAMA 259:3433, 1988

20. Shabot MM: Standardized acquisition of bedside data: the IEEE P1073 medical information bus. Int J Clin Monit Comput 6:197, 1989

21. Andrews RD, Gardner RM, Metcalf SM, Simmons D: Computer charting: an evaluation of a respiratory care computer system. Respir Care 30:695, 1985

22. Gardner RM, Clemmer TP: Selection and standardization of respiratory monitoring equipment. Respir Care 30:560, 1985

23. Clemmer TP, Gardner RM: Data gathering, analysis, and display in critical care medicine. Respir Care 30:586, 1985

24. Andrews BS, Gardner RM: Portable computers used for respiratory care charting. Int J Clin Monit Comput 5:45, 1988

25. Elliott CG, Simmons D, Schmidt CD et al: Computer-assisted medical direction of respiratory care. Respir Manage 19:31, 1989

26. Elliott CG: Computer-assisted quality assurance: development and performance of a respiratory care program. QRB 17:85, 1991

27. Joint Commission on Accreditation of Healthcare Organizations: characteristics of clinical indicators. QRB 15:330, 1989

28. Weissman C, Mossel P, Haimet S, King TC: Integration of quality assurance activities into a computerized patient data management system in an intensive care unit. QRB 16:398, 1990

29. Sue DY: Development of an ICU patient care monitoring and evaluation system in a teaching hospital. QRB 17:97, 1991

30. Luce JM: Improving the quality and utilization of critical care. QRB 17:42, 1991

USE OF MONITORING INFORMATION IN DECISION MAKING

ALAN H. MORRIS, MD[†]

The explosion of medical information has found clear expression both in the proliferation of medical publications and in the staggering amount of information collected from critical care patients. A recent morning rounds review of a critically ill patient in the Shock Trauma/Intermountain Respiratory ICU at the LDS Hospital produced a list of 236 different variables in the following categories: hemodynamics (14), blood gases (15), ventilatory management (20), hemogram (20), urinalysis (20), electrocardiograph (11), blood chemistry (20), special blood chemistry (12), urine chemistry (4), bacteriology (10), bone marrow (17), nutritional balance (20), coagulation (7), temperature (1), weight (1), and medications (44). Although many variables changed as a function of time, repeated (serial) measurements were not included. Nor did the list include information from physical examination, radiograph, special studies (eg, CAT scans, ultrasound, angiography, endoscopy, etc), physician consultation notes, nurses' notes, respiratory therapists' notes, physician progress notes, operating room notes, anesthesia notes, or pathologist reports. A plethora of data such as this brings to mind a recent quotation of Dr. David Eddy: ". . all confirm what would be expected from common sense: The complexity of modern medicine exceeds the inherent limitations of the unaided human mind."[1] One wonders whether a mere mortal could effectively assimilate all these variables and come to the "right clinical treatment decision" for a severely ill patient. Even acknowledging that all variables are not necessary for every treatment decision and that all the data are not independent, it still seems likely that most

The explosion of medical information has found clear expression both in the proliferation of medical publications and in the staggering amount of information collected from critical care patients. A recent morning rounds review of a critically ill patient produced a list of 236 different variables.

---

† Director of Research, Pulmonary Division, LDS Hospital, Professor of Medicine, University of Utah, Salt Lake City, Utah

physicians would have difficulty dealing systematically with this large mass of clinical data. In fact, dealing with as few as four variables has prevented experienced pulmonary/critical care physicians from systematically managing a mechanical ventilator in the inverse ratio ventilation mode (see section headed *Inverse Ratio Ventilation*). The physician who attempts to integrate knowledge from the pertinent literature with all of the patient data, including results of the physical examination, frequently faces a nearly impossible task.

Patient monitoring in the intensive care unit (ICU) is traditionally viewed in terms of identification of problems, prevention of problems, and the generation of a rapid therapeutic response in an individual patient.[2,3] This chapter takes a more global perspective and includes the impact of monitoring upon community practice as well. This seems justified by the paucity of documentation that individual patient monitoring achieves the favorable clinical goals that have been its objective, and the recognition that the interventions that may be caused by continuous monitoring constitute a potential nosocomial ICU hazard.[3,4] The failure of continuous fetal heart rate monitoring[5] and the controversy surrounding the use of flotation pulmonary artery catheters[6-8] are two examples of the challenging need to couple individual patient monitoring with the development of medical practice policy on a community level.

PROBLEMS PARTIALLY RESOLVED BY MONITORING

Problems that benefit from patient monitoring fall into the two general areas of individual patient care and medical policy formulation (community-wide medical practice).

INDIVIDUAL PATIENT CARE

Individual patient care suffers directly from input information overload,[9] which is a the frequent consequence of the complex clinical data sets faced by physicians grappling with modern patient care problems. Such input information overload impairs the physician's ability to generate a systematic therapeutic program. Digital computers have been utilized as a means of aiding physicians and other clinical care personnel in the management of large volumes of data. In the field of Critical Care Medicine, computer applications have made multiple contributions, from co-ordinating data to assisting in medical decision making. In most of these applications, the digital computer system has

Individual patient care suffers directly from input information overload, which is a the frequent consequence of the complex clinical data sets faced by physicians grappling with modern patient care problems.

been used as a tool to aid in the management and interpretation of large amounts of information. Computers can be expected to play an increasingly important role in medical practice,[10] although there is some controversy over the exact role computers should fill.[3] Although ICU computerization began at the LDS hospital 20 years ago, only about one fourth of the average LDS hospital medical chart is currently computerized.[11] It is of note that the fraction of the total medical record occupied by specific types of data seems unrelated to the frequency with which the data is used for decisions by the medical staff.[11,12]

COMMUNITY MEDICAL POLICY

Improvement of community medical care, through reformulation of medical policy, is in large part dependent upon the analysis of patient outcomes. Unfortunately, because of ill-defined and unstandardized care much noise is associated with patient outcomes data. As a result, the signal-to-noise ratio is poor and the interpretation of clinical outcomes is severely compromised. Of the three major elements involved in clinical research—the content of clinical care, patient selection, and the process of clinical care (Fig. 1)—only the content is clearly defined in most clinical research publications. The content represents the "what" we do for patients. It is usually easy to assess whether the study in question involves penicillin, gentamicin, or other drugs, extracorporeal support, mechanical ventilation, or some other therapeutic modality. The patient selection, that is, the "to whom" the "what" is delivered, is much more difficult to identify. For example, no uniformly accepted definition of adult respiratory distress syndrome (ARDS) exists at present. Nevertheless, there is usually some useful information concerning patient selection in most medical publications. In contrast, the process of medical care, the "how" we deliver the "what" "to whom", is almost never articulated. Therefore, the two most important goals of a Methods section in a scientific publication, that is, the provision of enough detail to allow a reviewer to critically evaluate the results of the work and its conclusions and enough detail to allow the interested investigator to duplicate the work, are usually not fulfilled. As a result, much "noise" is introduced into clinical settings from which medical publications are derived, making the interpretation of the outcomes of such work much more difficult for the medical community. It is informative to examine the relationship of these three elements (content, patient selection, and process of medical care) with the two major determinants both of the intensity of care to which

Because of ill-defined and unstandardized care, much noise is associated with patient outcomes data. As a result, the signal-to-noise ratio is poor and the interpretation of clinical outcomes is severely compromised. Of the three major elements involved in clinical research—the content of clinical care, patient selection, and the process of clinical care—only the content is clearly defined in most clinical research publications.

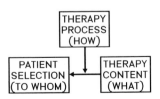

FIGURE 1 Three major elements involved in the delivery of clinical care.

Our focus in medicine for both clinical care and for clinical research is patient outcome, the most important of which is survival with resumption of a productive life. Unfortunately, the signal-to-noise ratio associated with outcome differences in clinical trials is frequently very low.

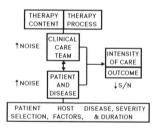

FIGURE 2 Determinants of the intensity of care and the ultimate patient outcome. The two major elements are patient–disease complex and the response to the patient–disease complex provided by the clinical care team. Both of these elements introduce noise that reduces the S/N ratio for outcome results.

a patient is subjected and of the ultimate patient outcome (the patient–disease complex and the response of the clinical care team [Fig. 2]).

Our focus in medicine for both clinical care and for clinical research is patient outcome, the most important of which is survival with resumption of a productive life. Unfortunately, the signal-to-noise ratio (S/N) associated with outcome differences in clinical trials is frequently very low. The noise in the clinical environment is both random and nonrandom (bias). Random noise can be dealt with by increasing the number of observations (or number of patients) made in a clinical trial. Since the S/N for random noise is proportional to the square root of the number of observations, increasing the number of observations (or patients) 100-fold would increase the S/N by 10. This is a difficult challenge in critical care medicine since the acquisition of large numbers of patients in clinical trials is not easy and is very costly. In contrast, nonrandom noise (bias), quite common in clinical settings, is not influenced by increasing the number of observations (or patients) and therefore must be reduced by other means. Both of the major elements that determine the intensity of patient care and the patient outcome (Fig. 2) are sources of both random and nonrandom noise. Noise is introduced in the patient–disease complex because of our inability to control host factors and disease etiology, extent, and duration. In addition, significant bias is introduced in patient selection, both in clinical care and, more pertinent to this discussion, in clinical trials. The patient identification and selection process is quite imperfect and incorporates much local bias due to the prejudices of individual clinical investigators and to the specific characteristics of their local clinical environments, as well as to the failure of the medical community to establish broadly accepted specific definitions of many diseases. Much work needs to be done and much improvement can be achieved in this regard. The other major element, the response of the clinical care team to the patient–disease complex, also introduces both random and nonrandom noise. Strong bias is injected into the response of the clinical care team as a result of many factors that play upon their behavior, including general and local cultural factors, local technical abilities, and experience—all of which affect the process of therapy. This process is usually poorly articulated. Frequently the rules behind decisions relating to important stages in the delivery of care cannot be uncovered. For both clinical trials and case reports, this deficiency means it is not possible to define "how" the investigation is actually conducted.

Few studies have dealt with the impact of controlling the

process of medical care, although it is clear that interpretations of outcomes will be difficult as long as the process of care is poorly defined. There is some evidence that control of the process of medical care is beneficial.[13,14] This contrasts with the more common emphasis in medical informatics on exploring how humans reason and on matching medical expert systems products to individual physician preferences.[15] Although it is generally believed that detailed protocols will not be able to replace individual physician judgment,[16] the minute-to-minute management demands of severely ill ICU patients provide an unusually fertile field for application of detailed protocols. My colleagues and I have attempted to reduce the noise associated with the clinical care team's response by defining, with computerized protocols, the process of medical care associated with the management of arterial hypoxemia in a clinical trial of two therapies for ARDS.[17,18] With more than 30,000 hours of application of computerized protocol control of clinical care, 24 hours a day, it is now clear that this approach is feasible and, with the appropriate computer infrastructure, is practical,[19,20] Such computerized protocol control of the process of care does appear to control the intensity of care of severely ill patients.[18] Whether it will be possible to generalize this approach is currently unknown. If it can be generalized, it may allow the performance of clinical trials that have the potential of significantly decreasing the noise introduced by the response of the clinical care team and thus increasing the S/N for outcome. This will very likely make a number of clinical studies more credible and more definitive.

Although it is generally believed that detailed protocols will not be able to replace individual physician judgment, the minute-to-minute management demands of severely ill ICU patients provide an unusually fertile field for application of detailed protocols.

MONITORING PURPOSES

The two general areas within which most monitoring activities fall are documentation and decision support.

The two general areas within which most monitoring activities fall are documentation and decision support.

DOCUMENTATION

Medical documentation serves many of the purposes of the airplane flight recorder ("black box"). Such documentation may add structure to the clinical database, and this in itself can produce favorable effects,[21] presumably through the "checklist effect".[22] Entry of data into a computerized database can occur either manually (via a keyboard) or by automatic entry through electronic connection such as the Medical Information Bus (MIB), which is being developed as an industry standard.[23–25] Manual (keyboard) data entry is routinely used by nurses,[26,27] physicians,[28] respiratory therapists,[29] and others in the LDS Hospital. Although in

The 18,000 data items recorded daily by our respiratory therapy department is a graphic expression of the enormous amount of data that must be reviewed for quality assurance purposes.

some institutions the keyboard seems to be an obstacle to medical computer use, at the LDS hospital the use of keyboards and simple screen menus has been readily accepted and routinely used as a bedside tool.

Documentation also provides the information base for quality assurance activities. Quality assurance, measures of outcome, and documentation of performance is a growing requirement of modern hospitals. Computer applications in critical care are an extremely valuable part of the response to the widespread demand for more cost effective care and for better documentation to justify clinical decisions. The 18,000 data items recorded daily by our respiratory therapy department is a graphic expression of the enormous amount of data that must be reviewed for quality assurance purposes. The quality assurance reviews of the Repiratory Care Department utilize data from the blood gas laboratory, the microbiology laboratory, and the respiratory therapists' clinical chart. Traditionally, manual surveys are typically limited to retrospective reviews and restricted to a small fraction of patients and to only a fraction of the hospital record data of these patients. Manual surveys are time-consuming and produce results that are frequently not available until months after the assignment is made. In contrast, off-line surveys of data by computerized review allow examination of all information and all patient records. Off-line computerized surveys are routinely carried out in our Respiratory Care,[30] Infectious Disease,[31,32] and Blood Bank[33] departments. Figures 3 and 4 display representative outcome data from Quality Assurance activities in the Respiratory Care Department.

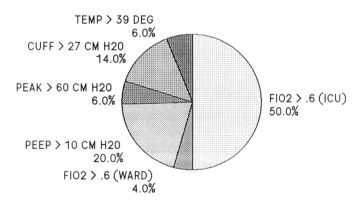

FIGURE 3   HELP System Alerts for the off-line computerized quality assurance program of the Respiratory Care Department. % distribution: 1987 monthly average (48 alerts/month). TEMP = humidifier temperature; CUFF = endotracheal tube cuff pressure; PEAK = peak ventilator pressure; PEEP = positive end-expiratory pressure; F_1O_2 = fraction of inspired oxygen.

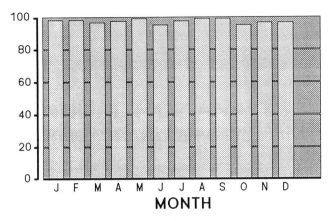

FIGURE 4   HELP System Alerts for the on-line computerized quality assurance program of the Respiratory Care Department. F_IO_2 analyses. Percent meeting respiratory care standard by month from January through December.

On-line computerized surveys provide an even more powerful tool for quality assurance in the clinical environment. The computerized database can be surveyed completely (all information of all charts and all patients) with all information reviewed on a real-time, daily, weekly, monthly, or yearly basis. Such surveys not only increase the power of our departments but also provide opportunities for outcomes research. An additional benefit is the possibility of comparing hospital performance with that of other centers and with historical LDS hospital data by referring to reference criteria such as the APACHE II score.[34] Figure 5 provides a representative example of results of such routine daily surveys from the Respiratory Care and Infectious Disease departments.

Documentation provides the database upon which decision support and outcomes analysis activities operate, and it provides the factual basis (and frequently the best defense) for medico-legal disputes.

DECISION SUPPORT

Decision support through patient monitoring can vary from the simple reminder intended to help medical care team members avoid careless mistakes, to complex protocols intended to provide specific instructions for therapy of seriously ill patients. Simple reminders can take the form of manual checklists for medication orders or the initiation of life-support equipment. Automated systems have the characteristics of consistency and attentiveness to detail at a level that is unachieveable by humans. Computers are capable of dealing with a large amount of information and

RESPIRATORY CARE ALERT

W 820 PATIENT   JJ
SPUTUM CULTURE   2/26/88 1045
PSEUDOMONAS AEROGINOSA

COMMON ORGANISM: WITH PATIENT AK E630
THERAPIST 23432 ALSO SAW PATIENT AK

FIGURE 5   HELP System Alerts for the on-line computerized quality assurance program of the Respiratory Care Department. JJ and AK are two different patients in rooms W820 and E630, respectively. Therapist 23432 is a specific respiratory therapist.

Decision support through patient monitoring can vary from the simple reminder intended to help medical care team members avoid careless mistakes, to complex protocols intended to provide specific instructions for therapy of seriously ill patients.

```
          L D S   H O S P I T A L   B L O O D   G A S   R E P O R T
                                                                        SEX  AGE   ROOM
        R        K.                  NO.          DR. L    P             F    48    DS

DEC 14 90  pH   PCO2  HCO3   BE    HB   CO/MT  PO2  SO2  O2CT  %O2  AVO2  VO2   C.O.  A-a  Qs/Qt  PK/ PL/PP  MR/SR
NORMAL HI  7.45 40.9  26.2   2.5  15.9  2/ 1                        16.1  5.5  300   7.30  22    5
NORMAL LOW 7.35 27.5  15.9  -2.5  11.9  0/ 1   62   90             16.1  3.0  200   2.90         0

14 04:16 V  7.32 52.0  26.3        11.7  3/ 1   49   82   13.5  100                             54/ 47/30   3/
14 04:15 A  7.34 48.2  25.5  -.2  12.0  3/ 1  162   95   16.4  100  2.55 212  8.30  383   35    54/ 47/30   3/
14 01:05 A  7.34 50.8  26.9   .9  12.3  2/ 1   59   89   15.3   40                 120          54/ 49/30   3/
        SAMPLE # 110, TEMP 36.1, BREATHING STATUS : IMV
        MODERATE MIXED CHRONIC AND ACUTE RESPIRATORY ACIDOSIS
        MODERATE HYPOXEMIA
        MILDLY REDUCED O2 CONTENT
        HYPOVENTILATION MARKEDLY IMPROVED
        PULSE OXIMETER SO2  93.0

13 17:35 A  7.36 57.9  32.2   5.8  12.1  2/ 0   70   92   15.7   60            222          53/ 50/30   3/
        SAMPLE # 109, TEMP 36.3, BREATHING STATUS : IMV
        SEVERE CHRONIC RESPIRATORY ACIDOSIS
        MILDLY REDUCED O2 CONTENT
        HYPOVENTILATION NOT IMPROVED
        PULSE OXIMETER SO2  94.0

13 13:31 V  7.42 53.3  34.2   8.9  12.0  2/ 1   49   84   14.2   80                             55/ 50/30  20/
13 13:30 A  7.40 56.4  34.5   8.7  12.3  2/ 1   71   93   16.1   80  1.46 158  10.80 345   57   55/ 50/30  20/
        SAMPLE # 108, TEMP 36.5, BREATHING STATUS : IMV
        SEVERE CHRONIC RESPIRATORY ACIDOSIS
        MILDLY REDUCED O2 CONTENT
        NORMAL O2 SATURATION AND PO2
        HYPOVENTILATION WORSE
        PULSE OXIMETER SO2  93.0

13 12:10 A  7.42 52.6  33.8   8.5  12.3  2/ 0   67   93   16.0   90            412          53/ 49/30   3/
        SAMPLE # 107, TEMP 36.3, BREATHING STATUS : IMV
        MODERATE CHRONIC RESPIRATORY ACIDOSIS
        MILDLY REDUCED O2 CONTENT
        HYPOVENTILATION NOT IMPROVED
        PULSE OXIMETER SO2  93.0

13 08:44 A  7.44 51.4  34.6   9.8  12.0  3/ 1   61   90   15.3  100            481          54/ 48/30   3/
        SAMPLE # 106, TEMP 36.6, BREATHING STATUS : IMV
        MODERATE MIXED RESPIRATORY ACIDOSIS AND METABOLIC ALKALOSIS
        MILD HYPOXEMIA
        MILDLY REDUCED O2 CONTENT
        PULSE OXIMETER SO2  92.0

13 06:05 A  7.43 51.6  33.9   8.9  12.1  2/ 1   54   88   14.9  100            487          56/ 51/30   3/
        SAMPLE # 105, TEMP 36.7, BREATHING STATUS : IMV
        MODERATE CHRONIC RESPIRATORY ACIDOSIS
        MODERATE HYPOXEMIA
        MILDLY REDUCED O2 CONTENT
        HYPOVENTILATION NOT IMPROVED
        PULSE OXIMETER SO2  87.0

13 04:59 O  7.53 35.0  29.3   7.5  12.3  1/ 1  412   98   18.1  100                             56/ 50/30   3/
13 04:57 I  7.41 55.0  34.5   8.9  12.3  1/ 1   34   72   12.4  100                             56/ 50/30   3/
13 04:56 V  7.43 50.3  33.1   8.2  12.2  2/ 0   38   78   13.4  100                             56/ 50/30   3/
13 04:55 A  7.42 51.3  32.9   7.9  11.9  1/ 0   47   86   14.3  100  1.28 156  12.20 495   74   56/ 50/30   3/
        SAMPLE # 104, TEMP 36.5, BREATHING STATUS : IMV
        MODERATE CHRONIC RESPIRATORY ACIDOSIS
        SEVERE HYPOXEMIA BREATHING OXYGEN **CONTACT MD OR RN!!!!
        MILDLY REDUCED O2 CONTENT
        HYPOVENTILATION NOT IMPROVED
        PULSE OXIMETER SO2  84.0
```

PRELIMINARY INTERPRETATION -- BASED ONLY ON BLOOD GAS DATA. ***(FINAL DIAGNOSIS REQUIRES CLINICAL CORRELATION)***
KEY: CO=CARBOXY HB, MT=MET HB, O2CT=O2 CONTENT, AVO2=ART VENOUS CONTENT DIFFERENCE (CALCULATED WITH AVERAGE OF A &V HB VALUES),
VO2=OXYGEN CONSUMPTION, C.O.=CARDIAC OUTPUT, A-a=ALVEOLAR arterial O2 DIFFERENCE, Qs/Qt=SHUNT, PK=PEAK, PL=PLATEAU, PP=PEEP
MR=MACHINE RATE, SR=SPONTANEOUS RATE.   *** SPECIMEN IDENTIFICATION: BLOOD (A=ARTERIAL, V=VENOUS, C=CAPILLARY, W=WEDGE;
                              FLUIDS (P=PLEURAL, J=JOINT, B=ABDOMINAL, S=ABSCESS); E=EXPIRED AIR;
                              ECCO2R (I=INFLOW, M=MIDFLOW, O=OUTFLOW)

FIGURE 6   HELP System Blood Gas Report. The patient's arterial-mixed venous oxygen content difference (AVO2) and machine (ventilator) rate (MR) are reduced because this patient is supported with veno-venous extracorporeal oxygenation and carbon dioxide removal.[17,18] The diagnostic statements for oxygenation, acid–base balance, and ventilation are derived from a standardized interpretative scheme.[37]

of applying a well-defined set of decision-making rules. Medical decision-making support is a major activity of the LDS hospital HELP hospital information system.[35,36]

Interpretation of a patient's laboratory test results is one of the simplest applications of computerized medical decision making. Blood gas (Fig. 6) and cardiac output (Fig. 7) measurements provide ready examples. The algorithms used to interpret these two sets of data are widely available in textbooks and publications.[37] Computerized interpretations provide uniformity and avoid common mistakes such as errors in computation, transcription, and incongruence of units. The rapid availability of the results and interpretations provides information that would not normally be obtained manually because of other demands that must be met by busy physicians and nurses.

The generation and presentation of alerts or warnings to physicians, nurses, therapists, and other members of the hospital staff represents another level of clinically valuable computerized decision making. Alerts are generated as a result of automatic interpretations of data from the clinical laboratories,[38,39] the respiratory care department,[40] the pharmacy department,[30] and other sites including the blood gas laboratory. Alerts are responses to recent and past patient medications and behavior, current medication administration, and medications ordered but not yet administered. Table 1 includes examples of alerts for severe hypoxemia, sepsis, electrolyte abnormalities, and drug incompatibility. The LDS hospital respiratory therapy de-

---

TABLE 1   Representative HELP Alert (Warning) Statements for Hypoxemia, Sepsis, Electrolyte, and Pharmacy Problems

Hypoxemia

Mixed venous PO_2 = 25 mmHg (critically low)

Severely reduced O_2 content (12.7 ml/dl) due to anemia

Severe hypoxemia breathing oxygen— Contact MD or RN!

Sepsis

Nosocomial infection probability = 0.91 due to age (79), diagnosis (upper GI bleeding, metastatic colon cancer, bowel resection), and urinary catheter

Electrolytes

Suggest that patient's potassium chloride therapy be changed to another form of potassium as patient's serum chloride is elevated at 120 mEq/l

Pharmacy

Concurrent aminoglycoside and vancomycin therapy may result in increased risk of nephrotoxicity

Antacids or Kaopectate (Upjohn) when given at the same time as digoxin will decrease the absorption of digoxin. Suggest that these two drugs be given at least 2 hours apart

Suggest that serum potassium be monitored daily as this patient is receiving a potassium-sparing diuretic and a potassium supplement

C A R D I A C   O U T P U T   R E P O R T

```
K       R       K.       NO. 2       DR L      P                    RM
HT    CM    WT 90.30  KG    BSA  1.97 SQM        AGE  48     SEX F
TIME          CO    CI   HR  SV   SI   MP  MSP   PA   RA  PW   PVR   SVR  RWI  LWI
NORMAL HI     7.30  3.50  89 101   48  105  123   19  5.0 12   1.0   18  11.0   85
NORMAL LOW    2.90  2.80  49  47   38   70   80    9  1.0  4   0.5   12   8.0   48
```

```
DEC 15 04:09  8.70  4.42  95  92   46   51   77   36  30.0M32   .5    2   3.8   28
        DEC 15 02:00  DOPAMINE (INTROPIN)   20 MCG/KG/MIN
        DEC 14 21:54  LEVOPHED (LEVARTERENOL)    0.143MCG/KG/MIN
        DEC 15 02:56  NEOSYNEPHRINE    0.710MCG/KG/MIN
        DEC 14 09:00  DIGOXIN 0.125 MGM, INJ
        SEVERE LV DYSFUNCTION

DEC 14 13:00  9.30  5.00  96  97   52   58   88   30  22.0M22   .9    4   5.7   47
        DEC 14 11:10  DOPAMINE (INTROPIN)   30 MCG/KG/MIN
        DEC 14 12:51  LEVOPHED (LEVARTERENOL)    0.057MCG/KG/MIN
        DEC 14 12:39  NEOSYNEPHRINE    0.710MCG/KG/MIN
        DEC 14 09:00  DIGOXIN 0.125 MGM, INJ
        MILD LV DYSFUNCTION

DEC 14 12:00  9.20  4.95 167  55   30   56   81   31  20.0M22  1.0    4   4.4   24
        DEC 14 11:10  DOPAMINE (INTROPIN)   30 MCG/KG/MIN
        DEC 14 11:49  NEOSYNEPHRINE    0.190MCG/KG/MIN
        DEC 14 09:00  DIGOXIN 0.125 MGM, INJ
        MODERATE LV DYSFUNCTION

DEC 14 04:10  8.30  4.46 107  78   42   50   73   26  10.0E18  1.0    5   9.1   31
        DEC 14 03:56  DOPAMINE (INTROPIN)    8 MCG/KG/MIN
        DEC 13 09:00  DIGOXIN 0.125 MGM, INJ
        MILD LV DYSFUNCTION

DEC 13 13:33 10.80  5.48 109  99   50   57   73   33  20.0M28   .5    3   8.9   31
        DEC 13 09:50  DOPAMINE (INTROPIN)   12 MCG/KG/MIN
        DEC 13 09:00  DIGOXIN 0.125 MGM, INJ
        SEVERE LV DYSFUNCTION

DEC 13 04:48 12.20  6.56 113 108   58   67   83   39  26.0M30   .7    3  10.3   42
        DEC 13 00:58  DOPAMINE (INTROPIN)    8 MCG/KG/MIN
        DEC 13 00:00  DIGOXIN 0.125 MGM, INJ
        MILD LV DYSFUNCTION

DEC 13 04:00 12.20  6.56 113 108   58   65   81   38  26.0M34   .3    3   9.5   37
        DEC 13 00:58  DOPAMINE (INTROPIN)    8 MCG/KG/MIN
        DEC 13 00:00  DIGOXIN 0.125 MGM, INJ
        MODERATE LV DYSFUNCTION

DEC 13 00:00 12.90  6.94 124 104   56  104  102   36  26.0M26   .8    6   7.6   58
        DEC 12 23:57  DOPAMINE (INTROPIN)    4 MCG/KG/MIN
        DEC 13 00:00  DIGOXIN 0.125 MGM, INJ
        LV PARAMETERS ARE WITHIN NORMAL LIMITS
```

FIGURE 7 HELP System Cardiac Output Report. CO = cardiac output; CI = cardiac index; HR = heart rate; SV = stroke volume; SI = stroke index; MP = mean systemic blood pressure; MSP = mean systolic blood pressure (systemic); PA = pulmonary artery mean pressure; RA = right atrial pressure; PW = pulmonary artery wedge pressure; PVR = pulmonary vascular resistance; SVR = systemic vascular resistance; RWI = right ventricular stroke work index; LWI = left ventricular stroke work index. The dates and starting times for the drugs indicated below the hemodynamic data sets indicate the time and date at which the particular drug therapy was begun.

partment alone generates and stores approximately 18,000 patient data elements in one day. Timely examination of this amount of information by hand is impossible. In addition, the low yield compounds the tedium that would be encountered with manual review. Alerts are generated in only about 5% of LDS hospital patients (Fig. 8).[28] The computerized monitoring automatically effects the review and examines every record so that all data from all patients are included.

A more comprehensive application of computers in medical decision making is the use of computerized protocols to aid and guide physicians in the conduct of a patient's therapy. The Total Parenteral Nutrition (TPN) protocol is an example of a broadly disseminated protocol applied throughout the LDS Hospital's wards and on different clinical services. It provides recommendations and a standard set of default orders that assure an adequate standard of care. The physician can, however, change the standard orders within constraints determined by patients' laboratory values. The options for tailoring an order to a particular patient's needs are therefore limited by the patient's state and the patient's laboratory values and the physician is thus constrained to choose among a set of options that appear to be appropriate for the patient. This prevents mistakes due to physician misinformation or oversight. Within the ordering program, education as well as guidance for therapy is provided to the physician interacting with the computer terminal. These computer-generated TPN orders are intended to guide, but not rigidly constrain, the physician and are available not only in the ICU but throughout the hospital.

The HELP protocol for management of arterial hypoxemia in patients with acute hypoxic pulmonary failure

A more comprehensive application of computers in medical decision making is the use of computerized protocols to aid and guide physicians in the conduct of a patient's therapy.

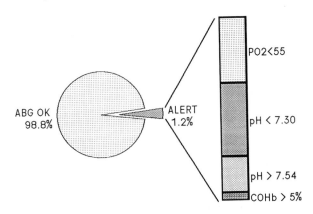

FIGURE 8   HELP arterial blood gas (ABG) alerts for the quality assurance program of the Respiratory Care Department. (Monthly average of 4,000 ABGs.)

(ARDS) is, in contrast, limited to ICU patient care.[17,19,20,41] It is an example of a more detailed computerized protocol, which, while providing specific and detailed instructions, imposes greater limitations on physician options. The protocols provide a standard therapeutic response to the severe arterial hypoxemia in mechanically ventilated patients with severe ARDS. These hypoxemia-focused protocols

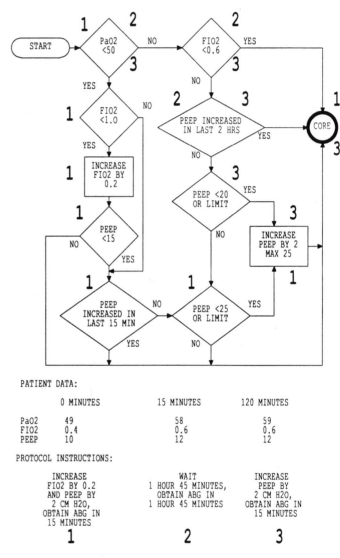

PATIENT DATA:

	0 MINUTES	15 MINUTES	120 MINUTES
PaO2	49	58	59
FIO2	0.4	0.6	0.6
PEEP	10	12	12

PROTOCOL INSTRUCTIONS:

INCREASE FIO2 BY 0.2 AND PEEP BY 2 CM H2O, OBTAIN ABG IN 15 MINUTES	WAIT 1 HOUR 45 MINUTES, OBTAIN ABG IN 1 HOUR 45 MINUTES	INCREASE PEEP BY 2 CM H2O, OBTAIN ABG IN 15 MINUTES
1	**2**	**3**

FIGURE 9   Selected elements of a protocol for the direction of management of arterial hypoxemia. Patient data and protocol instructions corresponding to numbers 1, 2, and 3 are those associated with the routes numbered 1, 2, and 3 in the flow diagram. CORE = continuous respiratory evaluation (diagnostic protocol) to which the patient is directed for reevaluation following the actions indicated in routes 1, 2, and 3.

have been generated using information in the published literature combined with that from local, national, and international experts. Involved physicians have agreed to abandon personal style and adopt a "standard" protocol therapy of arterial hypoxemia, ventilation, weaning, and extubation. While the physician is free to decline to follow a protocol instruction, he or she must provide a defensible reason (other than personal style or preference).

The protocol management of arterial hypoxemia is achieved primarily by manipulation of oxygen concentration and positive end-expiratory pressure (PEEP) during mechanical ventilator support of patients with severe pulmonary failure. This acceptance of protocol-controlled therapy has required a high level of collegiality and commitment from physicians, nurses, and respiratory therapists. The computerized versions of these protocols have been used for about 30,000 hours in routine around-the-clock care of about 70 patients with ARDS, and have proved to be much more easily applied and more accurate than manual paper-based flow-diagram versions.[19,20] Computerized protocol instructions control the therapy of arterial hypoxemia in patients with severe ARDS 94% of the day (23 of 24 hours) in our ICU.[18,42] In addition, they provide an audit trail that permits a detailed review of the performance of the protocols in the clinical environment. Figure 9 illustrates a simplified and selected portion of 1 of approximately 30 pages of protocols used for the control of arterial oxygenation in these patients. Three sets of representative instructions generated during routine application in one patient are also shown.

Acceptance of protocol-controlled therapy has required a high level of collegiality and commitment from physicians, nurses, and respiratory therapists. The computerized versions of these protocols have been used for about 30,000 hours in routine around-the-clock care of about 70 patients with ARDS.

INVERSE RATIO VENTILATION: AN EXAMPLE OF INTERDEPENDENCE OF INDIVIDUAL PATIENT CARE, MEDICAL POLICY FORMULATION, DOCUMENTATION, AND DECISION SUPPORT

While many publications deal with inverse ratio ventilation (IRV), there is no well-defined method of employment, and descriptions of the technique lack essential details.[43] Information gained from visits to domestic and international medical centers has confirmed our local experience that IRV is usually applied by trial and error, with changes in

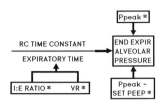

FIGURE 10 Conceptual diagram of inverse ratio ventilation or "controlled air trapping" protocol. End-expiratory alveolar pressure is adjusted by regulating the four variables indicated by asterisks. I:E ratio = inspiratory to expiratory ratio; Ppeak = peak ventilator pressure; VR = ventilatory rate; SET PEEP = external PEEP setting (either with the ventilator knob or with a water column).

ventilator settings based on pathophysiologic principles. All of this means that the application of IRV is not systematic and is, therefore, not reproducible in the clinical setting.

The results of the application of a computerized IRV protocol is particularly instructive because of implications regarding the limited number of variables that physicians are capable of managing.[44,45] The IRV protocol operates in a dedicated personal computer linked to a mechanical ventilator. It produces "controlled air trapping" that is reflected by the end-expiratory alveolar pressure. The desired end-expiratory pressure is entered into the IRV personal computer as the new target value. Four variables (inspiratory/expiratory ratio, (I/E) ventilatory rate, (VR) peak ventilator pressure (Ppeak), and PEEP setting (set PEEP) determine the end-expiratory alveolar pressure (Fig. 10). The computerized IRV protocol displays instructions for changing the four determining variables by small increments or decrements. Following the initial application of the computerized protocol in our ICU, the use of IRV has been markedly simplified, and it is now seen as a technique that can be used systematically, predictably, and reproducibly. This dramatic change in perception of IRV performance was noted by physicians, nurses, and respiratory therapists alike. It was concluded that the four determining variables (I/E, VR, Ppeak, setPEEP) had not been managed in a systematic manner before the computer protocol was applied, even though IRV had been used by experienced pulmonary/critical care physicians within an academic training program. This suggests that, faced with the challenge of adjusting four variables, experienced physicians were not able to develop a systematic response to ventilatory support problems. We do not think we are unique in this inability and suggest that others likely have similar limitations in their ability to manage clinical problems that have at least four variable determinants. Within the more than 236 different categorical variables noted in one ICU patient (discussed previously in this chapter), there are a number of clinically important problems involving more than four adjustable variables, including cardiac output (intracavitary pressures and pericardial or intrathoracic pressures on both the right and left sides of the heart, heart rate, ventricular septal position, electrical conduction and rhythm, arterial oxygenation, and medications), renal output (cardiac output, arterial oxygenation, venous pressure, abdominal pressure, intrathoracic pressure, and medications), and "tissue oxygenation" (cardiac output, arterial oxygen content, arterial oxygen pressure, oxygen consumption, bacteremia or infection, temperature, activity, and medications). These observations led us to question our ability to arrive at the "right therapeutic decision" when dealing with multivariate problems in severely ill patients.

SUMMARY

The availability of the computerized, fully integrated database from a hospital information system allows the performance of a number of monitoring tasks, which, in the absence of such a system, would be prohibitive because of the large investment of resources required for manual achievement of the same goals. Among these tasks are the acquisition and integration of data and the generation of appropriate reports. The decision-making support, which is now becoming more widely available in the HELP computer system, extends the impact of computers upon medical practice and provides the potential for much greater influence upon ultimate patient outcome. The application of computerized databases to quality assurance questions addresses an extremely important and highly visible area of concern in the current medical climate of the United States.

Available evidence dealing with the ultimate impact of such systems upon cost and cost-benefit ratios in hospital practice suggests a favorable impact of computers in hospital pharmacy[30] and infectious disease[32] departments. Carefully controlled randomized clinical trials dealing with patient outcome, especially survival, are sorely needed in order to provide the information base necessary for appropriate medical policy formulation relative to the future role of computerized data management systems in critical care medicine and in medicine at large. Nevertheless, the preliminary information currently available indicates the great potential for computer applications in critical care medicine.

The availability of the computerized, fully integrated database from a hospital information system allows the performance of a number of monitoring tasks, which, in the absence of such a system, would be prohibitive because of the large investment of resources required for manual achievement of the same goals.

Available evidence dealing with the ultimate impact of such systems upon cost and cost-benefit ratios in hospital practice suggests a favorable impact of computers in hospital pharmacy and infectious disease departments.

References

1. Eddy D: Clinical decision making. JAMA 263:1265, 1990

2. Hudson: Monitoring of clinically ill patients: conference summary. Respir Care 30:628, 1985

3. Gardner RM, Shabot MM: Computerized ICU data management: pitfalls and promises. Int J Clin Monit Comput 7:99, 1990

4. Ayers S et al: NIH consensus conference: critical care medicine. JAMA 250:798, 1983

5. Freeman R. Intrapartum fetal monitoring: a disappointing story. N Engl J Med 322:624, 1990

6. Robin ED: The cult of the Swan-Ganz catheter. Ann Intern Med 103:445, 1985

7. Shaver JA: Hemodynamic monitoring in the critically ill patient (editorial). N Engl J Med 308:277, 1983

8. Wiedemann HP, Matthay M, Mathay R: Cardiovascular-pulmonry monitoring in the intensive care unit. Part 2. Chest 86:656, 1984

9. Miller JG: Living Systems. p. 121. In: Information input overload. McGraw-Hill, New York, 1978

10. Rennels GD, Shortliffe EH: Advanced computing for medicine. Sci Am 257(4):154, 1987

11. Kuperman GJ, Gardner RM: The impact of the HELP computer system on the LDS Hospital paper medical record. p. 673. In: Proc 14th Annual Symposium on Computer Applications in Medical Care. Los Alamitos, California, IEEE Computer Society Press, 1990

12. Bradshaw KE, Gardner RM, Clemmer TP et al: Physician decision-making: Evaluation of data used in a computerized ICU. Int J Clin Monit Comput 1:81, 1984

13. Wirtschafter DD, Scalise M, Henke C, Gams RA: Do information systems improve the quality of clinical research? Results of a randomized trial in a cooperative multi-institutional cancer group. Comput Biomed Res 14:78, 1981

14. Dawes RM, Faust D, Meehl PE: Clinical versus actuarial judgment. Science 243:1668, 1990

15. Rennels GD, Miller PL: Artificial intelligence research in anesthesia and intensive care. J Clin Monit 4:274, 1988

16. Flanagin A, Lundberg GD: Clinical decision making: promoting the jump from theory to practice. (editorial) JAMA 263:279, 1990

17. Morris AH, Wallace CJ, Clemmer TP et al: Extracorporeal CO_2 removal therapy for adult respiratory distress syndrome patients. Respir Care 35:224, 1990

18. Morris AH, Wallace CJ, Clemmer TP et al: Extracorporeal CO_2 removal therapy for adult respiratory distress syndrome patients: a computerized protocol controlled trial. Réan Soins Intens Méd Urg, 6:485, 1990

19. Henderson SE, Crapo RO, East TD et al: Computerized clinical protocols in an intensive care unit: how well are they followed? p. 284. In: Proc 14th Annual Symposium on Computer Applications in Medical Care. IEEE Computer Society Press, Los Alamitos, California, 1990

20. East TD, Morris AH, Clemmer T et al: Development of computerized critical care protocols: a strategy that really works. p. 504. In: Proc 14th Annual Symposium on Computer Applications in Medical Care. IEEE Computer Society Press, Los Alamitos, California, 1990

21. Sutton GC: Computer-aided diagnosis: a review. Br J Surg 76:82, 1989

22. Wyatt J, Spiegelhalter D: Evaluating medical decision aids: what to test, and how? p. 1. In Talmon J, Fox J (eds): System engineering in medicine. Springer Verlag, Heidelberg, 1989

23. Shabot MM: Standardized acquisition of bedside data: the IEEE P1073 medical information bus. Int J Clin Monit Comput 6:197, 1989

24. Hawley WL, Tariq H, Gardner RM: Clinical implementation of an automatied medical information bus in an intensive care unit. p. 621. In: 12th Annual Symposium on Computer Applications in Medical Care. IEEE Computer Society Press, Los Alamitos, California, 1988

25. Gardner RM, Tariq H, Hawley WL, East TD: Medical information bus: the key to future integrated monitoring. (editorial) Int J Clin Monit Comput 6:205, 1989

26. Bradshaw KE, Sitig DF, Gardner RM et al: Computer-based data entry for nurses in the ICU. MD Comput 6:274, 1989

27. Gardner RM, Bradshaw KE, Holingsworth KW: Computerizing the intensive care unit: current status and future directions. J cardiovasc Nurs 4:68, 1989

28. Pryor TA, Gardner RM, Clayton PD, Warner HR: The HELP System. J Med Sys 7:87, 1983

29. Andrews RD, Gardner RM, Metcalf SM, Simmons D: Computer charting: an evaluation of a respiratory care computer system. Respir Care 8:695, 1985

30. Gardner RM, Hulse RK, Larsen KG: Assessing the effectiveness of a computerized pharmacy system. p. 668. In: Proc 14th Annual Symposium on Computer Applications in Medical Care. IEEE Computer Society Press, Los Alamitos, California, 1990

31. Evans RS, Burke JP, Pestotnik SL et al: Prediction of hospital infections and selection of antibiotics using an automated hospital database. p. 663. In: Proc 14th Annual Symposium on Computer Applications in Medical Care. IEEE Computer Society Press, Los Alamitos, California, 1990

32. Evans RS, Pestotnik SL, Burke JP et al: Reducing the duration of prophylactic antibiotics use through computer monitoring of surgical patients. DICP Ann Pharmacother 24:351, 1990

33. Gardner RM, Golubjatnikov OK, Laub RM et al: Computer-critiqued blood ordering using the HELP system. Comput Biomed Res 23:514, 1990

34. Knaus WA, Draper EA, Wagner DP, Zimmerman JE: APACHE II: a severity of disease classification system. Crit Care Med 13:818, 1985

35. Shortliffe EH: Clinical decision-support systems. p. 466. In Shortliffe EH, Perreault LE (eds): Medical informatics: computer applications in health care. Addison-Wesley, Reading, Massachusetts, 1990

36. Pryor TA: Development of decision support systems. Int J Clin Monit Comp 7:137, 1990

37. Morris AH, Kanner RE, Crapo RO, Gardner RM: Clinical pulmonary function testing: a manual of uniform laboratory procedures. 2nd ed. Intermountain Thoracic Society, Salt Lake City, UT, 1984

38. Bradshaw KE, Gardner RM, Pryor TA; Development of a computerized laboratory alerting system. Comput Biomed Res 22:575, 1989

39. Tate KE, Gardner RM, Weaver LK: A computerized laboratory alerting system. MD Comput 7:296, 1990

40. Elliott CG, Simmons D, Schmidt CD et al: Computer-assisted medical direction of respiratory care. Respir Manage 19:31, 1989

41. Sittig DF, Gardner RM, Pace NL et al: Computerized management of patient care in a complex, controlled clinical trial in the intensive care unit. Comput Methods Programs Biomed 30:77, 1989

42. Morris AH, Wallace CJ, Beck E et al: Protocols control respiratory therapy of ARDS (Abstr). Clin Res 38:138A, 1990

43. Kaczmarek RM, Hess D: Pressure controlled inverse-ratio ventilation, panacea or auto-PEEP. Respir Care 35:945, 1990

44. Boehm SH, Peng L, East TD et al: Computerized protocol management of pressure control inverse ratio ventilation (Abstr). Chest 98:77S, 1990

45. East TD, Böhm SH, Peng L et al: Exquisite management of pressure control inverse ratio ventilation by a computerized protocol (Abstr). Am Rev Respir Dis 141:A240, 1990

COST-EFFECTIVENESS OF RESPIRATORY MONITORING

BRUCE P. KRIEGER, MD[†]

Because of escalating health care costs and ever-expanding technology, the medical profession has been forced to confront issues of health economics,[1] specifically cost-effectiveness analysis.[2,3] This issue is very pertinent to critical care since intensive care unit (ICU) costs can be 3.0–3.8 times more expensive than routine hospital care[4] and mortality is much higher. In addition, studies have shown that up to 77% of admissions to an ICU were for monitoring only, of which only 10% subsequently required intensive care.[5] The costs incurred by institutions caring for patients who require mechanical ventilatory support (MVS) are nearing crisis proportions, as recently reviewed by Rosen and Bone.[6] Despite the monetary outlay, only approximately 50% of patients who required long-term MVS were eventually discharged,[7] and only half of these patients were alive 1 year later.[8] Therefore, the impact of health care economics, especially in the ICU, has far-reaching moral, monetary, and practical implications.

This chapter will explore the cost-effectiveness of various respiratory monitoring techniques. First, working definitions of the terms "cost-effective" and "monitoring" will be developed. These concepts will be applied to invasive techniques, such as pulmonary artery flow-directed catheters and continuous mixed venous oxygen saturation monitors. The growing array of noninvasive techniques will then be explored. Lastly, the future of respiratory monitoring in relationship to our expanding concerns and knowledge about burgeoning costs and difficult-to-prove benefits will be addressed.

Up to 77% of admissions to an ICU were for monitoring only, of which only 10% subsequently required intensive care.

[†] Associate Professor of Medicine, University of Miami School of Medicine, Chief, Pulmonary Intensive Care, Mount Sinai Medical Center, Miami Beach, Florida

DEFINITIONS

Monitoring is a continuous, or nearly continuous, evaluation of the physiologic function of a patient in real time to guide management decisions.

"Monitoring is a continuous, or nearly continuous, evaluation of the physiologic function of a patient in real time to guide management decisions—including when to make therapeutic interventions—and assessment of those interventions."[9] A monitor that requires insertion through a patient's integument or through an orifice is considered "invasive," whereas "noninvasive" monitors generally are placed onto the skin or next to an orifice. Table 1 lists the respiratory monitors that are commonly used in ICUs today; intermittent measurements (eg, pulmonary mechanics, arterial blood gas analysis) are not included in Table 1 because they fail to provide continuous evaluation of the patient as the definition for "monitoring" requires.

Cost-effectiveness analysis for nonmedical products requires simple rules of market operation with easily defined endpoints.[1] In medicine, this type of analysis is much more difficult because it often involves trade-offs between patient health, economics, and the physician's responsibility to the individual patient. As recently pointed out, the term "cost-effective" is often misused in medicine.[3] This chapter will follow a guide to cost-effectiveness analysis (Table 2) that Detsky and Naglie recently proposed,[2] which involves the following steps: (1) demonstration of efficiency or accuracy; (2) assessment of effectiveness, that is, the demonstration that a technique does more good than harm in the setting in which it is being utilized; and (3) the availability and resources required for using a specific monitor. When new monitors are compared to existing technology, they can be viewed as being cost-effective if they are less costly and equally or more effective.[3] This does not presuppose that the technique with the lowest cost-effectiveness ratio is the most desirable, since the added costs may be worth the added benefits when dealing with health care issues.

Robin and Lewiston[10] perceived two systematic errors

TABLE 1 Common Respiratory Monitors

Invasive	Noninvasive
Pulmonary artery flow-directed catheter	Pneumotachygraph
Systemic arterial pressure catheter	Inspired and expired gas analysis
Esophageal pressure catheter	Pulse oximetry
Airway pressure catheter	Transcutaneous and transconjunctival gas analysis
Pulmonary artery catheter with fiberoptic oximetry (SvO_2)	Impedance pneumography
	Respiratory inductive plethysmography

in medial practice, which they referred to as type 3 and type 4 statistical errors. In essence, these statistical errors describe a failure of appropriate cost-effective analysis. A type 3 error occurs when the risks involved with a technique have been underestimated, while a type 4 error refers to the underutilization of an intervention because of overestimation of the risks or perceived variability. Indeed, the "carte blanche" acceptance of many invasive techniques may have involved a type 3 error, while the reluctance to accept some noninvasive monitors may be a form of type 4 error. Both of these reflect an inadequate cost-effective analysis.

INVASIVE MONITORS
PULMONARY ARTERY FLOW-DIRECTED CATHETERS

Since Swan, Ganz et al.[11] introduced the pulmonary artery (PA) flow-directed balloon-tipped catheter into clinical medicine over two decades ago, it has been considered the gold standard for critical care and respiratory monitoring. Recent investigations and editorials emphasizing risk-benefit[12–15] and cost-effective analysis[16,17] have tarnished this image. Opinions vary widely, from calling for a moratorium,[13] to halt the "cult"[18] of the PA catheter to reviews in defense of its continued[19] or increased use. This controversy highlights the problems of accepting technology without first establishing its cost-effectiveness, specifically an objective assessment of its risk-benefit ratio. This is a "type 3-B error" according to Robin and Lewiston.[10] Although the PA catheter is generally considered a mainstay for respiratory and critical care monitoring, only the PA pressure readings are continuous and therefore meet the strict definition of monitoring as described earlier. Nonetheless, its widespread use requires that it be included in this discussion.

When calibrated and maintained appropriately, pulmonary capillary wedge pressure (PCWP) readings from the PA catheter accurately reflect left atrial pressure.[20] Technical problems occur one-third of the time,[21] and even when technically accurate, the PCWP may not reflect transmural pressure.[22] These concepts are often not appreciated by those who use the technology.[22] Another hemodynamic parameter that is attainable with most PA catheters is the thermodilution cardiac output (CO). This measurement is often interpreted by the clinician at face value without realizing that a thermodilution CO may vary up to 12.3% compared to a simultaneous CO by the gold standard (Fick)

TABLE 2   Definitions of "Cost-effective Analysis"

Demonstration of efficacy (accuracy)
Assessment of effectiveness (more good than harm)
Availability in specific area or indication
Less costly and equally or more effective than existing technology

Data from Detsky AS, Naglie IG: A clinician's guide to cost-effectiveness analysis. Ann Intern Med 113:147, 1990 and Doubilet P, Weinstein MC, McNeil BJ: Use and misuse of the term "cost effective" in medicine. N Engl J Med 314:253, 1986.

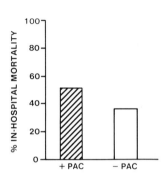

FIGURE 1 In-hospital mortality for patients with acute myocardial infarction and persistent hypotension (systolic blood pressure <90 mmHg) without shock. Total n = 1,281 patients; 388 managed with pulmonary artery catheter (+PAC) and 893 managed without pulmonary artery catheter (−PAC). Data from Gore JM, Goldberg RJ, Spodick DH et al: A community-wide assessment of the use of pulmonary artery catheters with acute myocardial infarction. Chest 92:721, 1987 and Zion MM, Balkin J, Rosenmann D et al: Use of pulmonary artery catheters in patients with acute myocardial infarction: analysis of experience in 5,841 patients in the SPRINT registry. Chest 98:1331, 1990

technique.[23] Therefore, a minimal difference of at least 15% between thermodilution determinations (mean of three injections) of CO is necessary before being clinically significant.[24] These problems do not reflect a poor product but rather a conceptual or interpretative misunderstanding.[17,25] Considering the widespread use of PA catheters, it is disturbing that a recent multicenter study[25] reported that physicians misinterpreted PA catheter-related questions one-third of the time.

The PA catheter itself is probably efficacious in various clinical situations,[19] therefore satisfying the first part of the definition of cost-effective (Table 2). However, its rapid acceptance by the medical community occurred prior to any demonstration that the technique does more good than harm in all of the situations in which it is used. Therefore, it has not satisfied the second requirement of being cost-effective as previously outlined.[2] Even the most recent exhaustive attempt[14] to support the continued use of the PA catheter in patients with acute myocardial infarction (which is one of the most frequently cited indications for its use) only demonstrated that the introduction of the catheter did not increase in-hospital mortality and failed to prove any benefit when it was used.[15] Figure 1 shows that the in-hospital mortality rates for patients with acute myocardial infarction and persistent hypotension (systolic blood pressure < 90 mmHg) but without shock were actually higher when a PA catheter was used. The data for Figure 1 were compiled from two studies (total n = 1,281), one favoring PA catheter use[14] and one questioning its use[12]; both studies attempted to control for severity of illness.

Analysis of the clinical efficacy of the PA catheter has been hampered by the lack of alternative methodologies, although recent techniques are being tested. Various studies have looked at the clinical assessment of patients' hemodynamic status using the PA catheter as "truth" with varying results.[19] A recent study[26] demonstrated that initial management without a PA catheter was possible, but only in selected cases. In a group of surgical patients, Shoemaker et al.[16] showed no significant differences between using central venous (CVP) vs PA catheters in mortality or organ failure when normal values were used as therapeutic goals, although the group earmarked for "supra-normal" values (as directed by a PA catheter) did fare better financially and medically. This investigation highlights that the real issue when evaluating the pulmonary artery flow-directed catheter is not the catheter per se, its indications, or its complications, but the proper collection and utilization of data for clinical decision making in yet-to-be-determined specific situations.[17] In conclusion, this monitoring technique is not cost-effective as it is being used in most critical care units today.

CONTINUOUS MIXED VENOUS O_2 SATURATION MONITORING

Measurement of mixed venous oxygen saturation (S_vO_2) is an indirect indicator of tissue oxygenation and cardiac output. Approximately 1 decade ago,[27] a fiberoptic reflectance system was incorporated into the flow-directed PA catheter that allowed continuous monitoring of S_vO_2 in critically ill patients. The premise was that continuous S_vO_2 recording would allow more rapid detection of a change in a patient's cardiorespiratory status.[28]

Using simultaneously obtained blood samples drawn from the PA catheter to determine S_vO_2 photometrically from a co-oximeter, Fahey et al.[29] showed a good correlation ($r = 0.95$, $n = 199$) between the fiberoptic catheter and simultaneous mixed venous blood samples over a wide range of S_vO_2 in 86 critically ill adults with respiratory failure. This correlation remained accurate over a period of 4 days. They also gave clinical examples of how changes in S_vO_2 heralded changes in a patient's clinical status (eg, when oxygenation or cardiac output was altered). In the same year, similar uncontrolled observations were reported in cardiac surgery patients,[30] medical cardiac patients,[31] and mixed patient populations,[32] which prompted one author[30] to suggest that the first indicator that mandated intensive hemodynamic tracking was the S_vO_2.

Boutros and Lee[33] tested the hypothesis that continuous S_vO_2 monitoring would predict a clinically significant change in a patient's status independent of standard observations (arterial pressure, PA pressure, PCWP, CVP, heart rate, CO, arterial blood gases, respiratory rate, ventilator settings, tidal volume, lab values, chest radiographs, and body temperature). They placed the S_vO_2 recorder in a box that was concealed from the staff caring for 15 patients in a surgical ICU and retrospectively scrutinized all instances ($n = 173$) when the S_vO_2 was less than 60% or greater than 80% or whenever a mixed venous O_2 sample was required by the team managing the patient. In 81.5% of the events, knowledge of the continuous S_vO_2 value would not have changed patient management; in 18.5%, the continuous S_vO_2 was at variance with clinical findings and the decisions based on these findings but actually was either misleadingly too high or too low. The authors concluded that awareness of the continuous S_vO_2 would not have altered their patients' management and never would have been the sole predictive signal for subsequent deterioration in their patients' status.[33]

Although insightful, this study addressed only one aspect of cost-effectiveness analysis, whether S_vO_2 monitoring does more good than harm (assessment of effectiveness, Table 2). It can still be considered cost-effective if it is less costly and equally or more effective[3] than existing technology. Indeed, one study[28] suggested a cost savings of $75.00 per catheter use compared to standard care (which included a PA catheter but no control group) but used perceived (not objectively measured) changes in ordering patterns without reporting specific data. In addition, S_vO_2 data was not useful in 45% of their patients because of sepsis. Rajput et al.[34] randomly assigned 51 medical ICU patients to receive a standard PA catheter (n = 26) or a fiberoptic catheter (n = 25) and found no decrease in the number of arterial or mixed venous blood gases that were ordered nor in the eventual outcome of their patients. Similar results were reported by Pearson et al.[35] in 226 adult postcardiac surgery patients, although charges (not costs) were used for comparison. Both of these studies concluded that routine substitution of the fiberoptic catheter for a standard PA catheter was not justified. In fact, the study by Pearson[35] questioned whether the PA catheter was even necessary in "low-risk" cardiac surgical patients.

The most detailed study concerning the economic and medical effects of continuous S_vO_2 monitoring involved 99 mixed medical and surgical ICU patients who were randomly assigned to a standard or fiberoptic PA catheter.[36] Statistical analysis by step-deletion multiple regression analysis was utilized for severity of illness (Acute Physiology and Chronic Health Evaluation, APACHE; Therapeutic Intervention Scoring System, TISS), number of arterial and venous blood gases, incidence of catheter-related problems, length of ICU stay, ICU mortality, and severity and outcome of adverse hemodynamic events. No difference in potentially adverse hemodynamic events, length of ICU stay, or mortality was noted. Statistically fewer ($P <$ 0.005) venous blood gases were performed in the fiberoptic catheter group, but this group experienced significantly more ($P < 0.025$) catheter-related problems. Overall *charges* were less for the patients managed with the fiberoptic catheter, but hospital *costs*, which are more pertinent in a fixed reimbursement system such as Medicare, were not lowered.

Although it is an accurate reflection of mixed venous oxygen saturation and is a valuable educational modality,[36] the fiberoptic catheter-derived continuous S_vO_2 monitoring system has not been shown to independently affect patient outcome. It has the potential to be less costly, but has not yet been shown to be cost-effective, nor does it avoid the known complications of invasive hemodynamic monitoring.[13]

ARTERIAL OXYGENATION

Miniaturization of the Clark electrode coupled with the recent development of fluorescent-based probes that are incorporated into fiberoptic strands allows continuous monitoring of the arterial oxygen tension (P_aO_2) with a 20-gauge arterial catheter.[37] Initial animal and human studies have shown good agreement with simultaneously drawn arterial blood gas (ABG) for pH and P_aCO_2, although P_aO_2 measurement requires further refinement.[38] No cost-effective data are available.

The availability of ABGs have revolutionized mechanical ventilatory care. Serial ABGs, although intermittent and therefore not a "monitor" in the true sense, are used as the gold standard to monitor arterial oxygenation and ventilation. However, no formal cost-effective analyses have been reported. Attempts have been successful in reducing the number of daily ABGs[39] without any adverse effects on medical care just by eliminating standing or repetitive orders, and encouraging better communication, closer administrative attention, and removal of arterial catheters as rapidly as possible. One study reported that the presence of an arterial line was the most powerful predictor of the number of ABGs eventually performed.[40]

Despite the ubiquitous use of the arterial blood gas and the fact that it is the most frequently ordered laboratory exam in the ICU,[40] many health care workers do not realize the variability and therefore limitations of the values obtained. For example, Thorson et al.[41] studied the variability of ABGs in 29 ICU patients who were clinically stable and found that the upper confidence limit for two P_aO_2 samples separated by 50 minutes was 23%. Appreciation of this natural variability will impact upon the following discussion concerning the accuracy of noninvasive oxygenation monitors.

Attempts have been successful in reducing the number of daily ABGs without any adverse effects on medical care.

Despite the ubiquitous use of the arterial blood gas and the fact that it is the most frequently ordered laboratory exam in the ICU, many health care workers do not realize the variability and therefore limitations of the values obtained.

NONINVASIVE MONITORS

PULSE OXIMETRY

Although the term "oximeter" wasn't coined until 1942, its basis dates back to 1666 when Isaac Newton began to study the nature of sunlight through a prism.[42] Development of an easy, simple pulse oximeter (S_pO_2 monitor) in the early 1980s precipitated an explosive acceptance of this technology for monitoring arterial oxygen saturation (S_aO_2), especially in the operating and recovery room where it has literally redefined the standards for anesthesia monitoring. However, it has only been in the past few years that researchers have investigated the accuracy, limitations, and indications for its use, despite it being dubbed the "fifth vital sign."[43] This is the first step in establishing that a new technique is cost-effective (Table 2).

It is essential that personnel who rely on pulse oximetry fully appreciate its strengths and its limitations. Because of the shape of the oxygen–hemoglobin dissociation curve, S_aO_2 or S_pO_2 measurements will be insensitive to changes in P_aO_2 at high levels of oxygenation (eg, above 80 mmHg) and will be affected by factors that shift the curve to the right or left (temperature, P_{50}, P_aCO_2, pH).[44] Dyshemoglobinemias, intravascular dyes, skin pigmentation, dark nail polish and ambient light have also been reported to interfere with accurate S_pO_2 readings.[42,45] The precision and bias[46] of most oximeters are less than 5%,[47] although accuracy decreases when the S_aO_2 is less than 70–75%,[48] and the response time of some systems can be as long as 27 seconds.[49] Perhaps the most distressing inaccuracy of the pulse oximeter during ICU utilization is motion artifact[45] and hypoperfusion states,[50] since continuous alarms eventually are "tuned-out" and thus ignored by the staff caring for the patient (Fig. 2).

The absolute accuracy of S_pO_2 for monitoring trends has been established in the research lab by Ries et al.[51] The 95% confidence limit for a single S_pO_2 reading compared to a co-oximeter-measured S_aO_2 is ±4%, which means that an S_pO_2 of 95% could equal an S_aO_2 ranging from 91% ($P_aO_2 = 60$ mmHg) to 99% ($P_aO_2 = 160$ mmHg).[45] A true change in the direction for S_aO_2 during exercise testing required an S_pO_2 change of greater than 3%.[51]

Although single S_pO_2 readings correlate well with S_aO_2 in critically ill patients,[52] precision, bias, and trend accuracy in the ICU have yet to be determined.[45] Cost-effectiveness analysis demands definition not only of accuracy but also of pulse oximetry's role in clinical decision making in the settings where the new technology is being applied. One of the first attempts to better define the utility of pulse oximetry in managing oxygen therapy in patients on MVS was by Jubran and Tobin.[53] They found that an S_pO_2 equal to 92% reliably predicted a $P_aO_2 \geq 60$ mmHg and avoided hyperoxia in white patients on MVS; the S_pO_2 readings were much less reliable in black patients. The efficacy of S_pO_2 and capnometry in monitoring postcardiac surgery

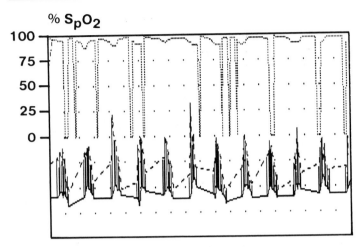

% S$_p$O$_2$

FIGURE 2   Ten-minute epoch showing continuous S$_p$O$_2$ readings on top. There are 12 periods where the pulse is lost, resulting in the S$_p$O$_2$ dropping to 0% and the occurrence of a false alarm. Cheyne Stokes respirations are seen on the bottom of tracing where each vertical bar is proportional to tidal volume as recorded by a respiratory inductive plethysmograph. When S$_p$O$_2$ was appropriately sensed, it ranged from 86% to 97%.

patients during weaning from MVS was studied by Neihoff et al.[54] They concluded that an S$_p$O$_2 \geq 95\%$ assured "adequate" oxygenation (P$_a$O$_2 > 70$ mmHg), but their data was limited by having the majority of patients hyperoxygenated (P$_a$O$_2 > 100$ mmHg) with only one arterial oxygen saturation < 90%. These investigators also prospectively compared the number of ABGs obtained from 12 patients, all of whom were weaned from MVS in less than 20 hours using noninvasive monitors (S$_p$O$_2$, capnometry), vs a control group and found a significant reduction in the number of ABGs (5.9 vs 10.5, $P < 0.0001$) in the group using noninvasive monitors. However, the precise role of pulse oximetry in aiding this reduction or whether this merely reflected more stringent order writing[39] could not be determined from their data. A much larger study (n = 842 admissions) of surgical ICU patients was unable to demonstrate any reduction in the number of ABGs or costs when pulse oximeters were used.[40]

Pulse oximetry is cost-effective when used as part of a protocol for tapering supplemental oxygen use in non-ICU patients.[55,56] When compared to a control group (n = 16), 13 patients for whom spot oximetry checks were utilized required fewer ABGs ($P < 0.005$) and fewer days on supplemental oxygen ($P < 0.001$).[56] This resulted in an estimated yearly savings to the hospital of $146,000, although details of how the authors derived the dollar estimates were not presented. Conceivably, a similar protocol using information from the Jubran and Tobin study[52] could be applied to patients on MVS as a cost-effective alternative to multiple ABG analyses in the ICU. The key to cost-effective use of pulse oximetry data is appropriate utilization, as alluded to during the discussion of resource management for noninvasive monitoring.[57] This may be why the studies that have investigated the cost-effectiveness of pulse oximetry[40,54] in the critical care setting have not been more positive.

TRANSCUTANEOUS AND TRANSCONJUNCTIVAL O_2 MONITORING

Oxygen and carbon dioxide that escape from the body's surfaces can be measured by placing miniaturized polarographic electrodes on the skin or palpebral conjunctiva, so-called transcutaneous and transconjunctival blood gas monitoring. The history and details of these monitors have been summarized recently.[58,59] The technology was first applied to neonates where the correlation between transcutaneous oxygen tension ($tcPO_2$) or transconjunctival oxygen tension ($cjPO_2$) and P_aO_2 was usually excellent (r > 0.90).[59] However, the correlation coefficient for $tcPO_2$ and P_aO_2 in adult patients was much lower, ranging from 0.06 in shock states to 0.89 in stable adults[60]; this correlation may also be worse in the elderly.[61] This phenomenon is expected since $tcPO_2$ actually measures oxygen delivery to the skin and conjunctiva and therefore is a function of both P_aO_2 and local perfusion as well as skin thickness.[58–61] Significant debate exists in the literature over whether the physiological basis of $tcPO_2$ (ie, oxygen delivery) offers an advantage or disadvantage to other noninvasive oxygenation monitors such as pulse oximeters.[61,62] In addition, since these monitors require heating of the skin to >40°C, local burns can complicate and limit their long-term use.

$tcPO_2$ monitoring appears to satisfy two parts of the definition of cost-effectiveness (Table 2)—it is accurate (but not equal to P_aO_2) and it is reported[63] in neonates at least to do more good than harm (although *not* proven in prospective, controlled trials). However, conflicting data[64,65] exist as to whether $tcPO_2$ was less costly than standard care (eg, serial ABGs). No cost-effective data on $tcPO_2$ or $cjPO_2$ monitoring exist for adult patients.

TRANSCUTANEOUS CO_2 MONITORING

Continuous monitoring of transcutaneous carbon dioxide ($tcPCO_2$) was made possible by a modification of Stowe's electromechanical sensor. $tcPCO_2$ and $tcPO_2$ monitors are often combined in one heated unit and were first evaluated in neonates.[58] Just as $tcPO_2$ is influenced by perfusion, the relationship between $tcPCO_2$ and P_aCO_2 becomes alinear during low perfusion states. However, in contrast to $tcPO_2$, the $tcPCO_2$ appears to reflect P_aCO_2 as well in adults as in neonates, with correlation coefficients as high as 0.89.[66] The $tcPCO_2$ is consistently higher than the corresponding P_aCO_2,[67] which reflects local CO_2 production. This is not an inaccuracy of the measurement, but a reflection of understanding exactly how the technology functions and what its limitations and "normal values" truly are.[58]

Healey et al.[68] investigated the accuracy of $tcPCO_2$ for the specific indication of tracking P_aCO_2 when switching 10 adult patients from mechanical ventilatory support to spontaneous breathing. The change in $tcPCO_2$ correlated well with the change in P_aCO_2 (r = 0.86), and changes in P_aCO_2 of ≥ 5 mmHg were accompanied by changes in $tcPCO_2$ in the same direction and vice versa. Even though the data was limited by the small number of samples (n = 20) and the short duration of the observations (30 minutes), it does suggest that $tcPCO_2$ technology could be cost-effective by being accurate for a specific indication in which savings could be realized (Table 2) by limiting the number of ABGs required in both intubated and nonintubated patients. However, there are no data on costs and therefore the cost-effectiveness of $tcPCO_2$ monitoring can only be suggested[63] at the present time.

END-TIDAL CO_2 MONITORING

Although end-tidal carbon dioxide ($P_{et}CO_2$) measurements have been used by physiologists for decades,[69] recent concerns about patient safety in the operating room spearheaded a rapid development and acceptance of commercial continuous $P_{et}CO_2$ monitors, especially by anesthesiologists. This enthusiasm has overflowed into the ICU[70] where it has been suggested that continuous $P_{et}CO_2$ monitoring could act as an early warning system for clinically significant changes in P_aCO_2[71] or as a noninvasive substitute for ABGs during adjustments and withdrawal of

MVS.[68,72] Unfortunately, the noninvasive nature of $P_{et}CO_2$ monitoring and therefore its perceived safety helped to launch its widespread use before its limitations were appreciated by clinicians. This is an analagous situation to what occurred with balloon-tipped PA catheters and pulse oximeters as discussed previously.

The first step in analyzing the cost-effectiveness of $P_{et}CO_2$ monitoring is establishing its efficacy (Table 2) compared to P_aCO_2 in intubated patients. Multiple studies using anesthetized[68,69,73] and spontaneously breathing adults on MVS,[68,75] including our own,[76] have shown good correlation between individual values of $P_{et}CO_2$ and corresponding P_aCO_2 with correlation coefficients ranging from 0.73[74] to 0.90[68]; our correlation coefficient was 0.78.[76] However, as Raemer et al.[73] pointed out almost 10 years ago, estimation of P_aCO_2 by $P_{et}CO_2$ "is not invariably reliable" because of the magnitude and physiologic changes that occur in the P_aCO_2 minus $P_{et}CO_2$ gradient [$P_{(a-et)}CO_2$]. In a study of 17 patients with respiratory failure,[77] no correlation between $P_{et}CO_2$ and P_aCO_2 was found since the $P_{(a-et)}CO_2$ varied from 0 to 39 mmHg. Interestingly, the $P_{(a-et)}CO_2$ correlated well (r = 0.80) with the dead space/tidal volume (V_D/V_T) ratio as determined by exhaled gas collection. This led the authors to conclude that although the $P_{et}CO_2$ was a poor estimate of P_aCO_2 in their patients with respiratory failure, the $P_{(a-et)}CO_2$ was helpful in assessing the efficiency of ventilation (ie, the V_D/V_T).[77]

This conclusion is expected if one appreciates that multiple physiologic conditions can alter the relationship between $P_{et}CO_2$ and P_aCO_2, such as changes in V_D/V_T, ventilation–perfusion ratios, positive end-expiratory pressure,[78] breathing pattern,[76,79,80] and cardiac output.[80] It is because of these factors that the precision and bias[46] of $P_{et}CO_2$ vs $PaCO_2$ is 15–20%[74] as opposed to only 5% for pulse oximetry. However, since the shape of the oxyhemoglobin is alinear, the absolute precision and bias of pulse oximetry expressed as mmHg may be worse than $P_{et}CO_2$.

If $P_{et}CO_2$ monitoring could be substituted for intermittent P_aCO_2 determinations for patients on MVS in the ICU or operating room, this technique would be cost-effective (Table 2). As outlined above, $P_{et}CO_2$ and P_aCO_2 may vary in individual patients. Therefore, authors proposed that the $P_{(a-et)}CO_2$ gradient be initially determined so that adjustments in $P_{et}CO_2$ would be made in the individual patient. Unfortunately, since the $P_{(a-et)}CO_2$ can vary even in individual anesthetized patients,[73] this correction is not reliable. A practical alternative is to show that trends in $P_{et}CO_2$ reflect trends in P_aCO_2, since this data could still

Estimation of P_aCO_2 by $P_{et}CO_2$ "is not invariably reliable" because of the magnitude and physiologic changes that occur in the P_aCO_2 minus $P_{et}CO_2$ gradient.

be useful in clinical decision making and therefore be cost-effective. Healey et al.[68] noted that rises in P_aCO_2 of ≥ 10 mmHg were correctly identified by similar changes (6–24 mmHg) in eight of nine postoperative patients. However, 25% of the changes in P_aCO_2 of ≥ 5 mmHg were accompanied by either no change in $P_{et}CO_2$ or a change in the opposite direction. In a larger study of 20 mixed medical and surgical ICU patients, we found similar disparities.[76] Five to six adjustments of ventilator settings were made in each patient, and changes in $P_{et}CO_2$ ($\Delta P_{et}CO_2$) were compared to changes in P_aCO_2 (ΔP_aCO_2). Only 18% of the $\Delta P_{et}CO_2$ were within 20% of the corresponding ΔP_aCO_2 (Fig. 3), and the trend in $P_{et}CO_2$ was opposite to the trend in P_aCO_2 in 20% of the patients. Similar inaccuracies were reported in postoperative cardiac patients in a preliminary study in which the change in $P_{et}CO_2$ incorrectly predicted the changes in P_aCO_2 42% of the time.[81] Therefore, in these studies it appears that $P_{et}CO_2$ is not cost-effective because it is not efficacious (Table 2) in patients with respiratory failure on MVS.

Given these restraints, $P_{et}CO_2$ monitoring may still prove to be cost-effective under other conditions. For example, one recent study[82] reported the usefulness of $P_{et}CO_2$ in adjusting hyperventilation in patients with head injuries early in their course of treatment. As mentioned

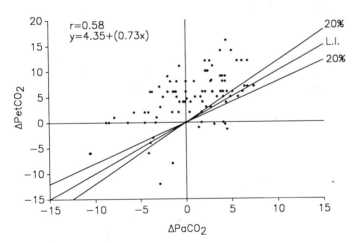

FIGURE 3 Identity plot showing the changes from baseline end tidal carbon dioxide ($\Delta P_{et}CO_2$) vs changes from baseline of simultaneously sampled P_aCO_2 (ΔP_aCO_2). Line of identity (L.I.) and 20% error lines are denoted. Only 18% of $\Delta P_{et}CO_2$ were within 20% of the corresponding P_aCO_2. From Hoffman RA, Krieger BP, Kramer MR et al: End-tidal carbon dioxide in critically ill patients during changes in mechanical ventilation. Am Rev Respir Dis 140:1265, 1989. With permission.

before, understanding the variability of a new technique ($P_{et}CO_2$) in relationship to the variability of the gold standard (P_aCO_2)[41] is necessary before rejecting the technique if one is to avoid committing a type 4 error.[10] Perhaps better education of the health care personnel who utilize $P_{et}CO_2$ monitoring will allow safe and cost-effective use of the technique in the future. Further studies are needed to address this question if we are to avoid the same pitfalls that are now haunting the use of the balloon-tipped PA catheter.[12,13,17]

IMPEDANCE PNEUMOGRAPHY

By placing two electrocardiographic electrodes on the chest and passing a low-amplitude alternating current through the chest, impedance can be calculated. As the thoracic cavity fills with air, impedance increases, which forms the basis for commercially available impedance pneumographic (IP) "apnea monitors." This technology was rapidly accepted by health care personnel prior to understanding or elucidating its limitations, which may have resulted in a type 3 error.[10] For example, a panel on infantile apnea monitoring[83] seriously questioned the utility of IP for detecting obstructive events in infants at high risk for sudden infant death syndrome (SIDS) despite its widespread use for this indication. This is not a malfunction of the IP monitor but a reflection of the limitations, and thus clinical utility, of the technique.[1] By measuring only rib cage excursions, it cannot reliably detect an obstructive event during which the rib cage continues to move but no effective ventilation is occurring (Fig. 4). Unfortunately, this is a serious shortcoming[84] as is the inability of IP to be quantitated for volume or timing information.

These questions concerning the efficacy of IP monitoring overshadow any possible cost-effective argument (Table 2).

A panel on infantile apnea monitoring seriously questioned the utility of impedance pneumography for detecting obstructive events in infants at high risk for sudden infant death syndrome.

RESPIRATORY INDUCTIVE PLETHYSMOGRAPHY

The inaccuracy of the impedance pneumograph can be eliminated by employing the Konno-Mead principle,[85] which states that the respiratory system can be approximated with two degrees of freedom, the rib cage (RC) and abdominal (AB) movements. Paradoxical thoracic or abdominal motion therefore cancel out so that an obstructive apnea is appropriately sensed (Figs. 4 and 5). This forms the basis for respiratory inductive plethysmography (RIP) as well as strain gauges, magnetometers, and bellows pneumographs.[86] Since RIP has undergone the most ex-

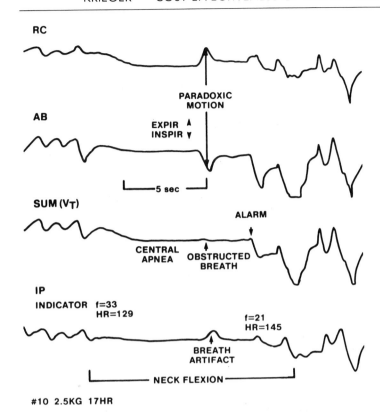

RC

**PARADOXIC
MOTION**

AB

EXPIR ▲
INSPIR ▼

└─ 5 sec ─┘

SUM (V$_T$)

ALARM

**CENTRAL
APNEA**   **OBSTRUCTED
BREATH**

**IP
INDICATOR f=33
HR=129**

f=21
HR=145

**BREATH
ARTIFACT**

└─── NECK FLEXION ───┘

#10 2.5KG 17HR

FIGURE 4 Simultaneous recordings from an impedance pneumograph (IP, bottom tracing) and a respiratory inductive plethysmograph (RC = rib cage; AB = abdomen; sum V$_T$ = tidal volume) of a 10-second mixed apnea in a 17-hour-old 2.5 kg neonate when neck flexion occurred. A 7-second central apnea is seen as depicted by no RC, AB, or V$_T$ movements. This is followed by two obstructed breaths (obstructed apnea) during which the RC and AB move in opposite directions without any significant tidal volume. Because RC motion occurred, the IP falsely registered two breaths rather than a continued apnea. The readout of respiratory rate (f) and heart rate (HR) from the IP are shown. An alarm sounded appropriately on the respiratory inductive plethysmograph after the 10-second mixed apnea but not on the IP. Expir = expiration; Inspir = inspiration.

tensive evaluation in clinical trials and is the only one that can be automatically calibrated[86-89] and used in the ICU, it will be reviewed.

The breathing pattern recorded by RIP can be analyzed in terms of volume, flow, timing, and thoracoabdominal (RC–AB) motion.[87] As opposed to almost all the other technologies discussed so far, RIP underwent laboratory and research evaluation before it was introduced into pulmonary medicine.[88] Because it is noninvasive it cannot exactly

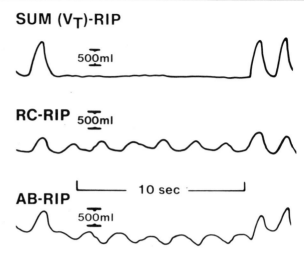

SUM (V$_T$)-RIP

500ml

RC-RIP 500ml

AB-RIP   └── 10 sec ──┘

500ml

FIGURE 5 Simultaneous recordings of abdomen (AB), rib cage (RC), and sum tidal volume (V$_T$) from a respiratory inductive plethysmograph (RIP) during an 11-second obstructive apnea (flat V$_T$ signal). Inspiration is depicted by upward movement of the V$_T$, RC, and AB signals. During the obstructive event, the RC and AB moved in opposite directions, which results in no significant respiration. This demonstrates the Konno-Mead principle[85] that the respiratory system can be approximated with two degrees of freedom and forms the basis for the isovolume and natural breathing calibration methods.[87] From Krieger BP: Respiratory inductive plethysmography. Prob Respir Care 2:156, 1989. With permission.

equal absolute measurements of volume, but it can estimate tidal volume (V$_T$) to within 10% of spirometric values when the patient does not move and within 20% despite changes in subject positioning and functional residual capacity.[87–89] The measurement of respiratory rate by RIP was within 10% of hand-measured spirometric waveforms recorded on a polygraph 98% of the time.[88] RIP can also detect thoracoabdominal asynchrony[86,88,90] and estimate changes in functional residual capacity (by recording changes in end-expiratory thoracic gas volume).[87–89]

Given these well-studied limitations, RIP is efficacious in the clinical setting and is available for use in the ICU[90–93] and for defined indications (described below). Therefore, it satisfies two of the criteria for being cost-effective (Table 2). Also, evidence indicates that when applied appropriately it is as (or more) accurate than available monitors. For example, both Tobin et al. and our group have shown that thoracoabdominal asynchrony as assessed by RIP may be one of the most sensitive indicators of the inability to successfully wean from MVS.[90,92] In this role, RIP acts as

Thoracoabdominal asynchrony as assessed by RIP may be one of the most sensitive indicators of the inability to successfully wean from MVS.

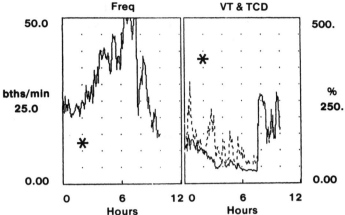

FIGURE 6 Ten-hour trend plots of respiratory frequency (Freq, left panel) in breaths/minute (bths/min), tidal volume (V_T, right panel), and the paradox index (TCD, right panel, dotted line). The asterisk depicts the point at which this 42-year-old quadriplegic patient was placed on a T piece during weaning from mechanical ventilatory support (MVS). Respiratory frequency progressively increased from 22 to 50 breaths/min, tidal volume decreased, and the paradox index worsened (dotted line elevated above the solid line in right panel). These trends indicated an inability to be successfully weaned from MVS.[90-92] Respiratory frequency decreased and V_T increased when the patient was placed back on MVS during the last 2 hours of the trend plot.

a more sensitive *extension* of clinical observation. By acting as a substitute nurse-observer and as a trend analyzer (Fig. 6), it can expedite weaning from MVS. In a preliminary uncontrolled study, the number of hours that patients were maintained on MVS was decreased from 63 ± 5 hours (mean $\pm$ SD) to 48 ± 4 hours ($P = 0.011$) without a change in the rate of reintubation after RIP was introduced into our institution in 1985.[93] This theoretically translated into a $40,000 cost savings for the hospital.

Whereas the previous study was retrospective and uncontrolled, a prospective trial was performed that utilized RIP as the mainstay of a noninvasively monitored intermediate care unit (NIMU) for pulmonary patients.[7] The NIMU is a four-bed unit in which each bed is equipped with continuous respiratory (RIP) and electrocardiographic (ECG) monitors that relay signals to a central station where a technician is located. Over a 1-year period, more than $173,000 in hospital costs (not charges) were saved with the use of NIMU in 94 Medicare patients while the quality of medical care was maintained as judged by the percentage of long-term mechanically ventilated patients who were weaned (64%) and discharged (58%) in comparison to other published figures.[7] The majority of the savings occurred because the nurse:patient ratio was 1:5.6 in NIMU vs 1:2 in the ICU where most of these patients would otherwise have stayed. There was also a small savings in ABGs and chest radiographs. This study satisfied all four of the criteria for proving that a new technology is cost-effective in that it was efficacious, effective, and available for a specific indications, and it was less costly but equally or more effective than existing technology (Table 2).

FUTURE OF RESPIRATORY MONITORING

PULMONOCARDIAC MONITORING

The pulmonary and cardiovascular systems function in parallel and in series, yet monitoring of these functions is often divided into separate categories. In a certain respect, this reflects the clinical perception that most catastrophes that occur in the ICU or operating room have a single underlying etiology. In some situations this is true, for example, the sudden development of ventricular tachycardia of fibrillation. However, many in-hospital "cardiac" arrests are the end result of pulmonary decompensation,[94] the "pulmonocardiac" arrest.[86] Schein et al.[94] recently reported that although no consistent abnormalities were present in laboratory tests obtained prior to in-hospital arrest in 64 patients, tachypnea was present in a majority of patients. This study highlights the need for combined pulmonocardiac monitoring.

One reason for the separation of cardiac and pulmonary monitoring was the lack of technology. The combination of respiratory inductive plethysmography for respiratory monitoring and a sophisticated ECG analysis system is now available and may herald an age of true noninvasive pulmonocardiac monitoring. In addition, inductive plethysmography has been adapted into a continuous, noninvasive monitor of changes in stroke volume[95] and can even be used for noninvasive measurement of central venous pressure.[96] Although attractive from a safety viewpoint, the efficacy and effectiveness compared to existing methods are just beginning to be reported. Therefore, this technology is too new to render a cost-effective analysis at this point.

Many in-hospital "cardiac" arrests are the end result of pulmonary decompensation, the "pulmonocardiac" arrest.

CONTROVERSIES

Recent articles have debated the issue of whether we monitor too much[97] or not enough.[98] Advocates of more monitoring expounded a cost-effective argument based mainly on the potential cost of a malpractice suit[98,99] and not on the principles outlined in Table 2. However, even these monitoring advocates appreciate the fact that the mere presence of monitors does not guarantee better patient care.[99] Every monitor requires a "human–monitor interface"; if the data is too difficult to interpret, or is wrong, or is taken out of context from the patient's clinical situation, then erroneous decisions may result. This represents a form of data overload that is a real concern in our high-tech ICUs and operating rooms. As highlighted at a recent conference,[9,57,63] noninvasive monitors have proliferated as a result of growing concerns over the complications of invasive techniques and the sense of security that monitors seem to provide when caring for critically ill patients. As outlined in this chapter, more monitoring is not necessarily better. Indeed, the most pertinent challenge to health care providers is how to monitor wisely.[97]

Every monitor requires a "human–monitor interface."

The most pertinent challenge to health care providers is how to monitor wisely.

References

1. Drummond M, Stoddart G, Labelle R, Cushman R: Health economics: an introduction for clinicians. Ann Intern Med 107:88, 1987

2. Detsky AS, Naglie IG: A clinician's guide to cost-effectiveness analysis. Ann Intern Med 113:147, 1990

3. Doubilet P, Weinstein MC, McNeil BJ: Use and misuse of the term "cost effective" in medicine. N Engl J Med 314:253, 1986

4. Spivack D: The high cost of acute health care: a review of escalating costs and limitations of such exposure in intensive care units. Am Rev Respir Dis 136:1007, 1987

5. Thibault GE, Mulley AG, Barnell GO et al: Medical intensive care: indications, interventions, and outcomes. N Engl J Med 302:938, 1980

6. Rosen RL, Bone RC: Economics of mechanical ventilation. Clin Chest Med 9:163, 1988

7. Krieger BP, Ershowsky P, Spivack D: One year's experience with a noninvasively monitored intermediate care unit for pulmonary patients. JAMA 264:1143, 1990

8. Witek TJ, Schachter EW, Dean NL et al: Mechanically assisted ventilation in a community hospital. Arch Intern Med 145:235, 1985

9. Hess D: Noninvasive monitoring in respiratory care—present, past, and future: an overview. Respir Care 35:482, 1990

10. Robin ED, Lewiston NJ: Type 3 and type 4 errors in the statistical evaluation of clinical trials. Chest 98:463, 1990

11. Swan HJC, Ganz W, Forrester J et al: Catheterization of the heart in man with use of flow-directed balloon-tipped catheter. N Engl J Med 283:447, 1970

12. Gore JM, Goldberg RJ, Spodick DH et al: A community-wide assessment of the use of pulmonary artery catheters with acute myocardial infarction. Chest 92:721, 1987

13. Robin ED: Death by pulmonary artery flow-directed catheter. Time for a moratorium? (editorial) Chest 92:727, 1987

14. Zion MM, Balkin J, Rosenmann D et al: Use of pulmonary artery catheters in patients with acute myocardial infarction: analysis of experience in 5,841 patients in the SPRINT registry. Chest 98:1331, 1990

15. Dalen JE: Does pulmonary artery catheterization benefit patients with acute myocardial infarction? (editorial) Chest 98:1313, 1990

16. Shoemaker WC, Kram HB, Appel PL, Fleming AW: The efficacy of central venous and pulmonary artery catheters and therapy based upon them in reducing mortality and morbidity. Arch Surg 125:1332, 1990

17. Shoemaker WC: Use and abuse of the balloon tip pulmonary artery (Swan-Ganz) catheter: Are patients getting their money's worth? Crit Care Med 18:1294, 1990

18. Robin ED: The cult of the Swan-Ganz catheter. Overuse and abuse of pulmonary flow catheters. Ann Intern Med 103:445, 1985

19. Matthay MA, Chatherjee K: Bedside catheterization of the pulmonary artery: risks compared with benefits. Ann Intern Med 109:826, 1988

20. Moser KM, Spragg RG: Use of the balloon-tipped pulmonary artery catheter in pulmonary disease. Ann Intern Med 98:53, 1983

21. Morris AH, Chapman RH, Goodman RM: Frequency of technical problems encountered in the measurement of pulmonary artery wedge pressure. Crit Care Med 12:164, 1984

22. O'Quin R, Marini JJ: Pulmonary artery occlusion pressure: clinical physiology, measurement, and interpretation. Am Rev Respir Dis 128:319, 1983

23. Taylor SH, Silke B: Is the measurement of cardiac output useful in clinical practice? Br J Anaesth 60:90S, 1988

24. Stetz CW, Miller RG, Kelly GE, Raffin TA: Reliability of the thermodilution method in the determination of cardiac output in clinical practice. Am Rev Respir Dis 126:1001, 1982

25. Iberti TJ, Fischer EP, Leibowitz AB et al: A multicenter study of physician's knowledge of the pulmonary artery catheter. JAMA 264:2928, 1990

26. Connors AF, Dawson NV, Shaw PK et al: Hemodynamic states in critically ill patients with and without acute heart disease. Chest 98:1200, 1990

27. Baele PL, McMichan JC, Marsh HM et al: Continuous monitoring of mixed venous oxygen saturation in critically ill patients. Anesth Analg 61:513, 1982

28. Orlando R: Continuous mixed venous oximetry in critically ill surgical patients: "high-tech" cost effectiveness. Arch Surg 121:470, 1986

29. Fahey PJ, Harris K, Vanderwarf C: Clinical experience with continuous monitoring of mixed venous oxygen saturation in respiratory failure. Chest 86:748, 1984

30. Schmidt CR, Frank LP, Forsythe SB, Estafanous FG: Continuous SvO_2 measurement and oxygen transport patterns in cardiac surgery patients. Crit Care Med 12:523, 1984

31. Gore JM, Sloan K: Use of continuous monitoring of mixed venous saturation in the coronary care unit. Chest 86:757, 1984

32. Birman H, Haq A, Hew F, Aberman A: Continuous monitoring of mixed venous oxygen saturation in hemodynamically unstable patients. Chest 86:753, 1984

33. Boutros A, Lee C: Value of continuous monitoring of mixed venous blood oxygen saturation in the management of critically ill patients. Crit Care Med 14:132, 1986

34. Rajput MA, Richey HM, Bush BA et al: A comparison between a conventional and a fiberoptic flow-directed thermal dilution pulmonary artery catheter in critically ill patients. Arch Intern Med 149:82, 1989

35. Pearson KS, Gomez MN, Moyers JR et al: A cost/benefit analysis of randomized invasive monitoring for patients undergoing cardiac surgery. Anesth Analg 69:336, 1989

36. Jastremski MS, Chelluri L, Beney KM, Bailly RT: Analysis of the effects of continuous on-line monitoring of mixed venous oxygen saturation on patient outcome and cost-effectiveness. Crit Care Med 17:148, 1989

37. Bratanow N, Polk K, Bland R et al: Continuous polarographic monitoring of intra-arterial oxygen in the perioperative period. Crit Care Med 13:859, 1985

38. Shapiro BA, Cane RD, Chomka CM et al: Preliminary evaluation of an intra-arterial blood gas system in dogs and humans. Crit Care Med 17:455, 1989

39. Civetta JM, Hudson-Civetta JA: Maintaining quality of care while reducing charges in the ICU. Ann Surg 202:524, 1985

40. Maukkassa FF, Rutledge R, Fakhry SM et al: ABGs and arterial lines: the relationship to unnecessarily drawn arterial blood gas samples. J Trauma 30:1087, 1990

41. Thorson SH, Marini JJ, Pierson DJ, Hudson LD: Variability of arterial blood gas values in stable patients in the ICU. Chest 84:14, 1983

42. Severinghaus JW, Astrup PB: History of blood gas analysis. VI. Oximetry. J Clin Monit 2:270, 1986

43. Neff TA: Routine oximetry. A fifth vital sign? (editorial) Chest 94:227, 1988

44. Schnapp LM, Cohen NH: Pulse oximetry: uses and abuses. Chest 98:1244, 1990

45. Tobin MJ: Respiratory monitoring. JAMA 264:244, 1990

46. Bland JM, Altman DG: Statistical methods for assessing agreement between two methods of clinical measurement. Lancet I:307, 1986

47. Severinghaus JW, Naifeh KH, Koh SO: Errors in 14 pulse oximeters during profound hypoxia. J Clin Monit 5:72, 1989

48. Chapman KR, Liu FLW, Watson RM, Rebuck AS: Range of accuracy of two wavelength oximetry. Chest 89:540, 1986

49. West P, George CF, Kryger MH: Dynamic in vivo response characteristics of three oximeters: Hewlett-Packard 47201A, Biox III, and Nellcor N-100. Sleep 10:263, 1987

50. Palve H, Vuori A: Pulse oximetry during low cardiac output and hypothermia states immediately after open heart surgery. Crit Care Med 17:66, 1989

51. Ries AL, Farrow JT, Clausen JL: Accuracy of two ear oximeters at rest and during exercise in pulmonary patients. Am Rev Respir Dis 132:685, 1985

52. Cecil WT, Petterson MT, Lamoonpun S et al: Clinical evaluation of the Biox IIA ear oximeter in the critical care environment. Respir Care 30:179, 1985

53. Jubran A, Tobin MJ: Reliability of pulse oximetry in titrating supplemental oxygen therapy in ventilator-dependent patients. Chest 97:1420, 1990

54. Niehoff J, Del Guercio C, La Morte W et al: Efficacy of pulse oximetry and capnometry in postoperative ventilatory weaning. Crit Care Med 16:701, 1988

55. Smoker JM, Hess DR, Frey-Zeiler VL et al: A protocol to assess oxygen therapy. Respir Care 31:35, 1986

56. King T, Simon RH: Pulse oximetry for tapering supplemental oxygen in hospitalized patients: evaluation of a protocol. Chest 92:713, 1987

57. Ritz R: Resource management for noninvasive monitoring. Respir Care 35:728, 1990

58. Tremper KK, Waxman KS: Transcutaneous monitoring of respiratory gases. p. 1. In Nocho-movitz ML, Cherniak NS (eds): Noninvasive respiratory monitoring. Churchill Livingstone, New York, 1986

59. Taylor W: Transcutaneous and transconjunctival blood gas monitoring. Prob Respir Care 2:240, 1989

60. Tremper KK, Shoemaker WC: Transcutaneous oxygen monitoring of critically ill adults, with and without low flow shock. Crit Care Med 9:706, 1981

61. Barker SJ, Tremper KK: Transcutaneous oxygen tension: a physiological variable for moni-toring oxygenation. J Clin Monit 2:130, 1985

62. Smith NT: Pulse oximetry versus measurement of transcutaneous oxygen. J Clin Monit 2:126, 1985

63. Martin RJ: Transcutaneous monitoring: instrumentation and clinical applications. Respir Care 35:577, 1990

64. Kibride HW, Merenstein GB: Continuous transcutaneous oxygen monitoring in acutely ill preterm infants. Crit Care Med 12:121, 1984

65. Peevy KJ, Hall MW: Transcutaneous oxygen monitoring: economic impact on neonatal care. Pediatrics 75:1065, 1985

66. Eberhard P, Mindt W, Schafer R: Cutaneous blood gas monitoring in the adult. Crit Care Med 9:702, 1981

67. Martin RJ, Beoglos A, Miller MJ et al: Increasing arterial carbon dioxide tensions: influence on transcutaneous carbon dioxide measurement. Pediatrics 81:684, 1988

68. Healey CJ, Fedullo AJ, Swinburne AJ, Wahl GW: Comparison of noninvasive measurements of carbon dioxide tension during withdrawal from mechanical ventilation. Crit Care Med 15:764, 1987

69. Nunn JF, Hill DW: Respiratory dead space and arterial to end-tidal CO_2 tension difference in anesthetized man. J Appl Physiol 15:383, 1960

70. Gothard JWW, Busst CM, Branthwaite MA et al: Applications of respiratory mass spectrometry to intensive care. Anesthesia 35:890, 1980

71. Marini JJ: Monitoring during mechanical ventilation. Clin Chest Med 9:73, 1988

72. Carroll GC: A continuous monitoring technique for management of acute pulmonary failure. Chest 92:467, 1987

73. Raemer DB, Francis D, Philip JH, Gabel RA: Variation in PCO_2 between arterial blood and peak expired gas during anesthesia. Anesth Analg 62:1065, 1983

74. Phan CQ, Tremper KK, Lee SE, Barker SJ: Noninvasive monitoring of carbon dioxide: a com-parison of the partial pressure of transcutaneous and end-tidal carbon dioxide with the partial pressure of arterial carbon dioxide. J Clin Monit 3:149, 1987

75. Weinger MB, Brimm JE: End-tidal carbon dioxide as a measure of arterial carbon dioxide during intermittent mandatory ventilation. J Clin Monit 3:73, 1987

76. Hoffman RA, Krieger BP, Kramer MR et al: End-tidal carbon dioxide in critically ill patients during changes in mechanical ventilation. Am Rev Respir Dis 140:1265, 1989

77. Yamanaka MK, Sue DY: Comparison of arterial-end-tidal PCO_2 difference and dead space/tidal volume ratio in respiratory failure. Chest 92:832, 1987

78. Blanch L, Fernandez R, Benito S et al: Effect of PEEP on the arterial minus end-tidal carbon dioxide gradient. Chest 92:451, 1987

79. Baker RW, Burki NK: Alterations in ventilatory pattern and ratio of deadspace to tidal volume. Chest 92:1013, 1987

80. Jones NL, Robertson DG, Kane JW: Difference between end-tidal and arterial PCO_2 in exercise. J Appl Physiol 47:954, 1979

81. Hess D, Schlottag A, Levin B et al: Use of capnography during weaning from mechanical ventilation following open heart surgery (Abstr). Chest 98:115S, 1990

82. Mackersie RC, Karagianest G: Use of end-tidal carbon dioxide tension for monitoring induced hypocapnia in head-injured patients. Crit Care Med 18:764, 1990

83. National Institutes of Health Consensus Development Conference Statement. Infantile apnea and home monitoring. U.S. Department of Health and Human Services, National Institutes of Health Publication No 87-2905, 1987

84. Shelly MP: Failure of a respiratory monitor to detect obstructive apnea (letter). Crit Care Med 14:836, 1986

85. Konno K, Mead J: Measurement of the separate changes of rib cage and abdomen during breathing. J Appl Physiol 22:407, 1967

86. Krieger BP: Respiratory inductive plethysmography. Prob Respir Care 2:156, 1989

87. Feinerman D, Krieger B, Belsito AS et al: Calibration of respiratory inductive plethysmograph during natural breathing utilizing principles of isovolume maneuver procedure. J Appl Physiol 66:410, 1989

88. Sackner MA, Krieger BP: Non-invasive respiratory monitoring. p. 633. In Scharf SM, Cassidy S (eds): Heart-lung interactions in health and disease. Marcel Dekker, New York, 1989

89. Werchowski JL, Sanders MH, Costantino JP et al: Inductance plethysmograph measurement of CPAP-induced changes in end-expiratory lung volume. J Appl Physiol 68:1732, 1990

90. Tobin MJ, Guenther SM, Perez W et al: Konno-Mead analysis of rib cage-abdominal motion during successful and unsuccessful trials of weaning from mechanical ventilation. Am Rev Respir Dis 135:1320, 1987

91. Tobin MJ, Perez W, Guenther SM et al: The pattern of breathing during successful and unsuccessful trials of weaning from mechanical ventilation. Am Rev Respir Dis 134:1111, 1986

92. Krieger BP, Ershowsky P: Noninvasive detection of respiratory failure in the intensive care unit. Chest 94:254, 1988

93. Krieger B, Shane D, Gazeroglu H et al: Timing of medical extubation: medical and economic implications (Abstr). Am Rev Respir Dis 133(Suppl):A352, 1986

94. Schein R, Hazday N, Pena M et al: Clinical antecedents to in-hospital cardiopulmonary arrest. Chest 98:1388, 1990

95. Sackner MA, Hoffman RA, Stroh D, Krieger BP: Thoracocardiography. Part 1. Noninvasive measurement of changes in stroke volume comparisons to thermodilution. Chest 99:613, 1991

96. Bloch KA, Krieger BP, Sackner MA: Non-invasive measurement of central venous pressure by neck inductive plethysmography. Chest 100:371, 1991

97. Hamilton WK: Do we monitor enough? We monitor too much. J Clin Monit 2:264, 1986

98. Block FE: Do we monitor enough? We don't monitor enough. J Clin Monit 2:267, 1986

99. Siegel LC, Whitcher C: Economics and monitoring. Int Anesthesiol Clin 27:200, 1989

INDEX

Page numbers followed by the letter f refer to figures; those followed by t refer to tables.